P9-DWB-779

# Success Stories

The Perfect 10 Diet has been around for years. Before the publication of this book, thousands of people lost weight and succeeded on the diet. Many blogged on the Perfect 10 Diet's website (www.ThePerfect10Diet.com) and shared their stories. Here is what many had to say:

"I am half my size after two years. I am down to 120 pounds from 220 pounds. I gained my health and figure back on the Perfect 10 Diet."

—*Jen C.*

"I am diabetic, and the Perfect 10 Diet helped me to get off my medications."

—*John O.*

"A diet that works better than cholesterol drugs is not a diet; it is magic."

—*Kelly C.*

"I lost 40 pounds, and I'm still losing."

—*Jimmy L.*

"It is not low-fat; it is not low-carb; it is unlike any other diet on the market. I love the Perfect 10 Diet."

—*Meghan B.*

"I am a man who wants to look his absolute best. The Perfect 10 Diet is getting me there."

—*Arthur M.*

"At age 44, I have the hormones of a 20-year-old woman thanks to the Perfect 10 Diet."

—*Tanya F.*

"As a senior citizen, I need to know everything new in the anti-aging arena. *The Perfect 10 Diet* is my bible."

—*Barry A.*

"I love the Perfect 10 Diet. I lost 44 pounds on this amazing, one-of-a-kind diet."

—*Sharon K.*

"Clear skin, more energy, feeling great; I can't ask for anything more."

—*Michael P.*

"As a woman in menopause, I am finally able to shed the pounds after learning about hormones."

—*Kelly A.*

"As a body builder, I love the Perfect 10 Diet. It helped me build chiseled muscles with the right supplements and more efficient workouts."

—*Michael I.*

"As a woman with a sluggish thyroid, the Perfect 10 Diet has helped me learn which foods I should eat to support my thyroid gland while shedding the pounds. Amazing."

—*Magda A.*

"I lost 45 pounds on the Perfect 10 Diet without missing any of the food I love. Now I know rich choices don't mean unhealthy."

—*Scott L.*

"I need a diet that is heart healthy, safe, and that keeps me in shape as I get older. The Perfect 10 Diet delivers."

—*Linda M.*

"A diet that tells a guy like me how to preserve his youth as he gets older is not a diet—it is the fountain of youth."

—*Ron R.*

"Delicious, easy, rich, and it delivers on all its promises. I love the Perfect 10 Diet."

—*Dominique S.*

"The Perfect 10 Diet is more than a hot-air diet with a sexy title; it is a diet with brains."

—*Peter C.*

"Forget plastic surgery. The Perfect 10 Diet is the closest thing to it without going under the knife."

—*Sabena F.*

"A diet that allows me to eat what I want and lose weight is not a diet; it is a miracle."

—*Jimmy V.*

"As a woman who tried to conceive for years with no success, I turned to the Perfect 10 Diet, and it helped me get pregnant."

—*Catherine P.*

"I am the kind of guy who can't live without carbs. Now, I eat carbs and lose weight."

—*Jason F.*

"Forget low-fat; forget low-carb. The Perfect 10 Diet is the diet that can change America."

—*Heather N.*

"Forget everything you think is healthy. *The Perfect 10 Diet* is an eye-opening book that will change your views on what is healthy."

—*Christopher M.*

"I went from a size 24 to a size 6, and I love it!"

—*Nancy A.*

"Understanding nutrition is a snap on the Perfect 10 Diet."

—*Oliver S.*

"Plain, simple, and easy: that's the Perfect 10 Diet."

—*Holly S.*

"Atkins, the South Beach Diet, Jenny Craig—now I know why these diets didn't work. They didn't balance my hormones. The Perfect 10 Diet did it for me."

—*David P.*

"My body fat is at 15 percent, down from 35 percent. I am a true believer."

—*Karen P.*

"American, Chinese, Thai, and Vietnamese cuisine on a diet…who can ask for anything more?"

—*Jonathan E.*

"Who needs Botox when the Perfect 10 Diet is a total face-lift?"

—*Melanie B.*

"The Perfect 10 Diet may not be popular at present, but it is absolutely the best in its class."

—*Ryan E.*

"As a senior citizen, I need to look after myself. The Perfect 10 Diet is my kind of a diet. I am back to eating the food I ate when I grew up."

—*Carol E.*

"Bread, rice, duck, fruit, and chocolate...what do I have to lose but the pounds? Sign me up for life."

—*Fernando J.*

"You can't go wrong with this diet."

—*Heather S.*

"As a woman who had breast cancer, I need to know which foods I should eat or avoid. The Perfect 10 Diet delivers."

—*Susan P.*

"All these fad diets out there don't stand a chance next to the Perfect 10 Diet. It will only be a matter of time before they are all history."

—*Paul N.*

"A diet that balances my hormones and speeds up my metabolism—I love it."

—*Maria B.*

"I am off my antidepressants just by following the Perfect 10 Diet."

—*Joseph A.*

"Weight loss, better health, delicious food. I'm a believer."

—*Lisa K.*

"I am a man living with HIV. I need a diet that boosts my immunity. The Perfect 10 Diet helps me stay healthy."

—*Sebastian A.*

"At age 50, I never thought I'd wear a bikini again, but I am living proof that the Perfect 10 Diet works."

—*Helen G.*

"No diet can top the Perfect 10 Diet. I guarantee it."

—*Jess O.*

"I look 10 years younger on the Perfect 10 Diet. I have the body I had in my teens and with no food deprivations. I feel I was given a new life on this amazing diet."

—*Julie L.*

"I am an actor and I have to look my absolute best. The Perfect 10 Diet is my diet."

—*John A.*

"I worked with a personal trainer for years, but I was never able to achieve results. The Perfect 10 Diet did it for me."

—*Karen L.*

"Who has time to prepare two sets of food? The Perfect 10 Diet is a plan for the whole family."

—*Georgette A.*

"At age 50, I feel like I'm 20 again on this amazing diet."

—*Ted S.*

"A diet that lets me eat anywhere is my kind of a diet."

—*Harold L.*

"Move over low-fat and low-carb diets: the Perfect 10 Diet has arrived."

—*Pearl L.*

"I used human growth hormone in the past to stay young, but I don't need it anymore on the Perfect 10 Diet."

—*Steven S.*

"At age 45, I am eating right for the first time in my life."

—*Linda D.*

"Ten fingers up—not two thumbs up—for the Perfect 10 Diet."

—*Keith A.*

"Who has time to read numerous books about insulin, thyroid, cortisol, leptin, growth hormone, and so on? All the juice is here, on the Perfect 10 Diet."

—*Rita V.*

"Call me superficial, but I want to be a 10. The Perfect 10 Diet got me there."

—*Craig B.*

"I lost more than pounds; I lost my baggy eyes and double chin."

—*Brittany A.*

"I have lots of energy. I found it on the Perfect 10 Diet."

—*Jamie B.*

"A complete makeover for my health and body."

—*Michelle A.*

"Forget fad diets; the Perfect 10 Diet is the ultimate answer."

—*Ethan P.*

"Eat anywhere, eat healthy meals, and enjoy the food I love? How easy is that?"

*—Carol Z.*

"The meal plan on the Perfect 10 Diet is nourishing, delicious, and healthy."

*—Barry H.*

"The Perfect 10 Diet is misnamed; it is a 100."

*—Tamara K.*

"An international diet with no counting calories is not a regular diet; it is a 10: the Perfect 10 Diet."

*—Brian M.*

"The Perfect 10 Diet addresses many diseases from A to Z."

*—Hope E.*

"All other diets I tried disturbed my hormones, but not the Perfect 10 Diet. I am finally able to achieve weight-loss results."

*—David H.*

"The Perfect 10 Diet is a century ahead of its time."

*—Keisha K.*

"A landmark in nutrition. A standing ovation for the Perfect 10 Diet."

*—Dean A.*

Thousands have been following the Perfect 10 Diet. Will *you* be the next to succeed on the Perfect 10 Diet?

# *The* Perfect 10 Diet

## 10 KEY HORMONES THAT HOLD THE SECRET TO LOSING WEIGHT & FEELING GREAT—*fast!*

Michael Aziz, MD

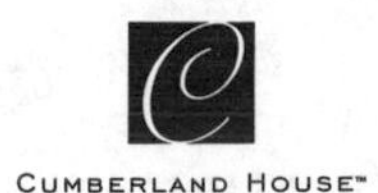

CUMBERLAND HOUSE™

Photos courtesy of Shutterstock, Fotosearch, and Mary Kate Wright, MS, CMI



The advice offered in this book is based on Dr. Michael Aziz's experience successfully treating thousands of patients over many years. The information in this book should not be used as a substitute for your physician's advice on hormone replacement, cholesterol, and diabetic drugs. Readers are advised to consult with their own doctors regarding the treatment of their medical problems. Neither the publisher nor the author takes any responsibility for any consequences from any advice, treatment, supplements, hormones, or medications to any person reading the information in this book. The initial stages of the Perfect 10 Diet are not appropriate for pregnant women or nursing mothers.



Published by Cumberland House, an imprint of Sourcebooks, Inc.
P.O. Box 4410, Naperville, Illinois 60567-4410
(630) 961-3900
Fax: (630) 961-2168
www.sourcebooks.com

Library of Congress Cataloging-in-Publication Data

Aziz, Michael
The perfect 10 diet : 10 key hormones that hold the secret to losing weight & feeling great—fast! / by Michael Aziz.
p. cm.
Includes bibliographical references and index.
1. Weight loss--Endocrine aspects. 2. Energy metabolism. 3. Reducing diets--Recipes. I. Title. II. Title: Perfect ten diet.

RM222.2.A975 2010
613.2'5--dc22

2009030763

Printed and bound in the United States of America.
LB 10 9 8 7 6 5 4 3 2 1

*To my family: Betty, Scott, and Jimmy*

"To know truly is to know by causes."
—Francis Bacon (1561–1626)

# Contents

**Part 3**



**Part 4: The Perfect 10 Diet Recipes**



**Part 5: Appendixes**

# Foreword

According to the World Health Organization, globally, there are more than 1 billion overweight adults, and at least 300 million are obese. People are becoming obese due to the availability of food, the changes in the kind of foods that are eaten, and decreased exercise. Industrialization, urbanization, and transportation have reduced physical activity; as a result, more than 60 percent of the global population is not sufficiently active. Because being overweight or obese makes people vulnerable to a variety of diseases (such as diabetes, heart disease, stroke, and cancer), a failure to maintain a healthy weight ultimately may compromise how long and how well you live.

In *The Perfect 10 Diet*, Dr. Michael Aziz thoughtfully presents the concept that diet and nutrition profoundly affect longevity by modulating hormone production. This book is filled with insightful science, presented in an accessible manner, to help you take action now—not only to lose weight, but also to significantly extend your life with years of productive vitality.

The American Academy of Anti-Aging Medicine (A4M) (www.worldhealth.net) is the world's largest professional organization dedicated to advancing research and clinical pursuits that enhance the quality, and extend the length, of the human lifespan. A4M comprises 22,000-plus physician, scientist, and health practitioner members from more than 100 nations. All of our professional members are keenly interested in practical ways to extend the healthy, productive lifespans of our patients. As such, the A4M is proud to have Dr. Michael Aziz, author of *The Perfect 10 Diet*, as a physician member.

—Ronald Klatz, MD, DO
President
The American Academy of Anti-Aging Medicine
Winter 2009

# Preface

What do you need to know to achieve total and "perfect 10" health? First, you need to understand nutrition in plain and simple English. The information I will share with you in this book is lifesaving. Although you may be unfamiliar at first with some of the medical terms I use, I strove to make this book easy to understand. Why? I've written this for everyone, so it doesn't matter if you're 18 or 80 years old, 15 or 150 pounds overweight—or not overweight at all. The knowledge you will gain from reading *The Perfect 10 Diet* will empower you to improve your overall health. I am confident that you, like my patients, will enjoy eating the foods included on the Perfect 10 Diet as much as you'll enjoy the diet's many benefits.

You may be wondering about the title of this book and diet. The Perfect 10 Diet is an ultimate makeover plan that works by balancing ten hormones, and it can change the way you look on the outside just as much as it changes the way you feel on the inside. I realized that the Perfect 10 Diet works better than all the other diets I'd ever reviewed before because it targets the ten hormones that keep us healthy and fit. It was a true reflection of how the diet really works and its endless benefits on health that go far beyond optimization of hormones.

But I have a confession to make: my true motive with the provocative title *The Perfect 10 Diet* is to get your attention.

When I first developed the diet, I had no title in mind. Naturally, *Dr. Michael Aziz's Diet* sounded good to me. But I quickly realized that it could take years for this diet to become popular. The health of the American public today is in dire straits, and we are simply running out of time.That does not mean, though, that this book is about superficial change. I was asked during a TV interview if I thought I was a "perfect 10." The interviewer went on to ask, "Isn't 'perfect 10' an exaggeration of what your diet can really do in terms of physical appearance?" I was offended and shocked by this question, which I thought reflected the superficiality of our modern society. But I quickly gathered myself together and replied, "Yes, I am absolutely sure I am a perfect 10. I am healthy, happy, and fit, and I have the energy of an 18-year-old." The Perfect 10 Diet will help you achieve your absolute best, in health and looks. But if you bought this book thinking like this interviewer, or if you're obsessed with the extreme beauty ideals of magazine models and movie stars that are enhanced by touched-up photos and plastic surgery, you're robbing yourself of happiness and joy. You are a perfect 10 when you're healthy, not sick. So love yourself, and love your body.

To make *The Perfect 10 Diet* fun to read, I've written this book with a positive tone and a fun style. But in truth, my heart is aching for my fellow Americans. I've only written *The Perfect 10 Diet* this way because I know that we doctors sometimes forget to speak to patients in simple language, thus leaving them clueless. The topic of hormones is also complex, and I don't want to lose your attention.

It took me over 8 years to write *The Perfect 10 Diet*, and I've done all the homework for you in this book. No other diet books or programs will ever come close or will be needed after you read *The Perfect 10 Diet*.

So can the Perfect 10 Diet change the health of people around the world? Can it help us move past all the erroneous information we've heard about nutrition for decades? Much of the information you already know about nutrition has been heavily influenced by the food industry and its lobbyists.

The Perfect 10 Diet is a rarity—a pleasant change from what we're used to hearing, past and present. The food choices may be old, but the Perfect 10

Diet puts them together in a refreshing, new way. *The Perfect 10 Diet* won't be the last diet book to hit the market, and I am sure that it will receive its fair share of criticism. But please don't let any attack on the Perfect 10 Diet derail you from your health goals. Whatever the reason for the criticism—ignorance, jealousy, or a perceived financial threat to the food industry or big drug companies—it's all meaningless. Any attention, negative or positive, will bring more people to the Perfect 10 Diet. So bring it on, critics—I am battle-ready. And I know we can correct this misinformation.

The Perfect 10 Diet is flawless. It's here to stay, and it will change lives. Big things are possible when everybody pulls together and does their part. I'm doing my part by talking to patients and doctors and giving lectures wherever I can. Let's all get loud and pass along the knowledge. Give this book to your family, friends, colleagues, neighbors, and doctors. Make a difference. Nothing should stop us. The word is out, and the message is now in your hands.

# Acknowledgments

I decided to write *The Perfect 10 Diet* after realizing that in order to really make a difference in people's lives, I must spread the news about the diet to the masses, rather than to one patient at a time. My vision was perfectly clear: I wanted to highlight the wrong and dangerous dietary path we've taken.

To accomplish this goal, a lot of people added fuel to my fire. I'm not a writer, nor did I ever plan to become one. However, my patients' constant encouragement prompted me to write every weekend and during rare breaks in my busy schedule.

No one publishes a book alone, and no one can do it without sacrifices and help from others. For this reason, I thank my family for putting up with me during the 8-plus years it took to complete this book.

I'm truly grateful to God for my wonderful parents who, early in life, taught me perseverance and determination and gave me the power to stand up for what is right.

Cathy Hemming, formerly of HarperCollins, was instrumental in giving me guidance when the book was just an idea.

My agent, Valerie Borchardt, is truly the finest agent in the literary world. She was there with me from the very beginning to the very end.

I thank you, Valerie, from the bottom of my heart, for believing in my message and the effect this diet may have on people's lives long before the writing was completed.

Dr. Ronald Klatz, MD, DO, president of the American Academy of Anti-Aging Medicine, I am forever grateful to you. I have learned a lot from your knowledge of hormones, and I admire your passion. You are truly an inspiration. You have changed my life and my patients' lives more than you will ever know.

Keith Berkowitz, I thank you for being a good friend. Doctors like you are hard to find. Lloyd Jassin, thanks for being a great lawyer during this lengthy project, and thanks for all the help with the paperwork.

Keith Olexa, Scott Rambova, Theresa Solimeo, Dr. Alex Eingorn, and my colleagues at Midtown Integrative Medicine are simply fantastic people. Their insight helped me improve my writing style by making it more straightforward and easier to read and understand.

My editor, Emily Heckman, was an enormous help in this massive undertaking. Her experience as both an editor and a writer makes me proud of the end result. Whenever I got overwhelmed, Emily was there offering brilliant suggestions to help me go on. Emily, I know I wouldn't have completed this book without you.

Also, many thanks to all the wonderful staff of my publishing house Sourcebooks, especially Dominique Raccah, Ron Pitkin, Paul Mikos, and Chris Bauerle, who were not deterred by the controversy about my mission to bring innovative and breakthrough information to the public. Special thanks as well to Peter Lynch, Regan Fisher, and Dawn Pope whose hard work and expertise in language and design helped bring the book to life. Your enthusiasm and vision to make *The Perfect 10 Diet* your number one book for the year is a delight after such a long journey—not to mention a pleasant surprise for a first-time author.

Heidi Krupp, you have my eternal gratitude for putting your veteran publicity skills and passion toward a project that can have a huge impact on public health beyond the borders of this country.

I have so many more people to thank, including Tina Thaisuriya, Mario Urgiles, Thomas Plunkett, Blake Kirby, Douglas Alexander, and Umberto

Rocca of Pongsri Thai, Maison, Nisos, Bice, the Russian Tea Room, and Armani restaurants in New York City. Thank you so much for contributing recipes to *The Perfect 10 Diet*. The richness and health benefits of your delicious recipes are nothing short of true perfection.

Michael Green and Michael Steinbrick, thanks for all your excellent exercise tips. I can't tell you how invaluable it has been to have you share the knowledge you've gained serving as veterans' personal trainers in New York City.

Finally, I owe it all to my patients. I have been humbled by your gratitude as you lost weight and triumphed over serious diseases without the use of drugs. Your collective weight losses and significant improvements in overall health are, undoubtedly, my life's greatest accomplishment.

—Michael Aziz, MD
New York, NY
Winter 2009

# Introduction

Do you want to be healthy, sexy, radiant, energetic, youthful-looking, thin, and wrinkle-free for a long time? Have you tried one diet after another and gotten no results at all? Are you tired of being overweight? How would you rate your health? If you can't stand starvation and food deprivation or hate spending hours at the gym, I am sure glad you selected this book. The Perfect 10 Diet can truly change your life. As you read on, you will discover the knowledge and power to achieve perfect 10 health and a perfect 10 physique. Really. I'm telling you the truth; it's that simple. The Perfect 10 Diet is more than just a diet. It's a way of life. By following my plan, you'll soon be on your way to becoming a perfect 10, ready to take on the world.

Starting a new diet often brings out the skeptic in us. It may raise some doubts or questions, such as:

- Will I lose weight on this diet?
- Will it help me lower my cholesterol level?
- Will it decrease my chances of developing heart disease and cancer?
- Will I be hungry or deprived of energy?
- Is it safe, and can it be followed on a long-term basis without any risks to my overall health?

- Is it easy to follow, or is it too restrictive?
- Is it the right diet for me?

These are all valid questions, and my answers will ease your mind. The Perfect 10 Diet is the right diet for you. It's so perfect that it can be followed by anyone, regardless of age, sex, background, physical build, or even disease state. The Perfect 10 Diet will benefit anyone who wishes to:

- lose weight
- balance hormones
- speed up metabolism
- lower cholesterol
- prevent heart disease
- reduce the risk of many cancers
- control diabetes
- lower blood pressure
- improve memory
- fight depression
- reduce stress and anxiety
- improve his or her sex life
- improve fertility
- increase energy
- strengthen bones
- have a glowing complexion
- improve his or her immune system
- live longer
- and much, much more

The Perfect 10 Diet is no ordinary diet, and you can really have it all in this breakthrough plan. The Perfect 10 Diet could have been easily called the fat-smashing diet, the hormone-fixing diet, the heart-healthy diet, the cholesterol-lowering diet, the diabetes-management diet, the anti-wrinkle diet, the fertility diet, the anti-aging diet, the sex diet, and on and on. But these titles don't do the diet justice, because the

Perfect 10 Diet covers every one of these health issues. The Perfect 10 Diet leaves no stone unturned as it shares nutrition information and the reasons behind it all.

It seems like a magical diet with all these promises, but it's true. The Perfect 10 Diet will truly liberate you from all the other yo-yo diets you've previously tried, and it will deliver on all its promised results. I guarantee it.

## What Is the Perfect 10 Diet?

In 1979, stunning Bo Derek starred in the movie *10*, and the number became associated with absolute physical perfection and beauty. If you already consider yourself to be a 10, you have no doubt been blessed with extraordinarily good genes. So why did I choose this provocative title that applies to so few of us? Well, I'm not really talking about beauty; I'm concerned with your health. When it comes to your health, anything less than a perfect 10 is not good enough. Your health is priceless.

But if you bought this book for its title and a desire to be sexually appealing, believe me, you've also come to the right place. The Perfect 10 Diet will make you look your absolute best, because when you're healthy, it shows in your skin, hair, nails, and physique.

It gets even better. What if I told you the Perfect 10 Diet can help you stay younger-looking, longer? You see, the Perfect 10 Diet does all its magic by improving many hormones that play major roles in weight and health. The Perfect 10 Diet focuses on the ten most important hormones in your body. Each of those hormones has a profound effect on others. And when these ten hormones are in perfect balance, you will not only lose weight, but you will also dramatically turn back the aging clock.

The Perfect 10 Diet has fewer rules and restrictions than other diets that leave you hungry, unsatisfied, or less healthy. Better yet, you won't ever have to count calories, fat grams, or net carbs again. The Perfect 10 Diet is designed to serve as an eating-for-life plan, not a quick-fix-and-fail diet.

Unlike diet books that limit food choices to one country's cuisine, the Perfect 10 Diet is about eating delicious, world-class choices from a variety of cultures, all the way from American to Vietnamese.

The food choices are rich, varied, and satisfying, including everything from fish poached in champagne to a decadent cheesecake. The Perfect 10 Diet takes into account the best aspects of myriad healthy cuisines and incorporates them into a single master eating plan that anyone can follow, maintain, and benefit from. Imagine that—an international diet that can be followed by people from all walks of life, with few rules or restrictions. Pick your adjective. Amazing. Astounding. Unbelievable. Unbeatable. All of them apply and give this one-of-a-kind diet a perfect 10 score.

## The Development of the Perfect 10 Diet

My journey as a doctor to develop the Perfect 10 Diet was a path that I'd never planned. In 1998 I started a private practice in internal medicine. I was enthusiastic about starting my career after many years of medical school and graduate training. But before long, my hope had turned to despair.

During my residency, I'd always assumed that seeing a large number of patients was just the nature of medical training, and it was the experience I needed to become a better doctor. But in private practice, nothing changed. In fact, it became worse. I found that I was caring for more patients in less time and drowning in paperwork from an ever-increasing bureaucracy. I was also seeing an increasing number of young people suffering from the onset of serious chronic illnesses, such as heart disease, elevated cholesterol, hypertension, diabetes, cancer, and obesity. All these conditions are traditionally treated with drugs and other medical interventions, but they also require extensive nutritional counseling to improve significantly.

Each day, I'd ask myself, "How can this be accomplished in a medical system that favors cost cuts rather than emphasizing prevention?" After less than 2 years in practice, I found myself questioning why I'd spent 12 to 13 years of my life training for *this*. Dealing with the bureaucracy and having only a few precious minutes to spend with each patient left me totally demoralized. I read countless stories in medical journals of doctors who shared my same frustration. The way medicine is practiced today, it's much easier to write a prescription for a specific drug than to spend hours counseling and correcting the cause or root of the underlying problem. "Next patient, please" was not the approach I wanted to take.

My own health under this workload wasn't any better. I was a little overweight. I had a touch of high blood pressure and high cholesterol, even though I was in my early thirties and hadn't changed anything in my diet. I was hungry all the time, and even though I exercised like a maniac after long days at work, I saw no results.

Naturally, and in good faith, I relied on nutritional guidelines put forth by the mainstream medical community and government guidelines (such as those by the USDA) to help me treat my patients. I believed wholeheartedly in the low-fat dogma because it was advocated by respectable organizations like the American Heart Association. But I found that something curious and quite discouraging was happening. Instead of losing weight or experiencing an improvement in their disease state and overall health, my patients continued to gain weight, and they became less healthy. It began to dawn on me that food is, in fact, medicine, and that my patients, who were following one low-fat diet or another, were being poisoned by their diets.

Here I was, a traditionally trained physician who was following the guidelines of my profession, yet I was watching helplessly as patient after patient failed to improve his or her health on low-fat diets. It was clear that the American Heart Association's low-fat guidelines were a failure for me and my patients, just like they were for the rest of the country. But like most doctors, I was not particularly knowledgeable in the field of nutrition. I wanted to learn what my patients were doing, so I went and bought all the popular diet books. It was a waste of time and money with lots of conflicting and inaccurate information.

I decided to go straight to the top, to the most well-respected institution in the country: Harvard University. Harvard researchers had developed an eating plan and designed a food pyramid that was in sharp contrast to the old USDA Food Pyramid, with its low-fat message (an abundance of grains at the base, few fats at the top). Fats were at the base of the Harvard food pyramid, or to be eaten in abundance, and refined carbohydrates were at the apex, or to be eaten sparingly. The Harvard Food Pyramid made perfect sense, because eating too many carbs translates into more sugar in your bloodstream, which leads to weight gain. Fats provide satiety. You are less likely to overeat when you include fats in your diet. That's why low-fat diets are so hard to stick to and fail you.

There is, however, a major problem with the Harvard food pyramid. At the base of this pyramid, olive oil, a healthy fat, got lumped together with manufactured polyunsaturated vegetable oils. The research is clear about the dangers of manufactured oils. I certainly wasn't going to tell my patients that fast-food oils should comprise a big part of their diets. It was time to find my own approach.

To help myself and my patients, I began to question why most diets fail, and I did research of my own. Was it possible that the dietary guidelines put forth by respected medical authorities could be outdated, misguided, or even wrong? I read all the research and epidemiologic studies I could get my hands on and I was amazed by what I found. To my astonishment, I found that there is a wealth of solid, conclusive research that directly contradicts what was—and still is—being promoted as healthy eating in this country. I read thousands of research articles that concluded that an aggressively low-fat diet is actually detrimental to health. This newfound knowledge led me to formally develop the Perfect 10 Diet.

Naturally, I was my own guinea pig for my new dietary plan. I noticed no cravings or hunger pains between meals. I lost all the weight I wanted to lose. My blood pressure and cholesterol dropped, and my energy level went through the roof. In turn, I shared this new plan with my patients, and they consistently enjoyed the same great results. The Perfect 10 Diet delivered an overall average of around 10 to 14 pounds of weight loss in the first 3 weeks alone. Finally—a diet that really works!

As I began to design the Perfect 10 Diet, I received input from experts who are the top specialists in their fields. I attended conferences all over the world. I reviewed countless scientific studies to lay the foundation for the diet and ensure its safety. All told, it took more than a few years to design the diet, building on a lifetime of medical knowledge.

I am so excited to share with you this groundbreaking and revolutionary way of eating. I created this plan for myself and my patients, who, just like you, were often confused by the mixed messages they received about healthy eating and nutrition from government agencies, the food industry, other physicians, nutritionists, major medical organizations like the American Heart Association, the media, and the constant stream of diet books vying for their attention. This great confusion motivated me to uncover the link between food and health and develop a lifelong eating plan.

## The Perfect 10 Diet Goes from an Office Pamphlet to a Media Sensation

Once I clearly understood why low-fat diets ultimately fail, my biggest challenge became figuring out how to convince my patients to let go of the belief that low-fat equals healthy, and instead follow a more balanced approach. Many of my patients were initially skeptical, but even the most resistant saw miraculous and rapid results when they followed the Perfect 10 Diet. While many of my patients were vaguely aware that not all fat is the same, and that there are both good and bad fats, most were shocked when I told them not to fear saturated fat, like butter and coconut. In fact, I told them, these healthy saturated fats do not raise cholesterol levels or promote heart disease, cancer, or obesity, as we've all been led to believe.

The Perfect 10 Diet started out as a series of informal handouts and pamphlets I gave to patients as I gathered and amassed research. Even with this minimal information in hand, my patients began to lose weight, improve their health, and see a reversal of disease states, often without the use of drugs or other medical treatments.

As a result, many patients stopped seeing me except for their yearly physicals. They no longer needed my services. After seeing these sensational results, I began to speak publicly about the restorative and healing effects of the Perfect 10 Diet.

As word of my patients' successful weight loss began to spread, it wasn't long before I was invited to speak about the Perfect 10 Diet principles on television and radio stations. People began to call my office, log on to my website, and share their success stories.

I was besieged with requests for more information about the diet, and so those few original pamphlets became the wealth of information in this book.

## How Is the Perfect 10 Diet Different from Other Diets?

Your body is a finely tuned machine. One way it keeps itself in balance is by using chemical messengers called hormones to regulate various functions. Hormones are complex chemicals that the body uses to send messages and information. Hormones stimulate or inhibit various functions in cells that, in turn, produce specific cell actions. Your body can't function properly if one or several of your hormones are missing or unbalanced, since hormones control everything, including weight. Hormones tell you when to eat and when to stop eating. Hormones also tell your body how to metabolize food and whether to use food for energy or storage. In short, hormones control your metabolism.

In a nutshell, the Perfect 10 Diet is a diet that balances hormones. This makes the Perfect 10 Diet quite unique, and very different from low-fat, low-carb, and other popular diets that disturb hormones. If hormones are disturbed, diseases develop.

The Perfect 10 Diet is the first of its kind because it works by improving your metabolism and optimizing the hormones that control health, weight, and aging. It will help you lose weight while also delaying the aging process. It's the perfect marriage of a diet and an anti-aging plan in a single comprehensive source.

In this book, I discuss ten hormones. You will learn where each of the ten hormones is manufactured in the body, the normal levels for those hormones, which foods help boost or balance hormone levels, and which foods disrupt or disturb hormone levels. The ten hormones are insulin and glucagon, which affect food storage; leptin, which affects satiety and gives you a feeling of fullness; growth hormone, which helps you grow and repair muscles and tissues; cortisol and thyroxine, which affect energy levels; dehydroepiandrosterone (DHEA), which relieves fatigue and improves your overall sense of well-being; and the sex hormones estrogen, progesterone, and testosterone, which affect weight, fertility, libido, and aging.

First, let's discuss a huge difference between the Perfect 10 Diet and low-fat diets. We're constantly advised that following a low-fat diet will help us become healthy and fit. We are also advised by the mainstream medical establishment to avoid natural fats, such as butter, and instead use highly processed vegetable oils for cooking. Following these recommendations has had a profound influence on public health. Take a look around: are we winning the obesity battle? Sadly, our health has deteriorated at an alarming rate, and we are facing an epidemic of illnesses such as type II diabetes, heart disease, cancer, hypertension, and obesity. Hmm...how can this be if we're all trying to follow the dietary guidelines we've been told are best for us?

Scientific research has shown that a low-fat/high-carbohydrate diet can dangerously raise the bloodstream's insulin levels. (Insulin is one of the hormones that the Perfect 10 Diet helps balance.) High insulin levels can lead to weight gain and increased hunger and can trigger disease development. Low-fat diets completely ignore the negative impact of excess insulin on health.

Low-fat diets also have a huge negative impact on other hormones that the Perfect 10 Diet addresses and helps to optimize. For example, recent research indicates that saturated fats and cholesterol-rich foods, which are condemned on low-fat diets, have no relationship to heart disease. In fact, saturated fats and cholesterol-rich foods actually play a role in the production of sex hormones, which maintain youth and prevent many of the old-age diseases.

Nonetheless, the "experts" tell us that healthy saturated fats such as butter are deadly, when research indicates the health benefits of these good fats. It's no wonder that heart disease, diabetes, and cancer are becoming increasingly common now that we are being given this kind of dietary misinformation. Casting fat as the enemy, despite the best intentions, has created a host of health problems. This simply means you need to put natural fat back in your diet, not eliminate it.

If you think I'm in the anti-carbohydrate camp, I assure you that I'm not. If, like me, you love bread, brown rice, and other carbs, the low-carb mania that swept the nation probably left you wondering if the real problem is in sugar. Low-carb diets advise you to stay away from oranges, grapes, and pasta. Not me. I love this food, and I am not about to give it up. And you shouldn't either. The truth is that low-carb diets are also unbalanced, and they are just troubling for your hormones and health. Low-carb diets do lead initially to weight loss because they balance insulin levels, but they send other critical hormones into disarray.

In addition, many low-carb diets are way too high in protein. Protein is a very necessary nutrient, but only in the right amounts. Eating too much protein can lead to kidney stones, gout, and osteoporosis. And let's get a reality check here: do you really think eating processed meat and little to no carbs on a daily basis is a healthy thing to do?

First, let's understand the connection between carbohydrates and good health. Fiber is the miracle nutrient that helps fight disease. Health experts recommend eating 25 to 30 grams of fiber a day. Some believe that 50 grams of fiber a day is a better target. When you load up on protein and fat, fiber gets shut out of your diet. On top of that, Americans eat comparatively few vegetables and fruits. We need to increase fiber in our diet, not eliminate it. And the best sources for fiber are vegetables, fruits, and whole grains—all of which are carbohydrates. Again, it's all about balance, and that's the focus of the Perfect 10 Diet.

Low-fat and low-carb diets are downright dangerous for your hormones and overall health, so I developed my own plan. Somebody's got to do it. Sure there have been many diets on the market that addressed obesity by targeting one specific hormone at a time, such as insulin, thyroid, or cortisol. But is obesity related to an imbalance of one hormone? I don't think so. Your body has hundreds of hormones. Targeting one hormone alone and ignoring others makes these diets fall short on delivering real or sustainable results.

## Low-Fat and Low-Carb Diets and Hormonal Imbalance

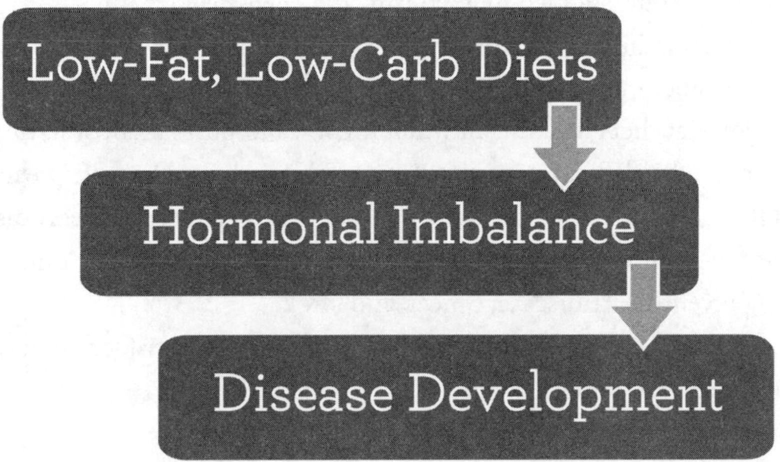


## The Perfect 10 Diet

The Perfect 10 Diet is unlike any other diet you'll ever hear or read about because its principles are new. The Perfect 10 Diet addresses all the major health issues that are currently plaguing Americans. So fasten your seat belt, because I am about to radically change your views about what is healthy. If there is anything at all controversial about the Perfect 10 Diet, it's that it finally sets the record straight about nutrition. This eating plan restores nutritional balance and promotes weight loss and overall good health.

The Perfect 10 Diet ensures that your body receives the right nutrient load, which is 40 percent carbohydrates, 40 percent fat, and 20 percent protein. The Perfect 10 Diet does not promote extremes, and it's certainly not another fad diet, since its principles exemplify what our bodies need for optimal health and weight. The Perfect 10 Diet will help you understand what foods your body needs to function optimally and make sense of all the conflicting information you've ever encountered.

The Perfect 10 Diet corrects erroneous information that continues to be spread, even by respected medical groups! In this book, you will learn the following:

- how to optimize the ten most important hormones in your body that control your health and weight

- how to eat rich and delicious food and still manage to melt away the fat
- how to fix your sluggish metabolism, and even speed it up
- how to make hormones work for you, not against you
- how to choose foods that can trigger weight loss
- why low-fat diets usually fail when it comes to permanent weight loss
- how a low-fat diet can actually raise a key blood lipid you never hear about (triglycerides) to dangerous levels, and how this can lead to heart disease
- how following a low-fat diet could deprive you of valuable vitamins that may prevent heart disease, cancer, and stroke
- how eating the right kind of fats may help lower your risk of heart disease and cancer
- how to tell good fats from bad fats
- how trans fats are formed, and how can they lead to disease
- why the USDA food pyramid is not nutritionally sound
- how to read and understand nutrition labels
- why popular low-carb diets can promote cancer by encouraging dieters to consume dangerous kinds of protein
- how to delay aging with hormone replacement
- how to shop at the supermarket with your health in mind
- how to establish an eating plan that's healthy and satisfying, with delicious recipes
- how to get exercise back into your life without becoming a gym rat
- how it is virtually impossible to achieve and maintain good health unless you follow a balanced diet

## A Sneak Preview

The Perfect 10 Diet addresses what other diets tend to ignore—balanced hormones. Too good to be true? On the contrary, the Perfect 10 Diet is based on the very latest discoveries about nutrition, health, and weight loss. Behind every recommendation is cutting-edge research that goes beyond the now-dated low-fat and low-carb approach.

As a matter of fact, the Perfect 10 Diet is not low in anything. On the Perfect 10 Diet, you will discover a nourishing, delicious, and sound way of eating—

one that is healthy for the whole family. That's important. The Perfect 10 Diet is about melting the pounds off the smart way. It works by speeding up your metabolism and ensuring that your hormones are optimized and balanced. That's really important when it comes to losing weight without feeling hungry.

*The Perfect 10 Diet* is divided into five parts:

**Part 1:** You'll learn how our modern diet failed us. You will read about ten important hormones and how they went into disarray with our modern diet. You'll understand the importance of balanced hormones on overall health and weight.

**Part 2:** The Perfect 10 Diet starts here. You'll learn about the nutrients your body needs to balance your hormones. You'll learn about the Perfect 10 Diet, its principles, and how to get started. The Perfect 10 Diet plan includes daily menus, shopping tips, stories you can relate to, and many chapters on how to make the diet work for you.

**Part 3:** As we get older, some of our hormones decline. In this part, the Perfect 10 Diet becomes an anti-aging diet as you'll learn how to optimize these hormones regardless of your chronological age. You'll learn how to balance hormones with supplements or hormone replacement if needed. You'll also learn how to overcome sluggish weight loss and pitfalls on the Perfect 10 Diet, and you'll find answers to common questions about the Perfect 10 Diet.

**Part 4:** You'll find over 70 recipes from famous New York City restaurants. They really hit the spot to make you enjoy the Perfect 10 Diet for life.

**Part 5:** Here, you'll find places to shop for organic food, and you'll learn about the huge differences between the Perfect 10 Diet and other popular diets.

The Perfect 10 Diet is both innovative and unconventional, and it is by far the best prescription I've ever given to any of my patients. I am proud to pass it along to you. So let's go, folks, you're about to star in this world premiere and become part of the revolution.

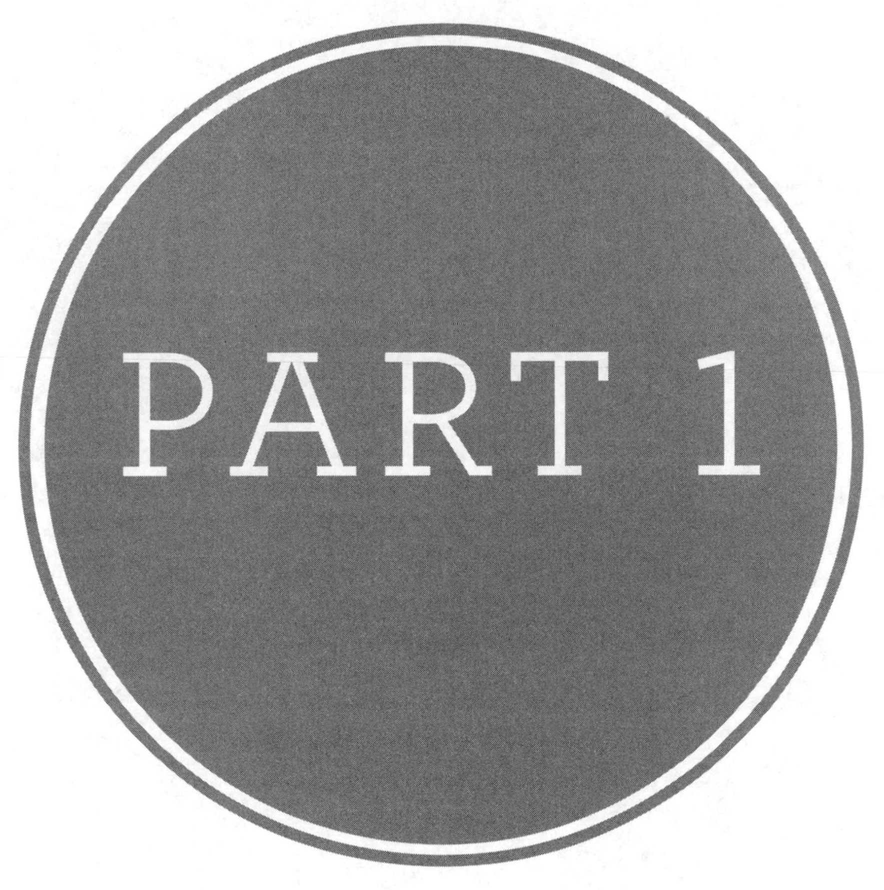
PART 1

CHAPTER 1

# How Our Modern Diet Is Failing

For a nation that spends more on health care than any other country, the United States certainly isn't very healthy. Did you know we are the sickest nation on the planet? As of this writing, 97 million Americans are overweight. Despite the huge success of many diet books, soaring sales of diet pills, and increased gym memberships, more Americans are overweight today than at any other time in history.

At present, nearly 62 million Americans suffer from cardiovascular disease, and many of them are permanently disabled. Heart disease is the number one cause of mortality for Americans, and cancer is second—despite tremendous medical advances in treating both diseases over the last several decades. Sixty million Americans are on the verge of becoming diabetic, and more than 25 million are already there. About 72 million people aged 20 years and older have high blood pressure. Osteoporosis is rampant. Arthritis, depression, and infertility are also on the rise. It's far from a perfect picture.

Today's generation is plagued by diseases. Never in history has there been such a surge in the number of people with so many serious illnesses. Why is such a developed nation losing its health despite tremendous medical advances? Conventional medicine can offer little help to reverse the onset of these diseases when our diet is contributing to it. The statistics are similar in many Western societies.

You've no doubt heard about the grandmother who ate three eggs a day, cooked only in butter or lard, drank whole milk daily, and lived a healthy life until she was 97 years old. *Gee*, you may be asking yourself, *how could this be possible if she followed a diet that's a perfect recipe for a heart attack or a stroke?* Was she simply lucky, or was she blessed with extraordinarily good genes? She did not take cholesterol or blood pressure drugs; she had not had bypass surgery. It is even more incomprehensible to hear that she never saw a doctor except when giving birth.

You might be tempted to ascribe her longevity to luck because most people who lived in her time died at a much younger age. But life expectancy was shorter then because there were no cures for infectious diseases like tuberculosis and pneumonia. Longevity, or the lack thereof, had much less to do with heart disease, stroke, and diabetes than it does today. These diseases were quite rare 100 years ago.

Nowadays, you hear young people discussing their high cholesterol levels or talking about their elevated blood pressure. You hear about women with breast cancer in their thirties or forties. You hear about men who have heart attacks in their forties, nonsmokers who undergo triple or quadruple bypass surgery, and people diagnosed with Alzheimer's disease in their 50s or 60s. What is going on here?

## What Changed in Our Diet?

Food is medicine. To understand this, we simply need to look at the dietary changes that took place in this country in the last century. Today's diet is certainly different from that of our grandparents. Our grandparents ate very little processed food, and they rarely consumed refined carbohydrates, sugar, and manufactured fats, such as refined vegetable oils or margarine. In their time, all food was organic, meaning it was not genetically modified and did not contain pesticides. Their diet included fresh vegetables, fruits, eggs from farm-raised birds, beef from grass-fed cows, raw whole milk delivered to their doors daily, healthy natural fats like butter and olive oil, and whole, unrefined grains. Unfortunately, today most food is processed, and much of the food we eat has been chemically modified.

Most people today eat too many low-fat, grain-based products and highly processed fats like refined vegetable oils. Our food is so modern that many of our grandparents wouldn't be able to recognize it. "Fat-free milk? What is that?"

This modern diet wreaks havoc on many of our hormones—and, in turn, our health. Now, we fear cholesterol-rich foods, including eggs, butter, whole milk, and other animal products. Many view fat (especially saturated fat) as poison and are obsessed with banishing it from their lives—a directive that stemmed from the erroneous belief that animal products and cholesterol-rich foods promote hardening of the arteries.

## How Our Modern Diet Is Failing

Probably the greatest dietary disaster that took our health downhill in this country has been the general recommendation to follow a low-fat diet. Surprised? I'll bet you are. "Have fruit juices, eat cereals, consume three servings of fat-free dairy daily, and always make low-fat choices" advises the American Heart Association. Official recommendations like these have led Americans down a path of obesity and disease.

If you are like most who listened to those guidelines or followed the low-fat dogma of the last few decades, you have unwittingly been set up for failure. You have also been misled and have greatly endangered your health. The truth is that low-fat diets embraced by most physicians, the American Heart Association, the National Cholesterol Education Program, and other medical authorities are just plain dangerous.

Did you know that the last time you drank skim instead of whole milk, you shortchanged yourself of valuable vitamins? Did you know that the fatty portion of eggs is where you find the highest concentrations of fat-soluble vitamins, such as D, E, and beta-carotene? Many of these vitamins are essential to make many of the hormones that preserve your health. But for most Americans fat-free milk and egg whites are believed to be the soundest choices.

Did you also know that on the Mediterranean diet, which is widely considered to be the healthiest diet in the world, fats constitute 35 to 40 percent of the calories consumed? Yet, people who live in the Mediterranean region have among the lowest incidences of heart disease and cancer in the world. I'm sure you've heard about the health benefits of incorporating extra-virgin olive oil, nuts, and fish into your diet. Even armed with this information, most are still buying into the low-fat myth.

## Lack of Willpower on Low-Fat Diets

Think about all the diets you've tried in the past. Chances are that every time you decided to lose some weight or eat healthy, you followed a low-fat diet. You switched from eggs to cereals, full-fat salad dressing to low-fat varieties, and whole milk to fat-free milk. I'll bet you felt miserable. You hated the taste of the bland food, felt hungry and exhausted, and perhaps gained more weight. Have you ever wondered why?

Don't spend another day racking your brain and beating yourself up about past failures. Fat is not the culprit in our diet: sugar is. Too few natural fats and too much sugar are causing a surge in many of the diseases that doctors, including myself, are treating today.

In countries where natural fats, such as olive oil, nuts, avocados, and butter are commonly consumed, heart disease, diabetes, and obesity are rare. Consider countries like Thailand, Japan, and France. The French maintain their health and slim physiques while consuming *foie gras* (animal livers, usually duck or goose), escargots (snails) dipped in butter, and rich, creamy dishes. Most Americans can't wrap their minds around the idea that these can be healthy choices that can be eaten on a daily basis, but the United States, and not France, is the country with higher rates of obesity, heart disease, and diabetes.

The results of the research are clear: eating fat does not make you fat. Rather, it's a *lack* of natural fats in your diet that makes you gain weight. This is information that the public desperately needs. Natural fats are essential for your cells to work properly. Fats slow down the absorption of food, stabilize blood sugar levels, decrease cravings, and make you feel full. Don't wait for the medical establishment to change its views about low-fat diets, because it's your health I'm talking about. Take action now and put natural fats back into your diet. You will eat less, lose weight, and feel more satisfied because fats balance insulin, your natural hunger hormone.

## The Effect of Low-Fat Diets on Insulin

One reason that low-fat/high-carb diets have failed us is that excess carbs quickly turn into sugar in the bloodstream. Sugar has no redeeming health benefit, wreaks havoc on the body's metabolic systems, and it's all down the supermarket aisle in low-fat or fat-free products, which are highly processed and loaded with sugar or high-fructose corn syrup. It's no surprise we were all destined to fail. On the other hand, consuming natural fats will make you feel full and satisfied.

Low-fat diets have failed us because when these diets came into vogue, scientists didn't fully understand the role insulin plays in general health maintenance. Insulin is one of the ten hormones that the Perfect 10 Diet helps balance. Insulin is the fat-storing hormone secreted whenever our bodies are called upon to metabolize food, and it's secreted in higher amounts when the food you consume contains sugar or your diet is high in bad carbs (Fig. 1.1). When you follow a low-fat diet, your pancreas will work overtime to secrete more and more insulin in order to deal with all that excess sugar. Why? Because sugar is damaging to your tissues, so your body must deal with it right away to expel it from your bloodstream. As your pancreas secretes massive amounts of insulin—more than you need—to store the sugars, your body forms triglycerides, or fat molecules, and you gain weight. When triglyceride levels rise, your risk for heart disease rises right along with them.

The low-fat diet craze was a real failure. When scientists figured out what went wrong, they also became aware of the satiety effect of fat consumption. You see, weight control is not only about calories, it's about hormones. When insulin is secreted in higher amounts, you feel hungrier, and you eat more. Certainly you've noticed that you end up adding more skim milk to your coffee than you would of whole milk, just to get a little flavor. Or that you feel fuller and more satisfied after eating eggs with cheese than after eating

**Figure 1.1:** Bad Carbohydrates, a Staple of the Western World

- Cake
- Candy
- Cereals
- Crackers
- Danishes
- Doughnuts
- Fat-free processed foods
- Fat-free yogurt with added sugar
- Fruit juices
- Jam
- Muffins
- Pancakes
- Pasta
- Pizza
- Potatoes (mashed or baked)
- Products made with white flour
- Soft drinks
- Table sugar
- Waffles
- White bread
- White rice

a big bowl of low-fat, commercially produced breakfast cereal. In the end, despite your best intentions, when following a low-fat diet you will end up consuming *more* empty calories from sugar, making *more* insulin, and gaining *more* weight. Willpower does not exist when insulin is high, and you just can't overcome this genetic wiring.

## A Nation on the Wrong Dietary Track

I don't want to scare you with the prospect of never eating another piece of cake or your favorite breakfast cereal, but I want to open your eyes to the dangers of being a carbohydrate addict or following a low-fat diet. The relationship between obesity and excess sugar in our diet is just the tip of the iceberg. Although you can see the effects on your waistline of too much sugar from increased insulin secretions, you can't see the damage it's doing to your cells and organs.

If you've ever dropped some jam or honey on your kitchen table, you know how sticky and difficult it is to clean up. The same thing happens inside your body when you eat sugary foods or follow a low-fat/high-carbohydrate diet. The metabolized sugar from excess carbs adheres to tissue and cells and destroys collagen. This leads to premature aging, among other things. Sugar also makes the cholesterol stickier, which in turn makes it adhere to the arteries. This leads to stiffening of the arteries and predisposes one to early cardiovascular disease. This is why diabetics are more likely to age rapidly and have an increased incidence of heart attack and stroke. When you follow a low-fat diet, you are, in essence, signing up for diabetes, since you will have an elevated sugar level in your bloodstream most of the time.

When the pancreas puts out more insulin, cells become insulin resistant because they're trying to protect themselves from the insulin's toxic effects and down-regulate their receptor activity. Some cells become more resistant before others—for example, the liver becomes resistant first, followed by muscle tissue, and, finally, fat. As all these tissues become insulin resistant, your pancreas puts out even more insulin. The link between high insulin levels and many diseases is now well established in the medical literature. High insulin levels have also been linked to heart disease, stroke, cancer, high blood pressure, elevated cholesterol, infertility, and even Alzheimer's disease. Years of following a low-fat diet will cause your pancreas to become strained, and it won't be able to produce enough insulin. When this happens, you'll be diagnosed with type II diabetes.

## The New Epidemic: Diabetes in Children

The increasing incidence of diabetes is disturbing and alarming (Fig. 1.2). A disease that should be very rare in young people is rapidly escalating, even among young children. The diagnosis rate for diabetes has shot up 100 percent in the last ten years. At present, 25 million people in the United States are diabetic, and 60 million more are prediabetic.

At one time, type II diabetes was called "senile" diabetes because it didn't usually affect people until they were well into their 60s or 70s. Obviously, no one wants to learn that he or she has developed an illness that's associated with old age. As more and more middle-aged people began to develop diabetes, its name was changed to "adult-onset" diabetes. Given the fact that so many children are now being diagnosed with this type of diabetes, medicine has once again bestowed a new name: "maturity onset diabetes of the young." Medicine is trying to keep up with the changing prevalence of this disease. You don't have

**Figure 1.2:** Diabetes in the USA

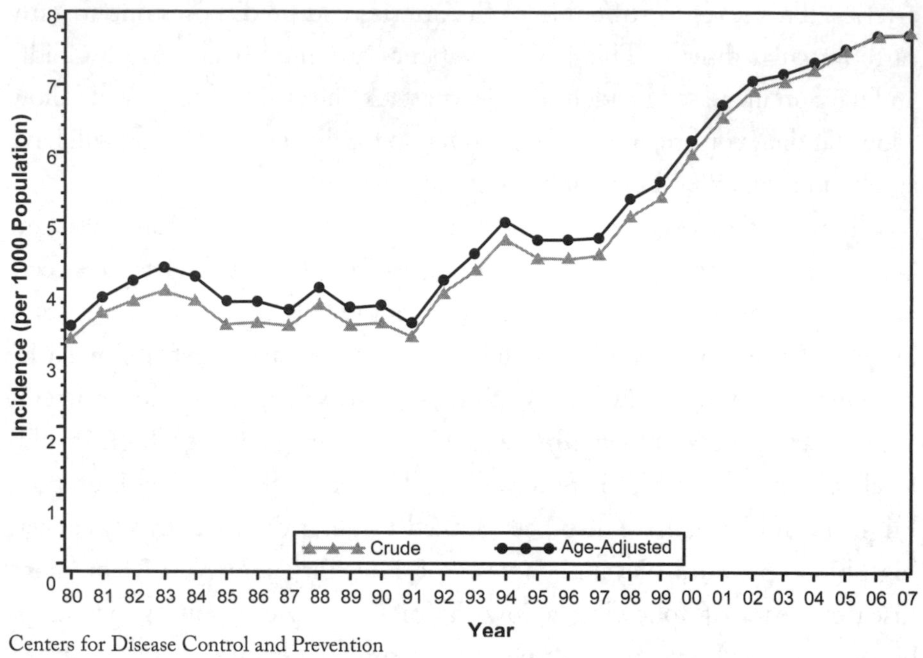


Centers for Disease Control and Prevention

**Figure 1.3:** The Effect of a Low-Fat Diet on Your Health

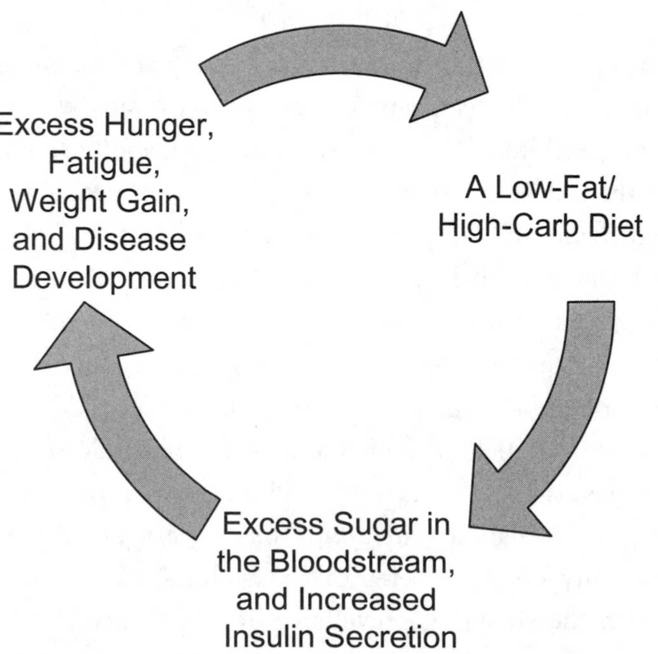

to be a rocket scientist to figure out that these changes are related to kids' massive—and escalating—sugar intake. They consume soda, jam, fruit juices, cereals, and fat-free products with loads of sugar. Is there a relationship? You bet there is.

## Effect of Low-Fat Diets on Other Hormones

If you think low-fat diets only have a negative effect on insulin, think again. Insulin is a master hormone that controls many other hormones. The damage also spills to growth hormone, estrogen, progesterone, and testosterone. I will talk more about these hormones in greater detail later in the book. When these hormones are disturbed or become unbalanced, a host of other illnesses can develop, such as osteoporosis, heart disease, anxiety, depression, infertility, and much more.

## A Low-Fat Diet Can Also Lead to Many Vitamin Deficiencies

Many Americans have eliminated natural fats from their diets as they've increased their carbohydrate intake, and in doing so they've become fat deficient. This means that they're also deficient in essential fatty acids (EFAs). According to recent research, EFAs have been shown to improve hormone functions and play a vital role in the prevention of degenerative diseases. When you follow a low-fat diet, your body will have a hard time absorbing the fat-soluble vitamins (A, D, E, and K). A deficiency in fat-soluble vitamins can lead to skin diseases and contribute to poor overall health.

## Are You Fat Deficient?

- Are you overweight or obese?
- Have you always been unsuccessful on low-fat diets?
- Do you feel you're hungry all the time, or do you have little to no control over your appetite?
- Are you tired and fatigued every time you eat pasta, pancakes, or waffles?
- Do you feel hungry one or two hours after eating a bagel or doughnut?
- Do you often crave sugary snacks?

If you answered "yes" to any of these questions, you may be fat deficient, which means that your body may be secreting too much insulin. If you have any of these symptoms, your body is telling you it needs help (Fig. 1.3). Please listen to this message, and take action by putting natural fats back into your diet. These symptoms are only one part of a bigger picture. Although these symptoms certainly indicate that you're not feeling well, the real damage is hidden away, at the cellular level. There is no way for you to know if your arteries are starting to clog, or if cancer is forming in your breast, pancreas, or colon. In contrast, disease does not develop when key hormones like insulin are in balance. If you understand all of these factors, you can definitely rule out a low-fat diet as a sound prescription for long-term health.

## Our Diet Includes Dangerous Amounts of Manufactured Oils

I have already discussed the dangers to your health and your waistline of exaggerated insulin secretions caused by low-fat diets and excess carbohydrates. But that's not all—low-fat diets go on to condemn many healthy natural fats needed to optimize sex hormones. Additionally, low-fat diets encourage dangerous amounts of manufactured or refined vegetable oils, which are horrible for your health. As a result, your diet may be low in essential fatty acids, such as the omega-3 fatty acids found in eggs, fish, and nuts. It may also be high in omega-6 fatty acids, found in highly processed vegetable oils like corn and soybean, which have been linked to cancer.

Why are we consuming so many manufactured fats? One big answer is lobbyists. Sadly, politics have played a major role in influencing nutrition organizations and government guidelines. As a result, Americans have been fed a great deal of misinformation about the relative virtues of the types of fats that are considered healthy, such as this statement from the American Heart Association: "Eliminate butter, coconut, and palm oil from your diet. Include polyunsaturated oils (corn, soybean, and cottonseed)." Let me be clear about this: these types of oils are highly processed, and should not be part of *anyone's* diet.

A century ago, the average person consumed less than 1 pound of these oils in a year. Today people in industrialized countries, including the United States, consume in excess of 67 pounds of polyunsaturated oils a year.

Fast-food chains' proliferation is playing a big role in this dramatic surge. Polyunsaturated oils are *truly* the heart-clogging fats. It's not surprising to see that the rate of heart disease increased right alongside the surge in consumption of these types of manufactured oils.

## How an Excess of Refined Polyunsaturated Oil Is Dangerous to Your Health

On average, we get as much as 30 percent of our daily calories from refined manufactured polyunsaturated oils, but research indicates this is too much. Omega-3 and omega-6 fatty acids are considered to be essential fatty acids. They are essential to our health because they cannot be manufactured in our bodies. For this reason, essential fatty acids must be obtained from food. Omega-3 fatty acids are found in eggs, fish, and nuts. In a healthy diet, the goal is a 1-to-1 balance of omega-3 to omega-6 fatty acids. The average American diet distorts this ratio to 20- or even 30-to-1 because of its massive amounts of omega-6s (vegetable oils) and low levels of omega-3s. This imbalance in the omega-3 to omega-6 ratio has contributed to a rapid increase in the incidence of many illnesses, such as heart disease, cancer, and depression.

When our bodies are overloaded with manufactured oils and deprived of healthy natural fats, such as omega-3 fatty acids, cells weaken and disease develops. Many refined polyunsaturated oils, such as corn and soybean, have been recommended by the medical establishment as healthy oils that can help lower cholesterol levels in the bloodstream. The truth is that the cholesterol is simply escaping from the bloodstream and being deposited in the tissues at higher levels in order to increase the stability of cellular walls. As a result, polyunsaturated oils are highly atherogenic, which means that they promote hardening of the arteries.

The dangers do not stop here. Polyunsaturated vegetable oils become even more toxic and unstable when they are heated due to the creation of free radicals, which are roaming electrons that damage cells. Free radicals also oxidize or damage cholesterol, which leads to premature aging (wrinkles), clogging of the arteries, and, potentially, cancer. I could write a 300-page book about free radicals alone, but I'll spare you the details here. Elimination of refined polyunsaturated oils from your diet should be a top priority.

**Figure 1.4:** Refined Polyunsaturated Oils (With Excess Omega-6 Fatty Acids) Have Been Linked To:

- Heart disease
- Cancer
- Stroke
- Asthma
- Oxidized cholesterol
- Thyroid disease
- Depression
- Aging skin
- Premature aging

## Too Much Trans Fat in Our Diet

Polyunsaturated oils are not the only bad fats we consume; it is also estimated that the average American consumes 10 to 14 grams of trans fats per day (Fig. 1.5). I'm sure you've heard some of the drama surrounding the dangers of trans fats. So what exactly are these hydrogenated oils or trans fats? I'll explain. In order to make an oil more stable, manufacturers add a hydrogen atom to it. They are literally altering the oil's molecular structure by adding this hydrogen molecule. This leads to the formation of trans fats, or damaged fats, which are particularly dangerous to health since they are completely foreign to the human body. Cells built in your body from hydrogenated oils and trans fats can become cancerous and impair hormone production.

One example of a hydrogenated fat is margarine. On the Perfect 10 Diet, it goes without saying that the consumption of margarine is completely forbidden. Here's why:

- It causes a disturbance in the hormone insulin, which can lead to weight gain.
- It creates a disturbance in the hormone leptin, which controls hunger.
- It is linked to allergies, as it interferes with the enzyme the body uses to make adrenal hormones.
- It interferes with the production of male and female sex hormones, which affect fertility and keep us young.
- It raises the level of bad cholesterol (low-density lipoprotein), which is bad.
- It lowers the level of good cholesterol (high-density lipoprotein), which is also bad.
- It increases your risk of heart attacks and stroke.

- It causes a wide variety of cancers.
- It contributes to infertility in women.
- It raises your chance of developing diabetes.

Ironically, hydrogenated margarine was recommended as a healthy fat by both the American Heart Association and the National Cholesterol Education Program well into the 1990s. It's no surprise that, even as a doctor, I ate margarine before I learned about its dangers. When I think of the years I did this as I listened to those so-called healthy recommendations, I can't help but think of the permanent harm I may have done to my body. Many Americans are beginning to learn about the dangers of margarine and have stopped using it in their own homes, but many still consume trans fats from other sources, like the fast-food industry.

Trans fats from hydrogenated oils and margarine are like plastics. Once you eat trans fats, they integrate into your cells and interfere with intracellular communications because your body cannot recognize their molecular structure. When cells can't communicate with each other, sugar and other nutrients remain in the bloodstream longer than they should because the damaged cells become unresponsive to hormones. As a result, the pancreas secretes more insulin to deal with the nutrients remaining in the bloodstream. Your insulin, which was already unbalanced because of your excessive sugar intake, is now totally screwed up. When an overabundance of insulin is circulating through your bloodstream, you are on your way again to becoming overweight. You also increase your chance of developing diabetes, heart disease, and cancer. You can thank trans fats for this vicious cycle.

**Figure 1.5:** Major Sources of Trans Fats in Our Diet

- Fast-food oils
- Margarine
- Frozen entrées
- Hydrogenated vegetable oils
- Processed low-fat food products containing hydrogenated oils
- Processed low-carb food products containing hydrogenated oils
- Vegetable shortening

## Low-Carb Diets and Hormonal Havoc

It's no surprise that Americans started to gain weight steadily since the low-fat diet dogma of the 1980s and 1990s, because we ate too many bad carbohydrates. Low-fat diets are simply out of balance. A fat-free muffin for breakfast has over 450 calories, which is plenty to give you the energy needed early in the day. But in no time you'll feel hungry since your body will quickly convert this white flour into sugar. You feel hungry because your insulin will go out of whack before it's even lunchtime. You overeat when you crave the same food that caused your insulin to go on a roller coaster in the first place. Low-fat diets also encourage the wrong types of fats, which leads to the disruption of other hormones. As a result, many Americans gave up on the low-fat message and turned to a different, or should I say opposite, approach: low-carb diets. Now you know why low-carb diet books became huge best sellers and helped millions lose weight: they balanced the insulin levels of dieters who had been encouraged to eat more fat and less sugar and bad carbs.

With the news all over the media, low-carb diets really took off. Diet industry watchers estimate that 30 million Americans are currently on low-carb diets. I admire the advocates of such diets, such as Dr. Robert Atkins and many of his successors, who fought conventional wisdom and realized the failure of the earlier low-fat approach. But if you are on the low-carb diet du jour, I have news for you: low-carb diets aren't any better for your hormones or health.

Have you ever been on one? Perhaps you've heard some positive research on low-carb diets. You've read that followers lost weight and their cholesterol went down, so you decided to give it a try. Maybe you lost some weight and felt a little better after giving your insulin a break, but ultimately you failed to achieve long-lasting results. If you failed on a low-carb diet, you may think there is something wrong with you. I can tell you this: there is nothing wrong with you. Low-carb diets create havoc with your hormones, too. Let me explain.

On the Atkins Diet, you eat eggs, bacon, and red meat, and you limit all carbs, including those from vegetables and fruit. On the South Beach Diet, you eat lean meat like veal and Canadian bacon, and you initially limit fruit. On Sugar Busters, you eat meat and cut out white flour, sugar, and starchy vegetables.

All of these diets initially reduce insulin, leading the body to rely on fat stores for energy. While on the surface this may seem logical, these diets are all fraught with other unseen dangers. There are no studies or long-term data that look at low-carb diet followers beyond two years. Yes, they show initial weight loss, but I suspect that if the studies were to go any longer, they would show low-carb diets to be a complete disaster on hormones and overall health.

If you're on the Atkins Diet, which is way too high in fat, this simply shuts down growth hormone, which is the hormone that keeps you young. Do doctors routinely check for growth hormone levels? Of course not. Do you want to do anything to shut down the hormone that is keeping you youthful? I don't know about you, but that's not for me. The Atkins Diet is also bad for your thyroid, as it encourages a high-protein lifestyle. Too much protein can shut down the thyroid hormone from converting to its active form. Thyroid hormone is a major hormone that keeps you fit. It controls your whole life, not just your metabolism.

If you're on the South Beach Diet, which favors manufactured polyunsaturated oils such as corn and soybean, the thyroid gland is also negatively affected. Polyunsaturated oils in their free fatty acid state also interfere with the conversion of thyroid hormone into its active form. And didn't you just read here how bad polyunsaturated oils are for your health? They can promote heart disease and cancer. Do you really want that?

Sugar Busters favors fake fats such as margarine. However, I just discussed the dangers of trans fats. This diet ends up messing up sex hormones. It is the sex hormones that keep you fit and young. This diet similarly disturbs leptin, the hormone that controls hunger.

The cellular damage and hormonal havoc of all these popular diets is immediate, although you may not feel it for a while. Hormonal havoc eventually leads to a sluggish metabolism. But the implications of hormonal imbalance go far beyond a sluggish metabolism. These are serious hormonal disturbances that come with grave consequences. Yes, you lose weight as you initially balance insulin, but you will pay dearly later—with your health.

Due to boredom and deprivation, I doubt that any person can really adhere to low-carb diets for any extended period of time. These types of diets can actually worsen carbohydrate cravings, and many people end up rebounding to a higher weight than where they started. I hear it from my patients all the time: "I lost 15 pounds on this or that low-carb diet, but I ended up gaining all the weight back and then some because I felt so deprived of carbs that all I eat now is potatoes and bread."

I get it: we want to lose weight. But at what price? If you knew the dangers associated with these popular diets, you would run for cover.

Who in their right mind would want to stick around with all these risks? Low-carb diets are a thing of the past because insulin is not the only hormone in play when it comes to weight loss. Your metabolism is controlled by other hormones. You have to support your whole metabolism, not wreck it.

## Weight Gain Is Not about Calories

Today, we have a greater understanding of the role hormones play when it comes to metabolism, health, and weight. The bottom line is that low-fat and low-carb diets failed us because they disturbed our hormones. Hormones are affected by everything you eat, whether it's fat, carbs, or protein. Your lifestyle, stress, and exercise play a role too. It happened to me in the past.

In my twenties, I was in perfect shape. Then came the big 3-0 and I gained 40 pounds in less than two years during my residency. I didn't understand how this happened since I really watched my calories. I look at my pictures now, and I know it wasn't pretty. At the time, I figured it all had to do with the fact that I worked 80 hours a week and exercised less than I used to. I couldn't do a thing to change my lifestyle because I worked 36-hour shifts every other day in the hospital, then went home to study.

Residency is like being jet lagged for years. I stayed awake during nights in the hospital by drinking coffee and sometimes eating a chocolate bar to give me energy. At home, I didn't cook; I ate TV dinners. I treated all food as calories, just like experts tell us. Who was I to question their knowledge at this early stage in my life? But now looking back, I realized why I easily gained weight. My hormonal balance was disturbed. My body was not able to cope with all the abuse inflicted on it with such tremendous stress combined with my poor eating habits. The pressures of residency probably raised my cortisol, the stress hormone, to the max, and that made me fat. Lack of sleep for years messed up my growth hormone, since it is secreted at night. Growth hormone is a fat-burning hormone that puts the brakes on insulin, the fat-storing hormone. Did I eat right to control insulin? Of course not. In fact, I raised my insulin level with my excessive coffee consumption and by eating bad foods such as sweets and frozen dinners. No wonder I gained weight.

## Too Much Processed Food in our Diet

It's not just sugar, polyunsaturated oils, and trans fats that made us sick. Our diet is also chock full of protein, artificial sweeteners, salt, dairy products, and chemicals galore. And let's not forget that there is too much processed food in our diet. This food is unrecognizable to our bodies and it is toxic to our endocrine systems.

Many think they eat healthfully, but in reality, they do not, since they eat processed food. Yes, processed food will fatten you up. Look at the ingredients in the salad dressing in the following box and ask yourself why on earth you would put this poison in your mouth. Do you think your body is going to say, "Great, I love artificial colors." Of course not. Your body can't recognize this food. Instead, it will secrete leptin, the hormone that controls satiety, to let you know you still need to eat. You'll feel hungry, and you'll overeat.

**Figure 1.6:** Ingredients of a Low-Fat Salad Dressing

Partially hydrogenated soybean oil, dye #5, high-fructose corn syrup, spices, xanthan gum, salt, natural and artificial flavors, preservatives to maintain freshness.

Contains trace soy ingredients

## Gender Benders

However, eating real food isn't the only answer to turn your health around and help you escape low-fat and low-carb hormonal horror. Our hormones are also negatively affected by gender benders. Gender benders are hormone impersonators that we're exposed to. Gender benders highjack your metabolism and negatively affect your natural hormonal balance.

For the most part, our bodies are amazingly resilient. But what our bodies are not designed for is exposure to the many endocrine disrupters found in the environment. These substances mimic our hormones. As result, they build up and interfere with the way our natural endocrine system works. These endocrine disrupters are known as gender benders, since they are causing males in many species to become feminized.

Pesticides, hormones found in nonorganic meat, and pollutants around us all act as gender benders. Did you know that handlers who spray insecticides over vegetables and fruits wear protective goggles and special gear to prevent any exposure since it can be life threatening? And we eat this food! What is this doing to us? Pesticides have been linked to insulin resistance and were found at higher levels in many diabetics. So when I tell my patients to eat a balanced diet with lots of organic food, some laugh and say, "Is this really important? And what does this have to do with my irregular periods or diabetes, Doc?" "It has a lot to do with your disturbed hormones," I reply as I show them their test results. The average American consumes one pound of pesticides each year!

I realized the importance of eating organic food years ago when I started waking up several times at night to urinate. I did a blood test on myself and found out that my estrogen level, the female sex hormone, was high, while my testosterone, the male sex hormone, was half of what it was supposed to be. How did this serious hormonal imbalance happen? The answer was probably in my diet. In men, a high estrogen level can compete with testosterone in the cells, rendering it useless, and can cause prostate issues, which led to my frequent nighttime urination. It can also lead to weight gain. As I ate more organic food, my hormones became balanced and the problem was resolved. In women, gender benders lead to what is called estrogen dominance. A disturbance of the estrogen to progesterone ratio in women is a serious condition and has grave consequences. Estrogen dominance can lead to irregular periods and an increased risk for breast cancer.

Another source of gender benders is growth hormones given to livestock and poultry, most of which contain fat-soluble estrogens. Again, hormones found in nonorganic food are highly estrogenic. Chemicals such as chlorine, cosmetics, and pollutants around us can cause hormonal imbalances too. Simply put, gender benders are now everywhere and create a disturbance in our natural hormonal balance. All these gender benders that mimic hormones act in several different ways to disrupt normal body functions.

Scientists have documented several disturbing human health trends from exposure to gender benders, including the following:

- **DECREASED FERTILITY:** In men, there has been a huge decline in sperm quantity and quality over the past 20 years. In women, there is also an increased incidence of endometriosis, a painful disease of the tissues lining the uterus that can result in sterility.
- **EARLY MENARCHE:** Doctors are seeing more and more young girls who are getting their periods before the age of 10.
- **INCREASED RATES OF CANCER:** The number of women who get breast cancer has greatly increased. In the 1960s the risk of getting breast cancer was 1 in 20, and now it is approaching 1 in 8. In cities with pollution problems, such as Los Angeles, the rates are much higher. Rates are also going up rapidly in Asian Americans, who have a low incidence of breast cancer to begin with. In men, testicular cancer rates have increased 4-fold in the last 40 years.
- **OBESITY:** Yes, gender benders are making us overweight, too.

## A Nation in Hormonal Chaos

When I look around, I don't see the obesity or the diabetes epidemic as others see it, as a problem of too much food and too little exercise, or calories in and calories out. It is too simplistic; that's not the whole story. I look deeper to the root of the problem, and what I see is a nation in hormonal chaos. It becomes very clear to me why many diseases are so prevalent today in our society.

- 75 percent of all Americans are overweight
- 25 million Americans have diabetes
- 60 million Americans have prediabetes
- 25 million Americans have an underactive thyroid
- 13 million American men have a low testosterone level
- 5 to 26 percent of women in their reproductive years suffer from polycystic ovary syndrome (PCOS), a condition of insulin resistance together with a high testosterone level, which can result in infertility

And the list goes on and on. I know some of you may be saying, "But I don't have diabetes, a thyroid problem, or irregular periods, Doctor! What do all these hormonal problems have to do with me? I just need to lose weight." The answer is that the Perfect 10 Diet is not a fad diet. It will help you lose weight, but it will not just put a Band-Aid on our serious health issues. Obesity is a condition of hormonal imbalance, and by balancing your hormones, the Perfect 10 Diet will fix your obesity as well as the other problems that your hormonal imbalance is causing. I think you're beginning to see how beneficial this diet is for you.

## Obesity

At present, the United States is number one in the world when it comes to obesity rates. Is obesity related only to disturbed hormones from low-fat, processed food and the toxins around us? Of course not. The truth is that many of us simply eat too much. Calories still count to a certain degree. Portion sizes have increased by 20 percent in the last three decades, both at home and in restaurants.

The answer to the obesity problem is not simple. Genes, hormonal imbalances, and even viruses are now acknowledged to play a role. Scientists suspect that there are lots of fat genes. Some of us simply have more fat cells than others, and the range is huge. Stress and a lack of sleep, as I mentioned earlier, fatten you up, too. But obesity in America has a lot to do with our modern diet and its relationship to hormonal imbalances.

I don't have all the answers for the obesity problem, but if you have the fat gene, you can offset the risk by exercising regularly and eating a diet that balances your hormones, not messes them up. You need a new plan that is balanced, easy, and has a sensible approach. I never found such a diet, so I developed my own. On the Perfect 10 Diet, I will give you a realistic plan with fabulous and rich foods that you should enjoy for life. The Perfect 10 Diet works because it allows you to eat the types of food that are consistent with a normal healthy metabolism. I'm glad to see that you are concerned about your weight, because obesity increases your chance of developing more than 35 major diseases. The list includes the following:

- arthritis
- cancer
- diabetes
- fatigue
- fatty liver
- gallstones
- hardening of the arteries
- heart disease
- high cholesterol
- high blood pressure
- infertility
- prediabetes
- sleep apnea
- stroke
- and much more

## A Lost Nation with No Guidance

The low-fat message made us sick, and the guidance from our medical authorities is misleading. It is no surprise that many of us are overweight and sick nowadays with all this hormonal chaos. When people gain weight from all the toxic food around us, many join one of the popular weight-loss chains for help. The problem is that their food is processed, too. I hear it all the time from my patients: "I am making a commitment to change my health, Doc. I am buying frozen meals now from this or that weight-loss chain. You will be proud of me." We need to wake up to what we think is healthy. It is an understatement to say that weight-loss chains that sell and promote processed food are simply wrecking hormones. They are wrecking health and lives. What price do you put on your health? The popular weight loss chains couldn't share the Perfect 10 Diet title because they are far from perfect. They promise you good health and ship processed food right to your doorstep. What a contradiction! Let me ask you, how long will you do that?

Some of us turned to the newest popular diet of the day. Just look at the list of the best-selling diet books over the last 40 years and you can see the tragic state we've reached when we have no good guidance from our medical organizations or when we act in desperation. In 1972 it was *The Atkins Diet*, a very high-fat/very low-carb diet. In 1979 the country moved to an opposite approach with *The Pritikin Diet*, a very low-fat/very-high-carb diet. In 1992, it was back to *The Atkins Diet*, with a new revised publication. Low-carb diets really took off big time with the low-fat approach showing all its ugly horrors. Many took notice. In 1999 *The Zone* was published. It is still a low-carb diet, but it's slightly more balanced. On the Zone, you can easily replace your meals with a processed Zone bar containing added chemicals. Isn't that an easy and practical diet that many can follow? In 2003 people embraced *The South Beach Diet*. Twenty million Americans are followers. *The South Beach Diet* recommends fake fats. In 2005 the country moved on to *Skinny Bitch*, a very strict vegetarian diet. If you happen to be man, don't despair; another fad diet will eventually come your way. And it did. In 2008 both men and women moved on to *The Flat Belly Diet*. Some fats were now acceptable on this diet, but so was processed food!

One thing's for sure: there is no shortage of fad diets. I heard that some 200 diet books hit the American marketplace every year. How come we have become so gullible? From one approach to another approach, and from one extreme to another extreme, what is happening? Our hormones are all over the place and can't figure out what to do with all the abuse we're doing.

The way I see it, we have truly been lost. I'm no longer surprised or even shocked by the diets my patients tell me they're following—the Latte Diet, the Grapefruit Diet, the Green Tea Diet, and so on and on. Without guidance from the medical establishment, we turn self-taught people into diet gurus. They appear regularly on TV and radio to dispense nutritional advice and detrimental recommendations. Would you bring your taxes to a doctor instead of an accountant? If you broke a tooth, would you see a mechanic or a dentist? What has happened to us? Did a lack of real food in our diet make us unable to tell the difference between real advice and fake advice?

## A Pharmaceutical Society

It's no surprise we've become a pharmaceutical society. I, for one, am sick of it. It is the twenty-first century, and our health is collapsing. Our medical system is broken. The information we are fed is influenced by lobbyists. Low-fat...low-carb...who knows what to believe or whom to believe? No wonder we are so sick. In the unlikely event that your doctor doesn't prescribe a particular drug to fix your ailing health during your all-too-brief 10- to 15-minute visit, you'll probably speak up about it. The pharmaceutical companies have taught people to ask for drugs themselves. It takes just a few minutes of watching TV for the viewer to learn the benefits of countless drugs. In the meantime, you'll be bombarded with commercials for sugary cereals, soda, margarine, and diet franchises advising you to buy processed food or low-carb products. As a result, we've become a sick society that thrives on drugs. Here's the truth: real, natural food is the miracle medicine Americans desperately need to improve their health.

Look at the older generation, many of whom are senile and even sick today—and they were not exposed to nearly as many toxic foods as we eat today! As a result, our generation will be in poorer health than this older generation. Take action and change your health. It is a fact; Americans work more hours than workers in other industrialized nations, and they have little time to cook. It's certainly easier and cheaper for us to grab a fat-free muffin, a doughnut, a slice of pizza, or a quick pickup from a fast-food restaurant instead of cooking in the kitchen for hours. Real food costs more money and takes more time to prepare. That may be true, but believe me: you don't need Martha Stewart's cooking skills to improve your health. Just eat real food and don't fear natural fats to get your diet balanced.

## Research That Contradicts the Low-Fat Approach Is Generally Ignored

I know that you've heard for most of your life that in order to stay healthy, you need to follow a low-fat diet. Perhaps your doctor has implored you to avoid cholesterol-rich food and choose cereals over eggs. Now you find yourself reading a book that tells you the exact opposite is true; that you shouldn't fear the natural fats in whole milk, butter, and cheese; and that you should cut anything that says "fat-free" on its label, including milk! A diet that dispels many mainstream recommendations can certainly send mixed messages. If you feel like Alice in Wonderland, you're not alone. But I am not here to confuse you; I am here to help you.

We are constantly confronted with lies, misconceptions, and myths about nutrition, but I've done all the homework for you with this book. Why isn't your doctor giving you the right information? He or she probably made it all the way through medical school without completing a single course on nutrition. Because of this lack of education, doctors today simply follow established guidelines, which are heavily influenced by the food industry and its lobbyists. As I explained in the introduction to this book, doctors have little time to spend with their patients in the age of HMOs. They're also trained to treat diseases with drugs instead of nutrition, and they're constantly inundated with propaganda from pharmaceutical companies.

Diabetic? Take this pill. Overweight? Take this pill. Depressed? Take this pill. There are pills for this and pills for that. If doctors took the time to check their patients' levels of insulin, growth hormone, thyroid, estrogen, progesterone, and testosterone instead of just treating their symptoms, they'd quickly learn that many health problems can be eliminated simply through diet changes or adjusting hormones to normal levels.

Some of my patients call me a holistic doctor, and others call me a diet doctor. Believe me: I'm neither. I practice medicine the way it is supposed to be practiced. There is a definite need for drugs, but drugs can't replace a healthy diet. Unfortunately, the medical system in the United States is broken.

## My Promises Are Huge Because the Perfect 10 Diet Delivers

I'm a firm believer in the curative power of food. Although I can't say with certainty that we can completely undo the permanent cellular damage caused by eating the wrong food, I say that I've seen the health of thousands of my patients improve dramatically once they followed the Perfect 10 Diet with its balanced approach. The secret to perfect 10 health and weight loss is hormonal harmony. Believe it or not, on the Perfect 10 Diet you will eat a lot of rich food and plenty of calories, and you'll still manage to lose weight. Sounds crazy? No, folks; your hormones will be working for you and not against you. That's why the Perfect 10 Diet is groundbreaking and earth shattering.

I know you have a hectic and busy life, so I will break it down and give you a sensible plan to make it easy to follow. I promise to give you all the information you need to improve your health. But you need to be an active participant. You have to be responsible for your own health because I can't baby-sit or supervise you. Everything you put in your mouth counts and ultimately affects your hormones and health. So forget low-fat, low-carb popular diets and everything else. We are starting fresh here. Balance and natural food is all it takes to be fit.

I realize that some of you just want to lose weight without knowing a whole lot about nutrition. "Tell me what to eat every day, Doctor. Give me a plan for breakfast, lunch, and dinner to lower my cholesterol because I have no time." I hear disturbing statements like this from many of my patients all the time, even from those who are quite sophisticated.

Look, I have to be brutally honest with you. I have written the Perfect 10 Diet for everyone, but here is the exception: this book is not for naïve people. If you don't want to know why you're overweight, why the scale is stuck, or why your cholesterol is high, or if you don't want to bother addressing or going to the roots of your health problems, the Perfect 10 Diet is not for you. I don't want to waste your time. Remember poor heath is not a good thing, and hospitals are not the place you want to be when you're older. It's your health, and it's your call to do whatever you think is right for you.

If you're ready to follow the Perfect 10 Diet, I have two specific requests before we get started. First, you need to listen to everything I say and trust me. The second request is to not get confused by contradictory messages about the Perfect 10 Diet. I don't care if this information is from our biggest fitness gurus, nutrition experts, fad diet authors, or even Uncle Sam. I hate to be controversial, but I have no choice because I want you to be healthy and not get derailed. Just because the government says three servings of dairy per day is essential does not really mean that that's right. Just because margarine manufacturers tell you in their commercials that margarine is good for you doesn't mean they're telling the truth. Get it? You need to eliminate fake food and restore nutrients. No more low-fat, low-carb, cabbage soup, or celebrity diets. Follow everything I say because I am not endorsed by anybody but myself. Believe me, you will be successful because you will get to the roots of the problems, and not shut your eyes to what is going on inside.

When you follow the Perfect 10 Diet to the core and balance your hormones, you:

- speed up your metabolism
- lose weight without going hungry
- eat more food and still lose weight
- are less likely to get diabetes
- are less likely to get prediabetes
- are less likely get heart disease
- are less likely to get cancer
- will be happy
- look younger
- improve your vision
- have radiant skin
- are less likely to get wrinkles
- strengthen your bones
- have shiny hair
- have strong nails
- get a higher sex drive
- have more energy
- delay the aging process
- prevent old-age diseases
- live a longer life

Are you ready to sign up? Are you ready to give your hormones a total makeover that will spill over to give you a sexy body and radiant skin? Great. Let's get to how the Perfect 10 Diet works.

## The Perfect 10 Diet Approach Is High-Fat/Low-Carb

Welcome to the future. No calorie counting here on the Perfect 10 Diet. Today, we have a greater understanding of how hormones affect weight, metabolism, and overall health. So it's time for a new slim-down mantra. Eat more fat and lose weight. No joke!

I am talking about moderation, of course, not the very high-fat/high-protein/low-carb extreme to shut down growth hormone, the youth hormone. The food choices on the Perfect 10 Diet help you drop the pounds and curb your appetite. So get ready to say, "Good-bye hunger, hello sexy body."

When you follow a more balanced diet, with less sugar and the right amount of natural fats, you'll slow down the absorption of food in your digestive tract. A slower pace of digestion delays the release of sugar into the bloodstream and stabilizes your sugar and insulin levels, which will make you less hungry. Your body will use the natural fats you eat for energy instead of all that sugar from carbs, and you'll end up eating less.

Many people fear that eating too much fat will make them fatter, and they believe that they're better off eating more carbohydrates. But there is a built-in safeguard when we eat natural fats: they do not trigger exaggerated insulin secretions. A stable insulin level promotes satiety, so our bodies do not crave an overabundance of food.

Here's an example: Avocados are a virtually perfect source of dietary fat, but how many avocados can you eat at a time? On the other hand, given the same level of hunger, how many cookies could you eat? Here's another example: How many pieces of fish, such as salmon, with a rich, creamy, buttery sauce could you eat for lunch or dinner? Compare that to the number of pizza slices you could eat for the same meal. You see my point? When you provide your body with healthy, natural fats as a source of fuel, you require fewer calories, produce less insulin, and in turn, you lose weight. No more processed food is allowed either—it will make your hormones go haywire. This means no more frozen dinners, diet soda, artificial sweeteners, and of course, trans fats. You will also avoid gender benders as much as you can to get all your hormones and your metabolism going at maximal speed.

**Figure 1.7:** Effect of a Balanced Diet on Your Health

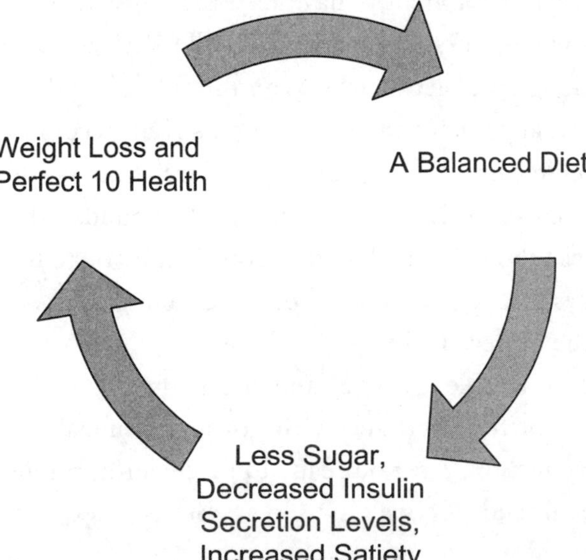

## How You Will Succeed on the Perfect 10 Diet

Numerous studies indicate that you can eat more fat and lose more weight than on the low-fat approach. You may even get away with eating an extra 300 to 500 calories a day and still manage to lose weight. Isn't that exciting?

Does this mean you can gobble thousands of calories from fat on the Perfect 10 Diet? Of course not. Moderation is the key to successful weight loss. On the Perfect 10 Diet, you will eat three meals and taper your calories throughout the day. By that I mean eating less as the day goes on: a large breakfast, normal lunch, and small dinner. This is specifically designed to support a healthy metabolism. I also want you to eat organic food as much as you can to limit pesticides and chemicals that can disrupt or mimic hormones.

I have included some snacks on the Perfect 10 Diet, but they're optional. I know you must be flipping out and saying, "Three meals a day? That's it, Doc?" You certainly should know by now that I am not going to sugarcoat anything to sell you my diet. No food is calorie free, except for water. Were you trying to lose weight or gain weight when you picked this book? I know that most nutritionists and health experts tell us to eat every three hours to lose weight, but look how overweight we've become.

Body builders came up with the frequent meal approach to gobble 4,000 to 5,000 calories each day in order to build muscles. Are you hitting the gym every day? If so, great, I have no problem with your snacking every day. That's why snacks are included on the Perfect 10 Diet plan. If you are not working out, keep snacks to a minimum. It is disturbing to see the frequent meal approach becoming a mainstream recommendation for the whole nation, regardless of age or activity level. Snacks add up to hundreds of calories and can easily make you put on the pounds. Three meals a day is plenty. Snacks should be included in your diet if you're hungry or diabetic, or on the days that you work out. You are encouraged to exercise 3 to 4 days a week on the Perfect 10 Diet.

The Perfect 10 Diet is here, and the party is over for fad diets. One hundred percent real food and with nothing artificial to enhance it: now that's true perfection. Are you ready to give your hormones a makeover to improve health and lose weight? Great. But is it too late for you to start the Perfect 10 Diet after decades on the wrong approach? Can you reverse the damage? I certainly hope so. Don't wait for the medical organizations and authorities to change their views on low-fat advice or manufactured fat. Please don't be tempted to get on the latest low-carb trend or order processed food from the big popular chains. Your health is at stake, and it is your most valuable asset, not to be treated like few dollars to throw away in Las Vegas when you have no chance of winning.

Make an effort now to save your life. We of this generation are on our own. We may have changed with the passage of time, but the biology inside us has not.

## *Mark's Story*

Mark is a 35-year-old patient who came to see me for relief from frequent and severe headaches. Mark is 5 feet, 9 inches tall. When he first came to see me, he weighed 260 pounds. His body mass index was a whopping 40 percent (30 percent is considered obese).

Mark was morbidly obese, almost twice his healthy weight, and his blood pressure was markedly elevated. In order to rule out a neurological cause for his headaches, I referred him for magnetic resonance imaging (MRI) of his brain. His MRI came back as normal, so it became clear to me that Mark's headaches were related to his elevated blood pressure—which was caused by his obesity.

Mark's blood work showed a markedly elevated triglyceride level (a risk for heart disease when high, and indicative of excessive carbohydrate intake). Mark had very low levels of high density lipoprotein cholesterol (C-HDL), which is another risk for heart disease when low. His examination and lab work indicated that he suffered from the metabolic syndrome, a disease of insulin resistance. His fasting insulin level was at 60, which is way too high.

I sat down with Mark and took an extensive dietary history. Mark told me that he had followed a low-fat and high-carbohydrate diet all his life. His weight constantly fluctuated, but it would always creep back up—no matter how vigilant he was.

Each morning, Mark ate cereal with fat-free milk and drank orange juice for breakfast. A typical lunch was usually a grilled chicken sandwich on white bread with fat-free mayonnaise, lettuce, and tomato, and a side order of a baked potato. He snacked on fat-free yogurts and pretzels. For dinner, he frequently ate pasta, a staple of his Italian background.

Mark's diet certainly followed the vague low-fat dietary guidelines we're all encouraged to follow, but I quickly realized that he ate practically nothing but sugar. Mark was shocked when I told him that following a high-fat and low-carbohydrate diet, a balanced diet, was the only way to improve his deteriorating health. I explained to Mark that the abundance of sugar and lack of natural fat in his diet were causing his health problems.

Desperate to feel better and lose weight, Mark began following the Perfect 10 Diet. Within ten months, he was down to 170 pounds, his headaches were gone, and his blood pressure, cholesterol, and insulin had all returned to normal levels. Mark reports that he's never felt better.

Like me at one time, and most other Americans, Mark was being poisoned by the massive amounts of processed food, sugar, refined carbohydrates, and low-fat products he ate.

## A Typical Day on the Perfect 10 Diet

**BREAKFAST:** Arugula Omelet with Rye Toast and 1 Apple
**OPTIONAL MIDMORNING SNACK:** ½ Cup Almonds
**LUNCH:** Grilled Chicken Salad with Extra-Virgin Olive Oil and Unsweetened Lemonade
**OPTIONAL MIDAFTERNOON SNACK:** Mixed Berries
**DINNER:** Grilled Salmon with Broccoli

### *Roberta's Story*

Roberta is a 32-year-old event planner. She is a statuesque 5 feet, 9 inches tall, but overweight at 205 pounds. Since her divorce 2 years ago, she turned to food for emotional support. Roberta is eager to lose weight since she is often before the public at prestigious events. Her usual effervescent spirit and zest is greatly diminished because of her weight gain. Roberta related her frustration with one of the popular low-carb diets that she is trying to follow. "I'm miserable. I have awful cravings for bread, and feel totally out of control, and I've lost only 4 pounds in 3 months," she said. I counseled Roberta about the risks associated with low-carb dieting. Her blood test revealed a sluggish thyroid. I placed Roberta on the Perfect 10 Diet and prescribed a thyroid hormone pill. She returned in 2 months; her thyroid was back to normal and she lost 17 pounds. Roberta continued to follow the Perfect 10 Diet and lost a total of 30 pounds in the following year. She regained her enthusiasm along with her self-confidence.

### A Typical Day on the Perfect 10 Diet

**BREAKFAST:** Whole-Wheat Bagel with Cream Cheese and 1 Orange

**OPTIONAL MIDMORNING SNACK:** ½ Cup Grapes

**LUNCH:** Grilled Tuna with Mixed Vegetables

**OPTIONAL MIDAFTERNOON SNACK:** Vegetable Juice

**DINNER:** Squash Soup and 1 Slice of Whole-Wheat Bread

CHAPTER 2

# The Evolution of the Human Diet: How We Got Here

In 1987 I was living in Spain as part of a medical school exchange program, and worked in the clinic of a major university hospital. During that time, I rarely heard a Spaniard of any age—male or female—talk about dieting. The Mediterranean diet, with all its health benefits, includes the cuisines of Greece, Italy, and Spain. In Spain, I didn't see the magnitude of health problems I see with my patients every single day in America. The Spaniards had no fear of food, whether it contained fat or carbohydrates. Spaniards eat well, and without guilt, until they are full. This experience in Spain taught me that the amount of fat a person consumes isn't the most important factor—the important contributor to obesity is "fake food."

So how did we get the idea that low-fat foods and manufactured fats are good for us in the first place?

## The Paleolithic Diet (2,000,000 to 10,000 BC)

I truly agree with those who say that if we ate like our distant hunter-gatherer ancestors, most of our health problems—including obesity—would disappear. During the Paleolithic period, our ancestors followed a low-carb diet and ate natural fats. They ate vegetables and nuts, but no grains. They ate fruit, but only seasonally. Rarely did humans eat sugar, except the natural sugars found in honey or fruit. Though sparse and primitive, this diet allowed our ancestors to survive on the earth for millions of years under very harsh conditions. In fact, we survived even when other animal species couldn't adapt and became extinct. Life for early humans centered on a constant struggle to obtain food. The average life expectancy was very short—probably not beyond age 30. This was not caused by a poor diet; rather, most succumbed to infections or predators.

During this time, our ancestors developed a taste for animal meat. The introduction of animal products into the human diet played a major role in our evolution. The fatty acids found in animal fat served as a new and potent form of brain food that spurred the development of the human brain. This animal fat also provided a longer sustained source of energy. Humans, like lions and tigers, no longer had to eat around the clock to keep up their energy, and they were able to focus on developing other skills. Unlike true carnivores, however, we retained our "sweet tooth" and continued to eat fruit. Until the discovery of fire, all food was eaten raw, which kept the delivery of nutrients to our systems very slow. This prolonged digestive time provided satiety and did not strain our metabolic or hormonal systems.

Exercise and movement were an intrinsic part of everyday life. Our ancestors walked long distances to hunt and find food. Chasing wild animals with clubs, climbing trees to collect nuts, and fleeing from predators were all part of daily life. Constant migration was also a fact of early human existence. As a result of this constant exercise, humans burned huge numbers of calories per day. This primitive diet provided us with the essential protein needed to build muscles and the natural fats we needed to promote satiety. The survival of early humans was aided by a diet that balanced the fat-storing hormone (insulin) and the fat-burning hormone (glucagon). When food was abundant, our ancestors ate lavishly. Then the food was converted to saturated fat by insulin and stored to be used for energy at a later time. When food was scarce, the stored fat would be converted by the fat-burning hormone (glucagon) into sugar and used for energy. Insulin and glucagon remain essential for our survival since they play a vital role in energy storage and usage (Fig. 2.1) and were in perfect balance in this time period.

**Figure 2.1:** Food Storage and Metabolism

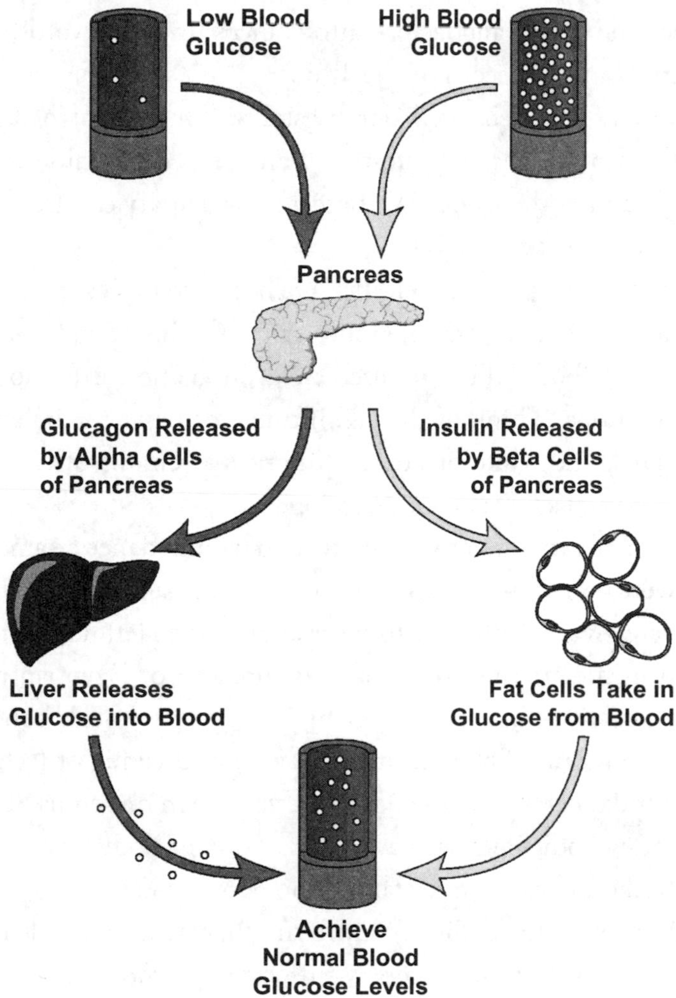


Wolters Kluwer Health, Inc.-Lippincott Williams & Wilkins.

## The Advent of Agriculture

The advent of agriculture challenged the integrity and harmony of our hormonal systems. Grains were added to the human diet about 10,000 years ago. This change radically shifted the dietary balance away from low-carb to high-carb eating. Until man domesticated cows about 8,000 years ago, humans never consumed milk beyond infancy. The addition of grains and milk brought a paradoxical shift. Although the human lifespan began to increase because people were no longer reliant on being part of the predatory food chain, a host of previously unknown diseases also began to arise, like allergies and gluten and lactose intolerances. In other words, we began to live longer, but not necessarily healthier.

This diet shift also changed our lifestyles. The advent of agriculture meant the end of a migratory lifestyle. Families, communities, and cities sprouted up around the world. We became a sedentary culture because we no longer had to chase our food.

As we added more grains to our diet, we began to eat less fat and protein from animal sources and consume more carbs. Grains provided a constant, ready source of food, which resulted in a population explosion. Grains became ubiquitous. Think of the significance of pasta for Italians, white rice for Asians, and white bread for Americans. Grains often meant the difference between survival and starvation.

In pharaonic Egypt, grains were cultivated in abundance around the Nile River and were part of the daily diet. Grains were so significant to Egyptians that they were given as offerings to the gods and even left next to mummies to be eaten in the afterlife. But close examination of Egyptian mummies reveals the negative impact of a diet high in grains—weak bones, rotted teeth, and other signs of poor health (that are not dissimilar to what people suffer from today). The statues and art we've seen in museums of Egyptian muscular young bodies were just an idealization of a body type. They are in direct contradiction to the true state of the population's health.

As we added milk to our diet, many found themselves not able to tolerate it. People who are lactose intolerant suffer such symptoms as abdominal pain and bloating when they consume dairy products.

## Our Modern Diet: The Last 200 Years

The human diet has changed more over the last 200 years than during the preceding 10,000 years. Following the introduction of sugar and refined vegetable oils into our diet, our health took a real nosedive. Many primitive societies did not change their diets following the onset of the Industrial Revolution, but many—especially ours—did. The United States certainly took to processed foods more aggressively than other industrialized countries, such as France and Japan. Yes, the French eat some refined carbs from pastries, but they still eat plenty of fresh vegetables and fruits. The same goes for the Japanese, who eat white rice, but always with abundant fresh fish and other seafood.

## Milk Pasteurization: A Good Thing or a Bad Thing?

Even milk, a recent introduction to our diet, changed from raw to pasteurized, and subsequently to pasteurized and fat-free. In moderation, whole-fat raw milk is quite healthy and provides nutrients and enzymes that promote health, but it must be consumed immediately to avoid spoilage. Things changed in the 1920s as health officials encouraged universal pasteurization, which kills bacteria. At the time, death rates related to infections were quite high. As improved sanitary conditions were implemented in the early 20th century, the death rate decreased, and pasteurization was wrongly credited as the key reason why.

As a result, pasteurization became big business. Gone were the days of small, family-run farms, which dairy farming replaced on a massive scale. Cows were no longer free to roam and eat grass; instead, they were confined to overcrowded stalls and fed soy, bakery waste, corn, grains, and other dead animals—anything *but* the fresh green grass essential to making healthy, nutritious milk. Cows are routinely injected with recombinant bovine somatotropin (rBST), a genetically engineered growth hormone that stimulates milk production. (The long-term effects of this hormone on our health are still unknown.)

Last, the cows' milk is pasteurized to promote shelf life. It's clear that pasteurized fat-free milk, which we are encouraged to consume on a daily basis, is not as nutritious as the full-fat raw milk humans consumed for thousands of years.

Research done on pasteurized milk reveals:

- Pasteurization destroys milk enzymes and forces the body to work extra hard to break down the milk nutrients.
- Pasteurization destroys and reduces many nutrients in milk, including vitamins A, C, and B complex.
- Pasteurization destroys many of the healthy bacteria present in milk.
- Pasteurization lowers calcium by 38 percent.

It's worth repeating: before pasteurization, adults consumed very little milk for thousands of years. Once pasteurization made dairy farming big business, milk began to be marketed as an essential food that should be consumed in the amount of three servings per day. Aggressive marketing led to an overconsumption of dairy and an upsurge in lactose-related illnesses. When saturated fats in dairy were condemned in the later part of the 20th century as atherogenic, simple sugars were at times added to many dairy products, such as yogurt, to replace the removed fat. This process took a further toll on our insulin secretions and other hormones.

## The Refinement of Whole Grains

In the late 19th century, mills started refining whole grains into nutritionally barren white flour. White flour has a long shelf life and makes fluffier breads and pastries. However, it's nutritionally empty. The taste of this new flour appealed to many people who viewed dark or whole-grain bread as "peasant" food, and in particular Americans were quick to embrace this new taste. The process of refining grains removes its fiber, which is actually the healthiest part of the grain and crucial for slowing digestion.

Carbohydrates in starches, such as white bread, are broken down upon digestion: first into maltose, and then into glucose, which quickly moves from the digestive system to the bloodstream. Maltose, which is made of two glucose molecules (glucose + glucose) and is present in white bread, is actually more harmful than pure table sugar, which has a different molecular structure. Table sugar (sucrose) is composed of two different molecules (glucose + fructose).

When table sugar is consumed, the glucose part moves into the bloodstream and raises blood sugar levels, but the fructose part is metabolized by the liver. In other words, table sugar has less impact on the glucose level in the bloodstream than refined carbohydrates have. This means that eating white bread or white rice is worse than eating a bowl of pure table sugar, since it has more of a negative impact on insulin secretion. Isn't it amazing that you think twice before putting 2 spoonfuls of sugar in your coffee, but you don't worry about eating a bowl of cereal or pasta? Never before in history have our bodies had to deal with this kind of sugar overload.

When you consume refined grains, blood sugar levels fluctuate erratically and dramatically, much more so than if you were eating pure table sugar alone (Fig. 2.2). The higher blood sugar levels rise, the lower they eventually fall, and those dips lead to hunger, which cause people to overeat. This leads to exaggerated insulin secretions and increased caloric consumption. These factors lead to weight gain and a downward spiral in overall health. It is not an overstatement to say that based on our overconsumption of refined grains, we are literally poisoning ourselves with sugar.

**Figure 2.2:** The Effect of Different Flours on Blood Sugar Levels

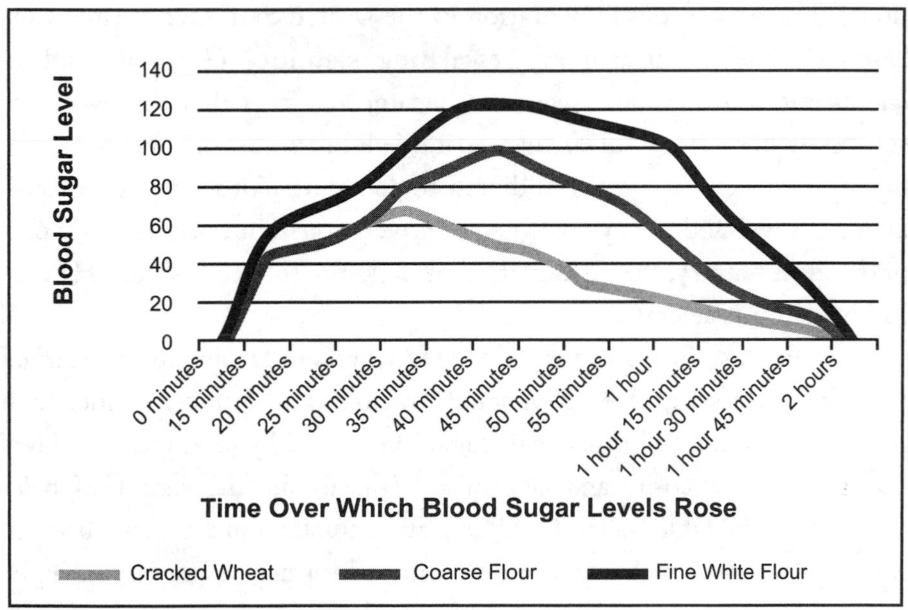


In addition, the nutritional deficiencies in refined grains have led to a spike in the incidence of a host of illnesses, such as beriberi, pellagra, and night blindness, during the last 200 years. It took years for doctors and scientists to connect these emerging diseases to nutritionally empty grain products. Once the connection was made, the food industry simply added vitamins and minerals to processed grain foods instead of promoting whole-grain foods. Ironically, this "enrichment" process was used to market these unhealthy products. Enriched carbs suddenly became the good guys—despite the fact that they are behind many of the plagues of modern society, like obesity, heart disease, diabetes, and cancer. Scientists who diagnosed patients with these diseases in the 19th and early 20th centuries hadn't even heard of the hormone insulin or the dangers of its excessive secretion.

## The Culture of Sugar and High-Fructose Corn Syrup

The process of producing granulated sugar by pressing the juice out of sugar cane and boiling it into crystals was developed in India about 500 BC. The Arabs introduced it to Spain, and from there it continued westward. Refining sugar was expensive, but by the end of the 19th century, sugar refineries were quite profitable. At that time, there were more than 30 sugar factories in operation in the United States, and Americans began to consume sugar in ever-escalating quantities. Given our biological affinity for fruits and sweets, it became apparent that the sweetness source—whether natural or man-made—didn't matter to our primitive brains. We were becoming addicted to the stuff. Although Americans' taste for sugar and honey remained relatively constant until the early part of the 20th century, the introduction of high-fructose corn syrup (HFCS-55) helped it accelerate.

High-fructose corn syrup was invented when food technologists learned to make sweet syrup from corn starch by boiling it with acid under high pressure. It is much cheaper than sugar and prized by food manufacturers because of its viscosity and lack of crystallization. Although HFCS-55 is identical to table sugar (sucrose), it's actually much worse because we consume it in such massive amounts. The fructose present in high-fructose corn syrup can also be used by the liver cells; however, if unused, it's converted into fat. Problems associated with high-fructose corn syrup include increased LDL (bad cholesterol) levels, leading to increased risk of heart disease; an altered magnesium balance, leading to increased osteoporosis; and an increased risk of diabetes.

Also at the turn of the 20th century, carbonated beverages, such as soda pop, became popular. Just 100 years ago, people drank only water when they were thirsty. A can of regular soda contains about 40 grams of high-fructose corn syrup, or approximately 9 teaspoons of sugar! How many cans of soda do you drink a day? The average American consumes

43 gallons of sugary soft drinks a year! According to the United States Department of Agriculture (USDA) figures, most Americans now consume about 160 pounds of sugar a year. These dramatic changes in our diet have taken a huge toll on our secretions of insulin and other hormones such as cortisol and leptin.

**Figure 2.3:** Foods that Contain High-Fructose Corn Syrup

- Apple sauce
- Barbecue sauce
- Bread
- Cereal
- Candy
- Canned fruit
- Cookies
- Chocolate Milk
- Crackers
- Fruit punch
- Fruit juices
- Ice cream
- Jam
- Jelly
- Ketchup
- Salad dressing

## The Introduction of Manufactured Fat into Our Diet

Before the Industrial Revolution, people ate vegetable oils (corn, cottonseed, and soybean) in very small quantities from natural sources (plants and seeds). In high doses, refined polyunsaturated vegetable oils, which are manufactured fats, promote the development of cholesterol deposits in the tissues; in turn, this causes clogged arteries and heart disease. In addition, refined polyunsaturated oils are at times hydrogenated (containing trans fats) which makes them even more deadly to us. As I mentioned previously, trans fats can't be recognized or even metabolized by our bodies.

In the 19th century, the Industrial Revolution spawned massive migrations to cities and manufacturing centers across Europe. This led to overcrowding and food shortages. A huge underclass of city dwellers found themselves living on the edge of starvation. Butter and other natural animal fats were scarce and costly, and they were available only to the upper classes.

In 1869 Emperor Louis Napoleon III of France offered a prize to anyone who could make a satisfactory substitute for butter suitable for use by the armed forces and the poor. In turn, hydrogenation was invented to create a butter substitute called margarine. Originally, margarine was manufactured by using an acid called margaric on animal products, an expensive endeavor. Later on, it was made from vegetable oil. After World War II, soybean oil became the major source of margarine and other hydrogenated oils (think of mixed vegetable oils). This manufactured fat certainly helped to feed the poor, but it also took a huge toll on the health of its consumers.

## Fat in the American Diet in the Late 19th and Early 20th Centuries

The typical American diet in the late 19th and early 20th centuries contained much more fat than most people eat today. Fat intake varied from 32 to 44 percent for the average American. At times, saturated fat constituted 36 percent of total calories consumed. Fats used for cooking were rendered from lard, beef, poultry, pork, coconut, and butter. Interestingly, heart disease was a rarity in those days, even though we are now told that these types of natural fats clog the arteries.

## Fat in the American Diet in the 20th Century

In 1911 Procter & Gamble launched Crisco, a hydrogenated vegetable oil that changed the cooking habits of virtually every American household. It was more economical to produce than butter, and no expense was spared to market it to the masses (Fig. 2.4). By 1938 Crisco was a household staple, and the consumption of refined vegetable oils in this country had tripled. Margarine consumption quadrupled between 1900 and 1950, and butter consumption plummeted.

However, by the 1950s, the American Heart Association reported that the United States was in the midst of an epidemic of coronary heart disease. The cause was then unknown. Many theories were suggested to explain this surge, including heavy sugar consumption, hydrogenated vegetable oils, and the flawed saturated-fat/cholesterol theory (more to come on that in the next section). It soon became clear that the switch from natural fats to hydrogenated polyunsaturated vegetable oils, coupled with rapidly escalating sugar consumption, had caused heart disease to become a full-blown epidemic by the mid-20th century.

**Figure 2.4:** An Ad Used to Market Crisco

Now it's oh, so easy to bake...
this lighter, richer Crisco cake
Enjoy real baking ease
with Crisco!
It's easier to blend, creamier than
other vegetable shortenings!
CRISCO'S CHERRY MINT CAKE
Crisco
use
Crisco
IT'S
DIGESTIBLE!

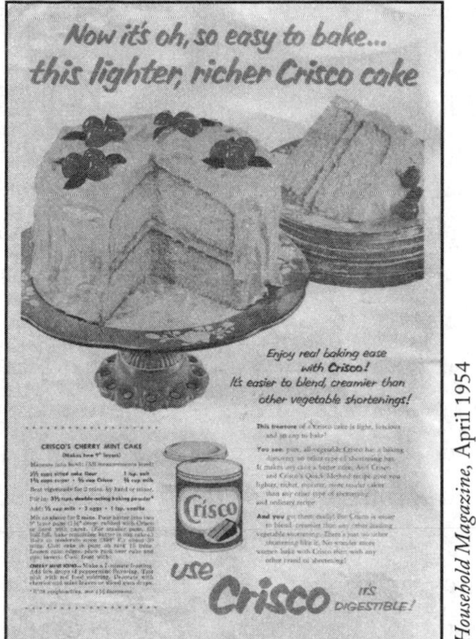

*Household Magazine*, April 1954

## The Saturated-Fat/Cholesterol Theory of Heart Disease

The saturated-fat/cholesterol theory was formally introduced to Americans by Dr. Ancel Keys, a research physiologist from the University of Minnesota. On a trip to Italy in the 1950s, Dr. Keys learned that heart disease was a very rare occurrence there. He also noted that many farmers in the region had a favorable cholesterol profile. He compared the Mediterranean diet to the American diet and found some striking discrepancies.

The Mediterranean diet included an abundance of vegetables, fruits, and whole grains. For the most part, the only oils consumed there were cold-pressed extra-virgin olive oil, and the people ate little sugar.

The Mediterranean diet was a balanced diet then, just as it is today. The American diet was pretty much the direct opposite. By the late 1950s, Americans were eating more refined carbohydrates, and much of the fats they consumed were hydrogenated, such as Crisco and margarine. Both refined carbs and trans fats have a profoundly negative effect on cholesterol. Dr. Keys, who had previously thought that both saturated and hydrogenated fats were behind the increase in heart disease, flip-flopped in his viewpoints and ultimately focused on hydrogenated fats and oils as the real culprit.

The edible oil industry quickly responded to this financial threat to its products by mounting a campaign to promote the belief that the *saturated* fat in hydrogenated oils was to blame and switched to a process called partial hydrogenation, claiming this would eliminate the problem. In truth, partial hydrogenation does not change the composition of manufactured oils or the amount of trans fats. It's just a gimmick.

As a result of these new industry claims, Dr. Keys ultimately concentrated on the saturated fats, such as butter, as a culprit behind heart disease.

Sadly, people bought this misinformation campaign wholesale, even though humans have consumed saturated fat in animal products and butter for thousands of years. How could we buy into the notion that saturated fats were bad for us, given that animal fat had fed our evolution and led to our brain development?

How could we buy into the notion that saturated fat causes heart disease when it is naturally produced in our bodies? Saturated fat is stored in our bodies to be used for energy when food is not available. It does not interfere with our hormones or cellular communication. However, this faulty theory gained so much momentum that large studies were conducted to support it. The most influential—and flawed—of these was the Seven Countries Study.

## The Seven Countries Study

After a World Health Organization (WHO) meeting in 1955, Dr. Keys introduced The Seven Countries Study, a 13-year comparative study of cardiac disease. The study included people in Greece (including Crete and Corfu), Finland, Japan, Italy, the Netherlands, former Yugoslavia, and the United States, and the study's findings showed that the lowest incidence of heart disease occurred in Greece, with Japan at a close second. There was a higher incidence of heart disease in all the other countries. An analysis of the countries' diets implicated saturated fat as the cause, and the misinformation began.

The advantages of the Mediterranean and Japanese diets should have been credited to the diets' relative absence of sugar, hydrogenated fats, and trans fats. Instead, it was wrongly credited to low consumption of natural saturated fats and animal products. Dr. Keys erroneously concluded that as people ate more and more saturated fat and animal products their cholesterol and their likelihood of heart disease would rise.

In retrospect, one can see that Dr. Keys carefully chose these seven countries to validate his faulty theory. Data were available for 22 countries. When researchers plotted other countries with a high saturated fat intake on the same graph, Dr. Keys's correlation simply vanished into thin air. For example, the raw data included Switzerland, a country with a high level of saturated fat intake from animal products and a relatively low incidence of heart disease, but Dr. Keys decided not to include it.

The edible oil industry, the beneficiary of these flawed findings, began funding further research designed to support this saturated-fat theory. Some of this funding came from Procter & Gamble (makers of Crisco), Mazola (makers of corn oil), and Fleischmann's (makers of margarine). Manufactured oils like margarine suddenly became good for our health, and natural fats like butter became dangerous.

After the dietary cholesterol theory of heart disease took center stage, it was not long before the American Medical Association, American Dietetic Association, and the National Academy of Sciences followed suit and began promoting manufactured vegetable oils over natural saturated fat. It is interesting to note that, at that time, Dr. Keys was on the nutrition advisory committee of the powerful American Heart Association (AHA). As a result, his biased research became the official basis for the AHA dietary guidelines published in 1961.

Although the relationships among refined polyunsaturated oils, trans fats, and cancer were emerging, endorsement by the medical establishment made us believe these manufactured fats were better for our health. The cholesterol/saturated-fat theory was here to stay.

But this dietary misinformation was just the beginning of a more radical change in the way Americans viewed all fats—both good and bad—with the advent of low-fat diets.

## Origin of the Low-Fat Diets

The steps to high-carb eating in this country were just the beginning of a radical change to eating more and more carbs with the advent of low-fat diets. In the 1950s, Nathan Pritikin, an engineer in his 40s, became interested in nutrition after he was diagnosed with heart disease. Believing that his own heart disease was caused by consuming too much fat, he devised an eating plan that consisted of a whopping 75 percent of total calories from carbohydrates. Pritikin's approach greatly influenced Senator George McGovern, who was interested in addressing the burgeoning obesity epidemic in this country.

This diet enjoyed immense popularity in its time, and its dominance led to the creation of the original United States Department of Agriculture food pyramid (Fig. 2.5), which featured grains (bread, pasta, and cereals) as its base. Furthermore, the pyramid didn't specify whether or not the grains should be whole or refined. These dietary guidelines were written by a reporter with no scientific background, and based solely on a single nutritionist's opinion. They were designed to make it simpler for the public to condemn all fats, placing them at the apex of the pyramid (which meant they were to be eaten only sparingly). The "preferred" diet was suddenly high in sugar, low in fiber, and low in all fats, whether they were good or bad.

Once the USDA made the low-fat dogma official, the food industry quickly began producing thousands of reduced-fat food products to meet the new recommendations. Fat was removed from foods like milk, crackers, and cookies, and replaced with something just as pleasurable to the palate. This meant added sugar or high-fructose corn syrup. These deadly foods were labeled and marketed as low-fat or fat-free. To make matters worse, much of this processed junk food received the approval of the American Heart Association (for a fee) since it met their criteria for a diet low in saturated fat and cholesterol. This disturbing new low-fat movement led to the rise of a new breed of doctors who took low-fat diets to low-fat extremes, such as Dr. Dean Ornish, who advocated no fish, nuts, or even olive oil in his original diet.

As people began to fear all fats—including healthy fats—they began to

**Figure 2.5:** The Original USDA Food Pyramid

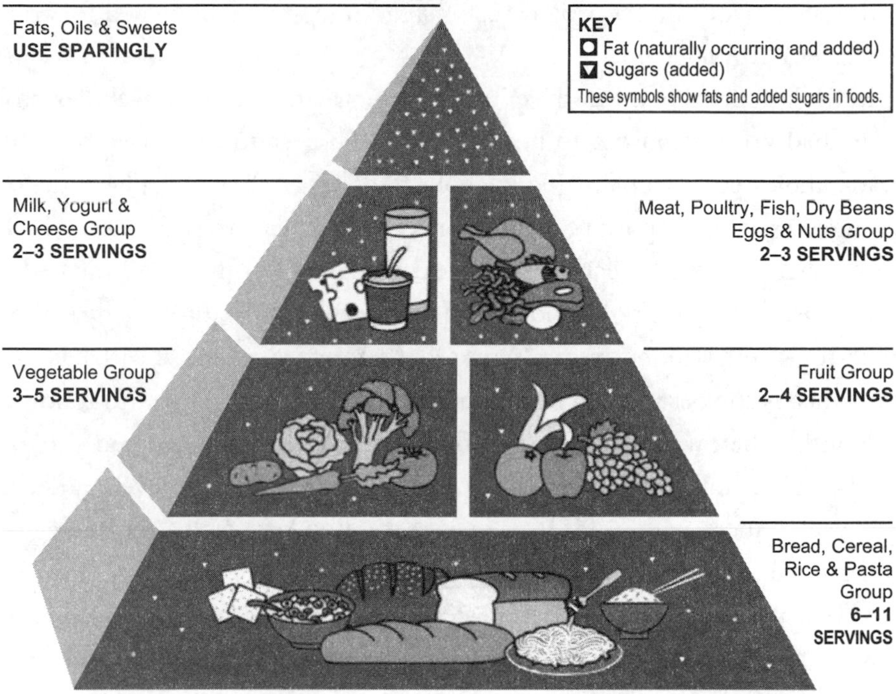

KEY
Fat (naturally occurring and added)
Sugars (added)
These symbols show fats and added sugars in foods.

Fats, Oils & Sweets
**USE SPARINGLY**

Milk, Yogurt & Cheese Group
**2–3 SERVINGS**

Meat, Poultry, Fish, Dry Beans Eggs & Nuts Group
**2–3 SERVINGS**

Vegetable Group
**3–5 SERVINGS**

Fruit Group
**2–4 SERVINGS**

Bread, Cereal, Rice & Pasta Group
**6–11 SERVINGS**

USDA website

gain weight at an alarming pace. In the 1970s, the percentage of fat in the American diet was about 42 percent, and carbohydrates made up another 40 percent. By the 1990s, the percentage of fat in the average American diet had decreased to about 30 percent, and consumption of carbohydrates had increased to about 50 percent. Because of this shift, people are experiencing epidemics of diet-related illnesses, such as obesity, heart disease, and diabetes. Many health experts now acknowledge that the low-fat message is radically oversimplified, and that it totally ignores the fact that some fats, such as olive oil and avocados, are good for us. Even saturated fats—also known as "bad" fats—are not deleterious at all. They are neutral to your cholesterol.

## The Exploitation of the Cholesterol Theory

With this radical shift in what is considered healthy, it was not long before the food industry began condemning cholesterol-rich foods. The experts labeled eggs and shellfish as bad for cholesterol, while they glorified cereals and pasta. If you think eating cereal instead of eggs is really good for your cholesterol, think again.

In the latter part of the 20th century, doctors learned that total cholesterol alone had no relationship to heart disease. Cholesterol subdivisions—the "bad" cholesterol (LDL), "good" cholesterol (HDL), and triglycerides—emerged as more important risk factors. In particular, triglycerides, which are greatly affected by eating sugar and refined carbohydrates, showed a strong relationship. Triglyceride levels go up when you eat too many carbohydrates; the hormone insulin works hard to store all those carbs as fat. This means the best way to lower your risk for a heart attack is to follow a Paleolithic diet, with no sugar or refined carbohydrates. The good cholesterol (HDL), another risk, appears to be protective at higher levels, and the best way to increase your HDL is to eat saturated fats, such as butter, eggs, and animal products, and to avoid sugar.

When it came to the bad cholesterol, or LDL, research showed it as a weak risk for heart disease. Many people who have heart attacks have normal LDL levels, while many people who do not develop heart disease have high levels of it. It's confusing, but it can be explained. You see, LDL is affected by both sugar and saturated fats. The French, for example, have higher LDL levels compared to Americans, but heart disease is much less common among the French.

Additional research concluded that LDL cholesterol has further subdivisions wrapped around proteins. The smaller subdivision of LDL is greatly affected by sugar and refined carbohydrates, and can clog the arteries (Fig. 2.6). The larger subdivision of LDL, which is affected by saturated fats (like whole-fat dairy), is fluffy and does not clog the arteries because it is too big to go below the arterial walls.

Aha, it all makes sense now. Here's the summation:

- A higher triglyceride level is bad.
- A higher HDL level is good.
- A higher small LDL level is bad.
- A higher large LDL level is harmless.

**Figure 2.6:** LDL Flow in the Arteries

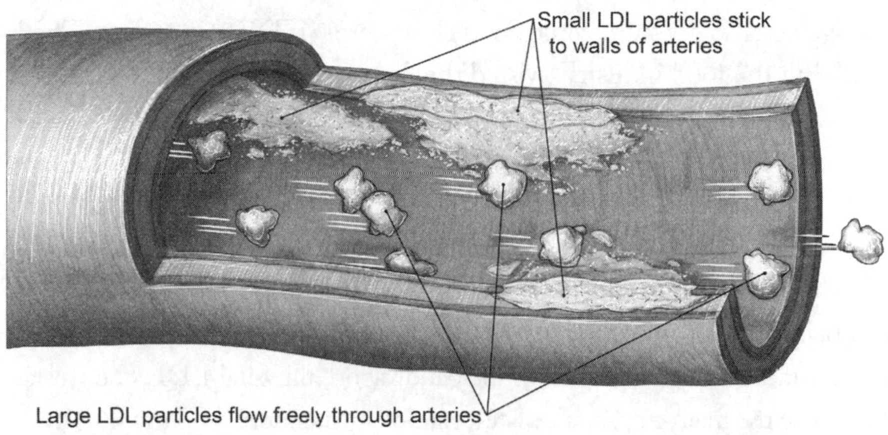


A healthy endothelium (arterial wall) acts as a barrier to LDL. When the endothelium is damaged by cardiac risk factors (high blood pressure, diabetes, smoking), it becomes porous. Small LDL particles penetrate the endothelial wall, and this leads to cholesterol buildup. Large LDL particles float freely in the bloodstream and are less likely to be deposited in the arterial wall.

Mary Kate Wright, MS, CMI

## The Effect of Natural Fats and Bad Carbs on Cholesterol

You've probably heard many times that eating a fatty steak is bad, and that LDL, or bad cholesterol, is the ultimate target to decrease your risk for heart disease. Let me explain how this information was twisted by the food industry to make us believe sugary cereals were good and porterhouse steaks were bad.

Consider a porterhouse steak, which many Americans view as poison after decades of recommendations that meat should be as lean as possible. Fifty percent of a porterhouse's total fat is monounsaturated fat, which has a beneficial influence on good cholesterol (HDL) and lowers the bad cholesterol (LDL). Saturated fat constitutes another 45 percent of its total fat, which also has a positive influence on HDL. Any rise in LDL is due to the large type of LDL, which does not clog the arteries. The remaining 5 percent of the fat in the steak is polyunsaturated, which lowers LDL but has no meaningful effect on HDL.

All these effects on cholesterol subdivisions are good. But no medical authority is willing to admit that eating steak has a positive influence on cholesterol. On the other hand, consider a sugary cereal, which most would view as a fairly healthy breakfast choice. After such a dense refined carbohydrate meal, triglyceride levels go up as your body converts the sugary cereal into fat. Then the smaller subdivision of bad cholesterol (LDL), the one that causes the arterial clogging, also goes up, while good cholesterol (HDL) plummets. That's all bad. But the food industry twisted the facts, and somehow a low-fat diet of cereals and fat-free milk became good for us.

The medical establishment's message for decreasing heart disease should have been to follow a high-fat/low-carb diet, not a low-fat/high-carb diet, but many official recommendations didn't want to contradict the USDA's food pyramid or the food industry claims. The food industry is big business. The triglyceride level, the most important part of the cholesterol equation, was left behind, and when the pharmaceutical industry jumped on the bandwagon, the total LDL, the weaker risk, became the main culprit. The latest cardiology literature is on my side.

Don't just take my word for it. Next time you watch TV, note the fine print in cholesterol drug commercials that clearly states, "This drug has not been shown to reduce the risk for heart attacks or stroke." Big Pharma isn't lying to you. The benefits of lowering LDL are minuscule, and two large clinical trials in 2008 found that lowering LDL to very low levels did not translate into measurable benefits that reduced the incidence of heart disease. But that doesn't mean they're going to dial back their nonstop commercials that reinforce the need for you to reduce your LDL. Despite the recent research that has shown LDL to be a weaker risk factor in heart disease, LDL remains the ultimate target to boost the profits of pharmaceutical industry.

## The Carbohydrate Theory for Heart Disease

Heart disease was a rarity a hundred years ago. The same goes for cancer. They were mostly observed in Western societies or in indigenous peoples who worked for Europeans and adopted their diet. As time passed, these diseases became increasingly prevalent in both colonial countries and nonindustrialized societies.

Sugar, molasses, white flour, and white rice are easily transported around the world without spoiling. Western diseases, however, soon follow.

First, societies see noticeable increases in dental cavities. Soon after, obesity, diabetes, heart disease, and cancer rates begin to rise. Scientists suggested that all these diseases had a single cause—sugar—because they were relatively uncommon in primitive societies, prior to the influx of sugar and refined carbohydrates.

Other scientists voiced a different viewpoint, saying that white rice is commonly eaten in many Asian countries and does not cause direct increases in the rates of obesity, diabetes, or heart disease. That's true. But in many Asian countries, people eat white rice out of necessity and it is used mostly for energy, since animal products are so expensive.

In the food-abundant United States and other Western nations, it's a completely different scenario. Both sugar and animal products are inexpensive and accessible. As a result, our bodies are faced with both animal products and excess carbs, and the excess sugar produced creates havoc.

In reality, our bodies are able to deal with sugar and utilize it quite efficiently, but the constant overconsumption of sugar pushes the body to the limit and ultimately ends up taxing the pancreas. In other words, if you eat a baked potato or a small cookie and follow it up with exercise, you'll be fine because your body will burn off the excess sugar. But if you consume cereals, fat-free milk, potatoes, and orange juice without burning off the excess sugar, you're on the road to straining your pancreas, gaining weight, and developing diseases by raising your insulin levels to dangerous levels.

I know some of you might be thinking, "But I know a girl who drinks soda all day, and she stays skinny!" Everybody is different. Why some of us become fat or develop diabetes, and some do not, depends on the amounts of sugar you consume, exercise habits, and genetics. I personally do not have the genes to be thin, and I seem to gain weight by just looking at food. But it's undeniable that sugar has pushed countless Americans to the limit and contributed to the rise in the rate of obesity, prediabetes, and diabetes. Take a look around. Believe me—all this obesity is not from eating shrimp, eggs, and other cholesterol-rich foods. It is from all the sugar, fat-free processed products, cereals, and soda we consume.

**Figure 2.7:** Modern Staples of Western Diets

- Refined carbohydrates (cereals, white flour, white rice, pasta)
- Low-fat dairy
- Refined vegetable oils
- Hydrogenated fats and oils (margarine and fast food)
- Fat-free processed food with added sugar and high fructose corn syrup
- Sugar

## The Current Mainstream Dietary Recommendations Are Outdated

In 2006 the largest study to look at the link between heart disease, cancer, and a low-fat diet found that a low-fat diet offers no benefits. The study, published in February 2006 in the *Journal of the American Medical Association*, was not just any ordinary study. It was so expansive that it's likely to be the final word on low-fat. Yet for some inexplicable reason, the respected medical authorities refuse to update their low-fat recommendations. Here are some other examples of current mainstream dietary recommendations we all bought into, despite the fact that new research has proven these recommendations to be completely false:

- Margarine is healthy. Butter is dangerous. Now research indicates that the exact opposite is true.
- Eating saturated fat can cause heart disease and cancer. Now research indicates that saturated fat has no relationship to these diseases.
- Eggs are bad because of their high cholesterol content. Now research indicates that eggs contain nutrients that may help lower the risk for heart disease.
- Cholesterol-rich food, such as shellfish, should be greatly limited since it may negatively affect blood levels. Now research indicates that cholesterol in food has little to no relationship to cholesterol levels in the bloodstream.
- Polyunsaturated vegetable oils, such as soybean oil, are healthy. Now research indicates that polyunsaturated oils may contain the deadly trans fats that can clog arteries and promote cancer.

### *The Mediterranean Diet*

All this misinformation about low-fat diets has certainly left you confused. Maybe you decided to follow the Mediterranean diet that everybody is raving about and that many fad diets try to imitate. Poultry, seafood, olive oil, 7 to 11 servings of whole grains a day, and a few drinks of alcohol a week, what have you got to lose? After all, health experts all seem to agree that the Mediterranean diet is the best diet for all of us to follow. I disagree.

If you follow the Mediterranean diet to its core, the heart benefits and cancer prevention are quite real. But the biggest difference between the Perfect 10 Diet and the Mediterranean diet is the goal. The Perfect 10 Diet is designed for you to lose weight. The Mediterranean is not. In fact, the Mediterranean diet will make you fat.

I mentioned earlier that the United States is number 1 in the world in obesity, but Greece is number 5 (Fig. 2.8). That's right, number 5. The Mediterranean diet is too high in grains. The Seven Countries Study I mentioned earlier that shone the light on the Mediterranean diet was done on farmers who worked in the fields all day long. So if you want to quit your day job and hit the gym 12 hours a day, 7 days a week, be my guest. If so, you should do just fine on the Mediterranean diet. If not, you are on your way to becoming fat.

The Mediterranean diet with its excess alcohol is also bad for your hormones. One to two alcoholic beverages a day is healthy? Really? Alcohol may be good for the heart, but I want you to stay sober, not get the chance to join AA. Alcohol interferes with normal sugar metabolism and impairs response to hypoglycemia. That's why people feel the need to binge the day after heavy drinking.

In men, alcohol lowers testosterone, the male sex hormone. It is toxic to the testicles and leads to decreased secretions of testosterone. It also increases the conversion of testosterone to estrogen, the female sex hormone. An imbalance of testosterone to estrogen ratio in men is a serious disturbance that will be addressed later on in this book.

In women, alcohol affects how estrogen is secreted. After one drink, estrogen levels can go as high as 300 percent within 30 minutes. And this surge in estrogen may be the factor responsible for the increased risk of breast cancer in women who are heavy drinkers. Alcohol also increases the secretion of the stress hormone cortisol, which can lead to a loss in muscle mass. Alcohol is also bad for growth hormone, the hormone that keeps you young and fit. How many hormones have been screwed up so far on this so-called perfect Mediterranean diet? I'm not sure. Unfortunately, I lost count.

That's not the only problem I have with the Mediterranean diet. I don't know about you, but I can't eat one country's cuisine every day for the rest of my life. I don't live in Greece or Italy. I live in the United States. The last time I visited those countries, I noticed that they had restaurants from all over the world, just like we do. We live in a global economy, and international restaurants are available even in the remotest reaches of the world. With this in mind, who can really follow just one country's cuisine? It's not only impractical, it's impossible unless you happen to live in a primitive tribe still undiscovered by civilization. For this reason, I developed the Perfect 10 Diet to be a diet that the whole world can follow. The Perfect 10 Diet does not limit your food choices to one country or one type of cuisine; the Perfect 10 Diet is international.

Do you like Belgian, Chinese, French, Japanese, Middle Eastern, Thai, or Vietnamese cuisine? Hey, it's all here on the Perfect 10 Diet. The Mediterranean diet is here, too—with some slight variations. The Perfect 10 Diet is world class all the way. You can follow any cuisine in the world you like on the Perfect 10 Diet as long the types of fat are natural. And that's the Perfect 10 Diet's superiority over all diets, including the one and only Mediterranean diet.

**Figure 2.8:** Ranking of Countries with the Highest Rates of Obesity

| RANK | COUNTRIES | PREVALENCE |
|---|---|---|
| # 1 | United States | 30.6% |
| # 2 | Mexico | 24.2% |
| # 3 | United Kingdom | 23% |
| # 4 | Slovakia | 22.4% |
| # 5 | Greece | 21.9% |
| # 6 | Australia | 21.7% |
| # 7 | New Zealand | 20.9% |
| # 8 | Hungary | 18.8% |
| # 9 | Luxembourg | 18.4% |
| # 10 | Czech Republic | 14.8% |

| | | |
|---|---|---|
| # 11 | Canada | 14.3% |
| # 12 | Spain | 13.1% |
| # 13 | Ireland | 13% |
| # 14 | Germany | 12.9% |
| # 15 | Portugal | 12.8% |
| # 16 | Finland | 12.8% |
| # 17 | Iceland | 12.4% |
| # 18 | Turkey | 12% |
| # 19 | Belgium | 11.7% |
| # 20 | Netherlands | 10% |

Percentage of total population who have a BMI (body mass index) greater than 30 kg./sq. meters. Data for Australia, Austria, and Portugal is from 2002. All other data is from 2003. Obesity rates are defined as the percentage of the population with a BMI over 30. The BMI is a single number that evaluates an individual's weight status in relation to height. For Australia, the United Kingdom, and the United States, figures are based on health examinations rather than self-reported information. Obesity estimates derived from health examinations are generally higher and more reliable than those coming from self-reports, because they preclude any misreporting of people's height and weight. However, health examinations are only conducted regularly in a few countries (OECD).

OECD Health Data 2005

## *Mary's Story*

I met Mary several years ago, when she came to see me because of her elevated cholesterol levels. "Since I got married 2 years ago, I've gone from a size 4 to a size 12. I don't take any drugs except for oral contraceptives." Mary was 37 years old, 5 feet, 4 inches tall, and weighed 160 pounds when I first met her. After taking an extensive history and doing a complete blood workup, I knew that Mary's elevated cholesterol was directly related to her diet. Her fasting insulin level was at 40 units, which is very high. Mary had been brainwashed into believing that all fat, except for margarine and refined manufactured vegetable oils, was bad.

She told me, "I don't understand it. I don't eat eggs or shrimp, Doctor, because of their high cholesterol content. I only eat cereals and pasta, and always make low-fat choices, from salad dressings to crackers."

Of course, most people with elevated cholesterol are advised to follow a diet low in saturated fat and cholesterol, and to use tub-margarine and other refined vegetable oils. My advice to Mary was to *increase* her intake of natural fat and to *eliminate* refined grains and processed foods from her diet.

My rather unconventional advice to improve her cholesterol levels and to lose weight alarmed Mary. "Wait a minute, Doctor. That's a first. I've never heard of a doctor advising his patients to follow a higher-fat diet, or to eat egg yolks," she said. "Are you sure you don't want to give me a cholesterol drug?"

"Mary, I'm positive," I replied.

Mary eliminated margarine from her diet and started to eat fiber-rich vegetables with each meal. Sure enough, within 3 months, she'd lost 23 pounds. Her fasting insulin level dropped to 4, and her cholesterol returned to a normal level without the use of any drugs or supplements.

## A Typical Day on the Perfect 10 Diet

**BREAKFAST:** Scrambled Eggs in a Whole-Wheat Wrap with Fresh Salsa
**OPTIONAL MIDMORNING SNACK:** Fresh Fruit Salad
**LUNCH:** Grilled Tuna with Baked Eggplant Parmesan
**OPTIONAL MIDAFTERNOON SNACK:** ½ Cup of Mixed Nuts
**DINNER:** Cauliflower Salad and 1 Pear

CHAPTER 3

# The Ten Hormones That Control Health and Weight

When your hormones are perfectly balanced, your body is ready to play the music of life. Like an orchestra with half the musicians taking the day off, your body can't make beautiful music without all its hormones present and playing together. When your hormones are there, playing in tune, you feel amazing. But let's see what happens when the pianist takes the day off, the violinist starts to play on his or her own, and the clarinetist can hardly play. How would that sound? Horrible, right? That's exactly what happens inside your body when your hormones aren't working together. Every bite you take influences your hormones.

It's no surprise that the dramatic dietary changes that we adopted because of our fear of fat and due to our increased intake of sugar have wreaked havoc on our hormones. In turn, we've become a sick society.

A hormone, by definition, is a substance that regulates bodily functions. The human body contains more than 100 types of hormones. Hormones regulate everything—your heartbeat, breathing, blood pressure, energy, weight, and so on. Hormones put you to sleep at night and wake you up in the morning. It's no exaggeration to say that hormones are crucial to every single function of survival.

The Perfect 10 Diet does its magic by improving your hormones. In this book, you will read about many hormones, but I only go into detail about the ten most important hormones. Some of these hormones are major hormones you can't live a single day without, such as insulin. Some are minor, such as sex hormones, which aren't critical to survival, but they affect how you age, look, and feel.

Our modern diet screwed up all the hormones that play a role in weight and health. Our ancestors did not consume soda, sweets, cereals, fat-free food, skim milk, refined vegetable oils, margarine, artificial sweeteners, or alcohol. Much of this food was never meant for human consumption, and we moved from a hormone-friendly diet to a hormone-unfriendly diet. Now let's learn more about these ten important hormones.

## INSULIN

SOURCE: Pancreas
NORMAL LEVELS: Fasting, micro 5 IU (International Units)/mL (milliliters)
FUNCTIONS: Food metabolism

Insulin, which was discovered by Frederick Banting and Charles Best in 1921, is secreted by the beta cells of the pancreas to regulate food storage and metabolism. If you have too much or too little of it, you won't live for long. In essence, insulin governs your body, and it has a profound effect on aging. Centenarians come from all countries and backgrounds. Some are even smokers, but they all have one thing in common— low insulin levels.

Your pancreas can store about 200 units of insulin each day. Insulin sweeps sugar inside cells, turns amino acids from protein into muscle, and transforms fatty acids into fat. Sugar is first stored in the liver and muscle. Excess sugar that can't be stored in the liver and muscles is converted to triglycerides to be stored as fat. Insulin secretion is promoted by all food groups. However, a low-fat diet full of excess carbohydrates causes the pancreas to overproduce insulin. The bad carbs of white bread, white rice, pasta, and starchy vegetables put you at risk.

The United States is a sugar nation. It's no surprise that excess insulin is our main hormonal problem. When you strain your pancreas with too much sugar, you gain weight and increase your chances of developing disease. If your pancreas becomes overwhelmed, it won't be able to continue making insulin, and it may even stop altogether. With not enough insulin going around, your blood sugar will remain elevated, and you'll develop diabetes. Your insulin levels must remain perfect, secreted just in the right amounts. If you're wondering whether or not you're producing too much insulin, just look at your belly. If you can't see your abs, your pancreas is secreting too much insulin. Get it?

FOODS AND FACTORS THAT HELP BALANCE INSULIN INCLUDE: chromium, a trace mineral that enhances insulin function, and is found in brewer's yeast, whole-grain breads, meats, eggs, and shellfish. Zinc is also important, and it is present in seafood and dark meats. Exercise is also essential to lowering your insulin levels and losing weight.

FOODS AND FACTORS THAT DISTURB INSULIN INCLUDE: sugar; low-fat products; artificial sweeteners; sweets; margarine; enriched, refined, and processed foods; and a sedentary lifestyle.

## GLUCAGON

SOURCE: Pancreas
NORMAL LEVELS: Varies, fasting around 60 pg (picograms)/mL or less
FUNCTIONS: Food metabolism

Glucagon is another hormone secreted by the pancreas. It performs the exact opposite function of insulin—it melts fat. Don't you love this hormone already? As I mentioned before, in the presence of glucose, your pancreas releases insulin. But in the absence of sugar (if your blood sugar is very low and you haven't eaten for 5 to 6 hours), glucagon is secreted. Why? Because your tissues need sugar and energy. In turn, glucagon pulls sugars out of storage—first, from the liver, and then from fatty tissues to raise your blood glucose level. If you have little glucagon, you will become fat. Excessive glucagon production can occur in the case of a pancreatic tumor, but that's another matter.

When glucagon metabolizes your fat into energy, you lose weight. When food is available, glucagon production is inhibited. In other words, you can never lose weight as long as you continue to eat, since your body has enough nutrients. How did our modern diet mess up glucagon secretion?

It's simple: glucagon production is inhibited every time insulin is present in your bloodstream. Insulin and glucagon are like night and day; they can't be present at the same time in the bloodstream because they have opposing actions.

Since most Americans overproduce insulin, their glucagon levels are also screwed up. Glucagon is always inhibited, and for this reason, many of us struggle with our weight. That's why low-fat diets won't keep you thin for long periods of time—because you'll always be hungry. Here's the good news: I will help you boost your glucagon levels on the Perfect 10 Diet.

Now you may be asking, "How am I going to do that, Doctor? Do I have to skip meals and starve myself to get some glucagon going in my bloodstream?"

Absolutely not. You see, when you eat natural fats and adequate amounts of protein, and avoid bad carbs, your insulin secretion is regulated. It follows that your glucagon will also be regulated, and you'll lose weight. It seems completely counterintuitive that eating fat will help you lose fat, but it's true. I realize you've been taught to fear fat all your life, but you have to change the way you think so you can start to melt the pounds the smart and easy way.

FOODS AND FACTORS THAT BALANCE AND INCREASE GLUCAGON INCLUDE: a diet low in sugar that features natural fats and sufficient protein. Skipping meals, which is not recommended on the Perfect 10 Diet, also increases glucagon, as does starvation (which, needless to say, is absolutely not recommended). Exercise also increases glucagon production.

FOODS AND FACTORS THAT DISTURB OR INHIBIT GLUCAGON INCLUDE: a low-fat diet leading to excessive insulin secretion, a sedentary lifestyle, and consumption of sugar and frequent meals.

## LEPTIN

SOURCE: Fat cells
NORMAL LEVELS: Fasting, 4 and 6 ng (nanograms)/dL (deciliter)
FUNCTIONS: Satiety

Do you have no control over your appetite? You may have a leptin problem. Leptin is secreted by the fat cells, and not an endocrine gland. When leptin was discovered in 1995, it was dubbed the "holy grail of weight loss." Leptin manages how much fat is stored around the organs and under the skin. When fat cells are filled with an abundance of food, more leptin is secreted, and the leptin enters the brain to curb your appetite. As a result, you feel full and satisfied. If your leptin levels are too low all the time, you're probably malnourished and have very little body fat. Or it may be a rare genetic inability to produce leptin.

Initially, scientists believed that if you gave leptin to overweight people, it would stimulate fat burning. Unfortunately, it had the opposite effect. When scientists measured leptin in overweight individuals, they were in for a big surprise. Overweight people were not leptin deficient; in fact, they produced *too much* leptin. It turns out that excessive levels of leptin often go hand in hand with high sugar and elevated insulin levels. You see, food without nutritional value, such as refined carbohydrates, low-fat products, foods containing high-fructose corn syrup and trans fats, and other fake foods, sends erroneous signals to the brain. The body interprets those signals as starvation, which makes the body burn fewer calories and store fat even in the presence of high leptin levels. When leptin is high because of all the fake food you eat, your satiety switch becomes broken. As a result, you gain weight, because you will be as hungry as a wolf and will have no control over your appetite.

If you have a high leptin level, that's not a good thing. High leptin levels appear to be associated with high blood pressure, heart disease, stroke, and obesity. How can you fix your unbalanced leptin? Again, eat real food, include more natural fats, and eliminate bad carbs.

FOODS THAT CAN HELP BALANCE LEPTIN INCLUDE: vegetables, fruits, whole grains, foods containing natural fats, and fish.

FOODS THAT DISTURB LEPTIN INCLUDE: low-fat foods, refined carbs, sugar, sweets, and foods containing trans fats.

## THYROID HORMONE

SOURCE: Thyroid gland

NORMAL LEVELS: Total T3 for adults 60 to 181ng/dL, total T4 for adults 4.5 to 12 mcg (micrograms)/dL

FUNCTION: Energy and metabolism

A discussion about metabolism must include the thyroid gland, one of the largest endocrine glands in the body. This gland is found in the neck just below the thyroid cartilage (known as the Adam's apple in men), and it is controlled by the brain's hypothalamus and pituitary.

The thyroid gland produces two types of hormones: triiodothyronine (T3) and thyroxine (T4). The "3" and "4" refer to the number of iodine molecules in each thyroid hormone molecule. Eighty percent of thyroid hormone is T4, and 20 percent is T3, the active part of the thyroid hormone. An underactive thyroid makes your metabolism slow to a crawl, which can make you gain weight even if you don't eat much.

Thyroid hormone has actions beyond metabolism and keeping you fit: it provides energy, improves thinking abilities, boosts the immune system against infections and cancer, decreases bad cholesterol, and lowers blood pressure.

Hyperthyroidism (overactive thyroid) and hypothyroidism (underactive thyroid) are the most common problems of the thyroid gland. Hypothyroidism occurs when your thyroid gland does not make enough thyroid hormone. It's estimated that about 25 million Americans have an underactive thyroid. Sufferers have an excessive slowdown in metabolism, low body temperature, fatigue, slow heartbeat, high triglyceride levels, dry skin and hair, hair loss, menstrual problems, depression, memory disturbances, and weight gain. Are you getting the picture? Thyroid hormone is involved in everything.

Hyperthyroidism can lead to bulging eyes, unhealthy weight loss, and even mania. But *The Perfect 10 Diet* is a diet book not a medical textbook, so let's concentrate on the dietary factors that can cause you to develop an *underactive* thyroid, and lead you on an uphill battle with weight. Why does hypothyroidism occur? Actually, it's an autoimmune disease, which means the body attacks the thyroid gland and you end up making less thyroid hormone. But how does this relate to our modern diet? Interestingly enough, our modern diet can contribute to a sluggish thyroid rather than support this important gland.

Low-fat diets lead to a disturbance in both high insulin and leptin levels. Leptin is the master hormone that helps regulate thyroid. In times of starvation, leptin levels fall, signaling the thyroid and other hormones to switch into conservation mode. Metabolism slows down, body temperature lowers, and vital nutrients are conserved. But leptin resistance from refined carbs and excess sugar distorts the signals this hormone sends to the thyroid gland and the rest of the body, and may direct well-fed, and even overweight, individuals into fat-storage mode. In turn, low-fat diets can lead to an underactive thyroid.

Also, polyunsaturated oils, such as soybean and corn oil, have made things worse. They can block the absorption of iodine, which is needed to make thyroid hormone.

Our diet is very high in salt. In most developed countries, iodine has been added to salt to prevent an underactive thyroid from developing in infants. However, research indicates that excessive levels of iodine are just as bad as low levels. Excess iodine blocks the enzymes that produce thyroid hormones.

If you've been following a strict low-carb diet, you're also out of luck. Low-carb diets are way too high in animal protein (meat, poultry, fish), which lowers the conversion of T4 to the active form of the hormone, T3, and, in turn, reduces thyroid function.

That's why both low-fat and low-carb diets are disastrous for your health and will never make you a perfect 10. All of these dietary changes could be related to the increased prevalence of hypothyroidism. Only the Perfect 10 Diet will help you support this important hormone with the right food choices. Isn't that exciting?

FOODS THAT CAN BALANCE THYROID HORMONE INCLUDE: sea salt (in moderation), fish, shellfish, and sea vegetables, particularly seaweed. The iodine that is naturally present in the right amounts in these food groups is essential for the proper function of the thyroid gland. When you also eat enough fruits and vegetables, the "safe" types of carbohydrates, you increase production of thyroxine.

**FOODS AND OTHER FACTORS THAT CAN LEAD TO THE DEVELOPMENT OF A SLUGGISH THYROID INCLUDE:** low-fat, low-carb, and low-protein diets; excess alcohol; vinegar; excess salt; fluoride in tap water; and polyunsaturated oils, such as soybean and corn oils.

## HUMAN GROWTH HORMONE (HGH)

SOURCE: Pituitary gland
NORMAL LEVELS: Adults <10 ng/mL
FUNCTIONS: Growth and repair of tissues

Human growth hormone (HGH) is the quintessential anti-aging hormone. For simplicity's sake, I will refer to it as either HGH or growth hormone. HGH is released from a small gland in the brain called the pituitary. Without HGH, we'd all be dwarfs. With too much, we'd all be giants. Doctors call HGH the fountain of youth, and they're right; it's the closest thing we have to it. HGH was first discovered in 1920. The medical community has long considered it to be necessary to help us grow to adult size, and unnecessary past age 21. Recent studies have overturned that notion. HGH gets a bad reputation because of its abuse by athletes, but this is unjustified.

HGH levels in our bodies start to decline gradually from age 21 forward, all the way until we die. That's why the body regenerates itself at a much slower rate as we age. Many Americans are deficient in HGH, mostly because of their body fat. Body fat is a great inhibitor of the HGH secretion. The more body fat you have, the lower your HGH will be. HGH keeps us fit, and that's why it's harder to lose weight when you're already overweight.

HGH puts the brakes on insulin, the fat-storing hormone. Let's see what happens when you get old. HGH declines with age, but insulin remains the same or rises if you are on a sugary diet. You'll start to accumulate fat even if you don't change your diet or physical activity. It is no wonder as a kid or a teenager, you could pig out on pizza and French fries without consequences, but as you've gotten older, you probably gain weight more easily.

HGH levels are also disturbed by frequent meals. In developed countries like the United States, we have an abundance of food, which keeps our HGH levels low. HGH levels rise when you fast, a response to the days when humans were dependent on an unstable food supply. Indeed, fasting has been used for centuries to promote longevity, and it is among the most potent ways to induce HGH secretion.

Symptoms of HGH deficiency include wrinkled, sagging skin; thinning bones; accumulation of body fat; thinning hair; depression; anxiety; fatigue; decreased libido; and lowered immunity. Why does HGH play a role in immunity? Because HGH helps grow the thymus gland, a gland in the chest that makes T-cells, the cells responsible for fighting infections.

People who take HGH for anti-aging swear by it. Their energy levels rise, their depression disappears, and their outlook on life becomes much more positive. They get more muscles and lose fat. You might be thinking, "But I can't afford HGH, Doctor." That's okay, because the Perfect 10 Diet will raise your HGH levels naturally. Once you begin to eat the right amounts of protein, incorporate exercise in your daily life, lose weight, and get adequate sleep, your HGH level will go up.

FOODS AND OTHER FACTORS THAT CAN HELP BALANCE GROWTH HORMONE INCLUDE: vegetables, fruits, poultry, eggs, fish, anaerobic exercise, weight loss, and fasting.

FOODS AND OTHER FACTORS THAT NEGATIVELY AFFECT GROWTH HORMONE LEVELS INCLUDE: low-protein diets, alcohol, vinegar, white bread, pasta, low-fat products, cereals, and a sedentary lifestyle.

## CORTISOL

SOURCE: Adrenal glands
NORMAL LEVELS: 180 ng/mL from 8 to 9 a.m., 45 ng/mL from 4 to 8 p.m.
FUNCTIONS: Energy and inflammation control

The adrenal glands, which are located on top of the kidneys, secrete a number of hormones. On the Perfect 10 Diet, I limit the discussion to two hormones, DHEA and cortisol, that play a role in weight.

The role cortisol plays in the shape of our waistlines is at times debated, but there is no doubt that it plays a role in abdominal obesity (the spare tire). If your waistline is wider than your hips, this central fat plays a role in the inflammation of the arteries and increases your chance to develop heart disease.

Cortisol, a stress hormone, gives us energy. Just as with insulin, we have a big cortisol problem; it's too high in many people, and too low in many others. If cortisol is too high or too low for too long, you won't live very long. This major hormone keeps us alive thanks to its three essential and powerful properties: it increases blood sugar levels (and thus energy levels), raises blood pressure, and neutralizes inflammation. In the 1990s I published a paper in a major medical journal on the strong anti-inflammatory effects of cortisol. It truly does wonders.

But how did cortisol get impaired by our modern diet? Again, the answer is excess sugar. Let me explain. You see, sugar, fruit juices, and just about anything else sweet releases sugar quickly into the bloodstream. That doesn't just impair insulin; it also has a negative effect on cortisol. Our bodies are not designed to deal with sugar overloads.

As insulin is secreted in higher amounts on a low-fat diet, blood sugar plummets. That's where the cortisol link comes in. In primitive times, cortisol was called upon only when we encountered stressful situations, such as running from predators. It gives us quick energy to run from danger. But today, cortisol is called upon each time your sugar levels plummet after eating a cookie, drinking soda, or consuming any other sugary food or drink. This creates chronic high levels of cortisol. This leads to insulin secretion to deal with the sugar; then, insulin resistance follows.

Insulin resistance is a condition in which cells become resistant to the effects of the hormone and higher and higher levels of insulin are produced to deal with the food. When you are insulin resistant or have too much insulin, you become fat. If you have excess cortisol in your bloodstream, this shuts down serotonin, a neurotransmitter that affects your mood. When serotonin levels drop, depression can result. Depression is now on the rise nationally, even in children.

Next, excess cortisol reduces your production of melatonin, the sleep hormone secreted by a small gland called the pineal gland. A drop in melatonin leads to insomnia. Hello, Ambien! If you don't get enough sleep, you won't make enough HGH, the hormone that keeps you fit and young, since it is produced mostly during sleep. It's no wonder we are so sick—excessive sugar, poor sleep, and stress are constantly traumatizing us.

If all the sugar and stress increases the demand on your adrenals too many times, they can eventually burn out. Many doctors don't diagnose adrenal fatigue because it's not recognized as a medical condition in textbooks, but it does exist in the literature. When the adrenals don't makc enough cortisol, you may look tired or have dark circles underneath your eyes. You're also less likely to be able to cope with stressful situations, and you may experience panic or anxiety attacks. Then, your doctor may put you on an anti-anxiety medication that can even make you gain weight. Here's the good news: the Perfect 10 Diet balances cortisol.

FOODS AND OTHER FACTORS THAT CAN HELP BALANCE CORTISOL HORMONE INCLUDE: vegetables, fruits, fish, eggs, poultry, and occasionally some red meat. Try your best to relax and avoid stressful situations.

FOODS AND OTHER FACTORS THAT CAN DISTURB CORTISOL HORMONE INCLUDE: sugar, alcohol, sweets, soft drinks, cookies, cereals, fat-free products, foods containing trans fats, and stress.

## DEHYDROEPIANDROSTERONE (DHEA)

SOURCE: Adrenal glands

NORMAL LEVELS: They vary with age, but DHEA sulfate for men is 400 to 500 mcg/dL, and for women it's 370 to 430 mcg/dL

FUNCTIONS: Numerous, including a possible role in weight

DHEA, another steroid hormone made in the adrenal glands and brain, is one of the most plentiful hormones in the body. Levels of DHEA decline with age; a 70-year-old produces about 10 percent of the DHEA levels produced by a 20-year-old.

First identified in 1934, DHEA is produced in greater quantities than other adrenal steroids. Since DHEA can be converted into other hormones, including estrogen and testosterone, scientists assumed DHEA was merely a reservoir the body could draw on to produce other hormones. However, identification of DHEA receptors in animals' livers, kidneys, and testes suggests that DHEA has specific physiologic functions.

The role DHEA plays in direct weight control is controversial. In the early 1980s, DHEA was widely sold in health-food stores, primarily as a weight-loss product. Until 1986, DHEA was a nonprescription drug, but the FDA reclassified it because its long-term risks were unknown. Today, the FDA still does not approve DHEA for any medical indication. But DHEA naturally increases serotonin, which tells your brain when you've had enough to eat and inhibits the conversion of glucose into fat. DHEA also protects against arteriosclerosis and lowers insulin.

Animal studies have shown that DHEA assists in the prevention of obesity, diabetes, cancer, heart disease, and even graying of hair. In humans, DHEA is gaining ground as a hormone that improves one's sense of well-being, relieves fatigue, fights depression, and plays a role in the prevention of osteoporosis in postmenopausal women. DHEA, like many of our other hormones, is not immune to the damaging effects of manufactured fats. Symptoms of DHEA deficiency include fatigue, anxiety, depression, low sexual desire, and lack of sexual satisfaction. On the other hand, adequate levels of DHEA are linked to longevity. If you overload on DHEA in the form of supplements, you may develop oily skin and acne.

FOODS THAT HELP BOOST DHEA PRODUCTION INCLUDE: vegetables, fruits, poultry, eggs, and saturated fats such as butter.

FOODS THAT CAN DECREASE DHEA PRODUCTION INCLUDE: sugar, sweets, alcohol, margarine, coffee, white bread, soy, and pasta.

## ESTROGEN AND PROGESTERONE

SOURCE: Mostly ovaries, but a small amount is produced in the adrenal glands

NORMAL LEVELS: In females, levels vary in relation to ovulation; in adult males, estrogen: < 130 pg/mL, and progesterone: < 1.4ng/mL

FUNCTIONS: Numerous, including weight maintenance

Estrogen and progesterone are the female sex hormones. Estrogen is primarily a female sex hormone, but both men and women make estrogen. Women, of course, have higher levels of it. Femininity is the essence of estrogen. Estrogen enlarges breasts and widens the pelvis, and it provides that curvy, sexy appearance. Estrogen also stimulates the sympathetic nervous system, increases alertness, lowers body fat, protects against heart and Alzheimer's disease, increases insulin sensitivity, and improves glucose tolerance.

During reproductive years, a woman makes estrogen every day of the month. The ovaries produce progesterone, the other female sex hormone, during the two weeks before a woman's period.

Although people often think of estrogen as a single entity, this hormone is actually three biochemically distinct molecules that the body produces naturally—estrone (E1), estradiol (E2), and estriol (E3). These three estrogen molecules have different activities that make them more or less "estrogenic." Estradiol is made from the ovaries, and it gives women their curvy appearance. Estrone is made from body fat. Estriol is present in small amounts and is mostly made during pregnancy. Around the age of menopause, the ovaries shrink. Estradiol (E2) decreases, but the body still needs estrogen. Estrone (E1), which is made in the adrenals, becomes the main type of estrogen present in postmenopausal women, and that's really bad. Estrone (E1) starts to shift fat from the buttocks to the belly, leading to a decrease in curves and an increase in belly fat. This abdominal fat starts to produce more estrone (E1), which just leads to more and more belly fat—it's a vicious cycle. As a result, it becomes difficult to lose weight. If you don't support estrogen production, you'll gain weight.

**Figure 3.1:** Levels of Ovarian Hormones Estrogen and Progesterone During the Menstrual Cycle

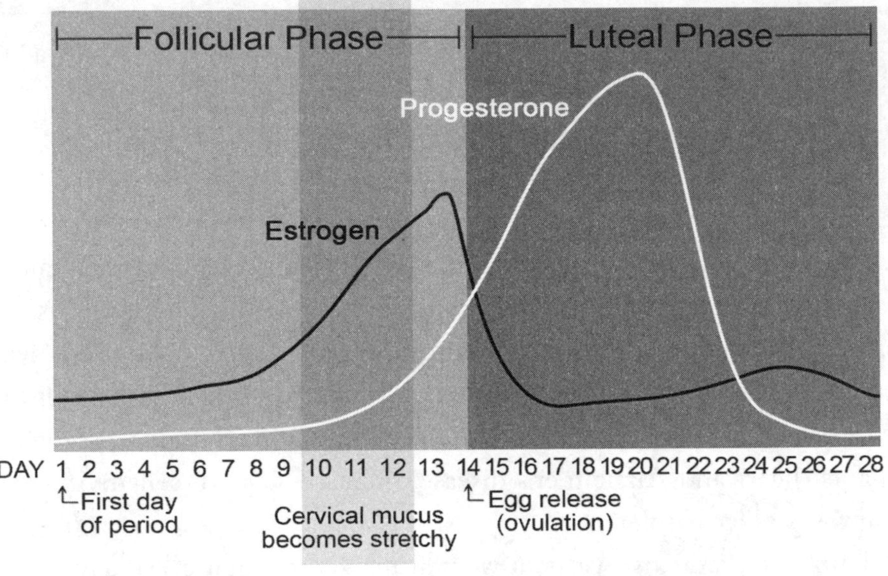


Mary Kate Wright, MS, CMI

Symptoms of low estrogen or estrogen deficiency can occur at any age, but they are more prominent in menopause. They include hot flashes, night sweats, headaches, vaginal dryness, mental fuzziness, frequent bladder infections, a decreased sexual response, and weight gain. You can end up with excessive amounts of estrogen if you take extra estrogen in the form of exogenous hormones or if your body makes too little progesterone. Symptoms of too much estrogen include depression, bloating, pounding headaches, breast swelling, and excessive vaginal bleeding. A good estrogen-to-progesterone ratio in young females is 20-to-1.

Progesterone, the other female sex hormone, downregulates estrogen activity. Progesterone is produced by the ovaries. It reduces anxiety and has a calming effect on mood. It makes women happy. Postpartum depression is caused by a rapid decline in progesterone levels. Progesterone increases sleepiness, helps to build and maintain bones, slows the digestive process, promotes appetite and fat storage (which is important in pregnancy), helps breast tissue mature, and prepares breasts to produce milk.

Low progesterone levels can happen at any age, but production especially plummets around menopause. Symptoms of low progesterone or progesterone deficiency include PMS-like symptoms, premenstrual migraines, irregular or heavy periods, and anxiety. Women can suffer from excessive amounts of progesterone if they take too many hormone replacements; these symptoms include: sleepiness, drowsiness, and depression.

Both estrogen and progesterone levels have suffered because of our modern diet. Excess sugar and elimination of natural fats led to serious disturbances in these important sex hormones. It is no wonder infertility and early menopause are now on the rise.

Researchers are also gaining new insights into the processes through which E1, E2, and E3 are metabolized, detoxified, and excreted. These molecules break down or are detoxified into estrogen metabolites. These metabolites can have stronger or weaker estrogenic activity—and thus increase a woman's risk of breast, uterine, and other cancers. Therefore, understanding estrogen metabolism and the things we can do to affect it are important to reducing the risk of cancer. Flaxseed, cruciferous vegetables, omega-3 fatty acids, and exercise can help with dangerous estrogen metabolites and can prevent cancer.

These female hormones are important for men as well. Estrogen sensitizes the male brain, and too little estrogen can effectively neuter a man. However, in men, excess estrogen is the real problem, especially as we get old. Too much caffeine and obesity can lead to overproduction of this female sex hormone instead of testosterone, the male sex hormone. Insecticides in our food chain have also contributed to the phenomenon of excess estrogen in men. Of course, a disturbance in the estrogen-testosterone balance in men can translate into weight gain.

Men also synthesize progesterone, which is the precursor of testosterone (the male sex hormone) in smaller amounts. The decline of progesterone in males plays a role in increasing the conversion rate of testosterone into another hormone, dihydrotestosterone (DHT). Excess DHT as we age stimulates the proliferation of prostate cells, which enlarges the prostate gland and narrows the urethral channel, leading to urination problems.

FOODS AND OTHERS FACTORS THAT BALANCE ESTROGEN AND PROGESTERONE INCLUDE: eggs, butter, fish, poultry, whole milk, and weight loss.

FOODS AND OTHER FACTORS THAT CAN DECREASE OR DISTURB ESTROGEN AND PROGESTERONE INCLUDE: sugar, fat-free foods, margarine, excess alcohol, smoking, drugs, a lack of sexual activity, fat-free dairy products, and obesity.

## TESTOSTERONE

SOURCE: Testes in men, and adrenals in men and women
NORMAL LEVELS: males, varies with age, 241 to 827 ng/dL; females, 60 to 76 ng/dL
FUNCTIONS: Numerous, including weight maintenance

Everyone knows that testosterone is the essence of maleness. Yes, testosterone makes men masculine, but testosterone is also present in small amounts in women, and aids libido in both genders. For years, the medical community has sent the message to men that testosterone is bad because it leads to heart disease and prostate cancer. That's simply not true. On the Perfect 10 Diet testosterone is positively worshipped. In men, adequate testosterone levels prevent heart disease, and testosterone has no link whatsoever to prostate cancer.

The male ideal is wide shoulders, a muscular chest and arms, a narrow waist, and strong legs. Well, let me tell you something man-to-man: you can't attain that ideal unless you eat foods that support this important hormone, such as animal products and cholesterol-rich foods. And testosterone is not just a sex hormone—it's a total body hormone. In adult males, testosterone is necessary to maintain muscle mass and strength, bone mass, normal hair growth, libido, and sperm production. It also keeps us fit and lean.

If you are a man interested in looking his best, I feel for you. Many experts with impressive credentials have steered you away from the foods you enjoy. The food industry has convinced you that in order to lose fat, you have to eat their processed products. As a result, you've gotten out of shape, weak, and perhaps even sick.

As a result of 40 years of the low-fat dogma, the average U.S. man is more out of shape than his 1960s predecessor. Low-fat diets lower testosterone, make it harder for you to build muscle, and make it easier for you to gain fat. In the 1980s the average testosterone level in men was around 600; now it's closer to 400. Insecticides, hormones in animal products, elimination of natural fats from our diet, and excess sugar screwed up this important hormone. Also, cortisol, the stress hormone that promotes fat storage, is testosterone's mortal enemy.

If you want to look like a god, eat like a man. That means plenty of animal products, butter, egg yolks, and whole milk—not margarine, skim milk, or soy milk—to support your testosterone production. Don't worry about making too much testosterone, because producing too much naturally is rarely a problem. Abuse of testosterone from unnatural sources, such as anabolic steroids, can lead to acne, oily skin, and decreased fertility.

Do you have low testosterone levels? Are you taking Viagra to get an erection? Don't despair—the Perfect 10 Diet will help you. Am I promising to transform you to one of those hulking figures on the cover of *Muscle and Fitness* magazine? Of course not. Those guys commit their lives to exercising regularly in order to look like Greek gods. But I do promise you will look your absolute best on the Perfect 10 Diet plan.

FOODS AND OTHER FACTORS THAT BOOST TESTOSTERONE PRODUCTION INCLUDE: eggs, liver, butter, fish, poultry, and frequent sexual activity. (Isn't that an added bonus?) Weight loss can also increase levels.

FOODS AND OTHER FACTORS THAT CAN DECREASE TESTOSTERONE PRODUCTION INCLUDE: sugar, fat-free foods, margarine, excess alcohol, tobacco use, recreational drugs, a lack of sexual activity, and obesity.

There are many other hormones that affect weight. The list includes epinephrine and norepinephrine (the stress hormones made by the adrenals); ghrelin (which is made in the gut and increases when you think of food); neuropeptide (which is found in the brain, is regulated by leptin and ghrelin, and tells you when to eat); adiponectin (which lowers blood sugar); and resistin (which plays a role in insulin resistance). While I limit this discussion to the ten most important hormones, the Perfect 10 Diet balances all hormones.

Many of these ten hormones are controlled by a specific area in the brain called the hypothalamus, which also regulates the pituitary gland. The pituitary gland releases other hormones that regulate many of these ten hormones. All of these hormones interact and are affected by one another. It's a lot of science, but you get the picture. In order to be a perfect 10, all of your hormones must be in perfect tune. The orchestra has to play together, or there won't be any music.

From breakfast cereal to fast food, today's culinary landscape has been disastrous to overall health and these ten hormones. Hormonal imbalance is not a joke. Diet, not drugs, is both the problem and the answer. Consuming a healthy diet enables one to be fit and to postpone aging. Hormonal imbalances accelerate the aging process at the cellular level and set you on the path toward disease.

If you want these ten hormones (Fig. 3.3) to be in perfect balance, forget about the USDA food pyramid, low-fat guidelines, and the latest low-carb trend. The Perfect 10 Diet is the only diet in the world that will help you balance these ten important hormones. In this book, I'll show you the foods to eat, foods to avoid, the rhyme and reason behind it all, and the exceptions to the rules. *The Perfect 10 Diet* also includes menus you can follow to make sure you're getting the best nutrition for your body.

Weight loss, better health, more energy, and balanced hormones, what're you waiting for? It's time to run away from all this hormonal havoc and get started on the Perfect 10 Diet right now.

**Figure 3.2:** Human Endocrine System

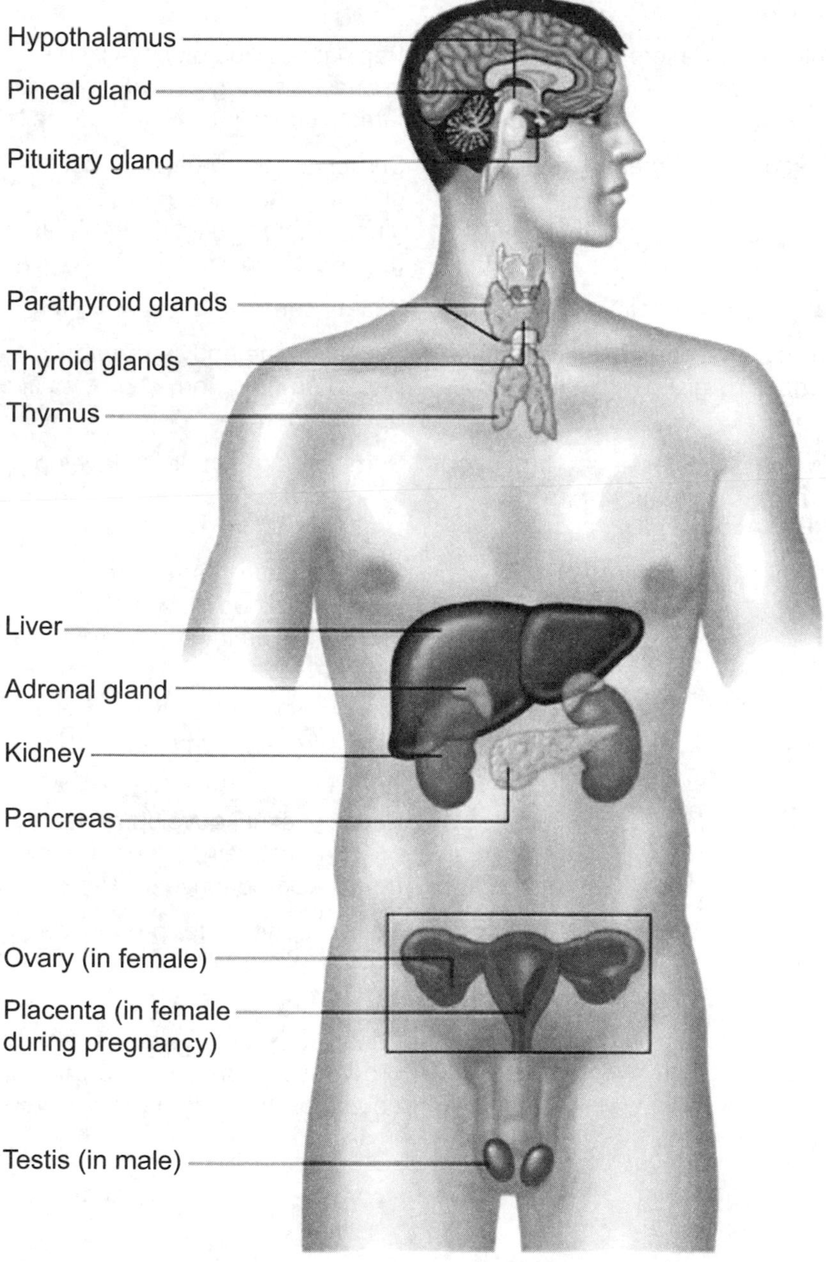

**Figure 3.3:** The Perfect 10 Diet Hormones and Their Functions

| HORMONE | SOURCE | TARGET TISSUE | FUNCTION |
|---|---|---|---|
| Insulin | Pancreas | Throughout the body | Regulates blood glucose levels; increases storage of glycogen; facilitates glucose intake by body cells |
| Glucagon | Pancreas | Liver | Stimulates the breakdown of glycogen (stored carbohydrate) into glucose (blood sugar); regulates glucose blood level |
| Leptin | Fat cells | Brain | Satiety control |
| Thyroid Hormone | Thyroid gland | Throughout the body | Increases the body's metabolic rate; promotes normal growth and development |
| Growth Hormone (HGH) | Anterior pituitary gland | Throughout the body | Stimulates growth and development |
| Cortisol | Adrenal gland | Throughout the body | Plays key role in stress response; increases blood glucose levels and mobilizes fat stores; reduces inflammation |
| DHEA | Adrenal gland | Throughout the body | Father of sex hormones |
| Estrogen | Ovaries | Female reproductive system | Causes sexual development and growth; maintains proper function of female reproductive system |
| Progesterone | Ovaries | Mammary glands Uterus | Prepares uterus for pregnancy |
| Testosterone | Testes | Throughout the body | Causes sexual development and growth spurt; maintains proper functioning of male reproductive system |

## *Sharon's Story*

Sharon, 54, who previously weighed 264 pounds, had struggled with her weight for 21 years. She'd tried her fair share of low-fat, low-carb, and other fad diets.

"With each diet, I'd lose weight, but I'd gain it back—and then some," Sharon explained. Her periods were irregular. Her lab levels indicated her thyroid was sluggish, her sex hormones were low, and her insulin level was sky high.

I put Sharon on the Perfect 10 Diet, and she followed it diligently. She focused on her goals, and each month, she achieved them. She gave up all the fake food she'd been eating, including low-fat muffins and skim milk, and started to eat eggs, shrimp, duck, and even butter. Within 2 years, Sharon lost 132 pounds, and that's not all; she managed to keep the weight off, a difference that has given her a new way of living that's filled with energy and confidence.

### A Typical Day on the Perfect 10 Diet

**BREAKFAST:** Sourdough Whole Grain Toast with Butter and Mixed Berries

**OPTIONAL MIDMORNING SNACK:** 1 Orange

**LUNCH:** Sardina Chicken Wrap (Chicken, Spinach, and Portobello Mushrooms)

**OPTIONAL MIDAFTERNOON SNACK:** ½ Cup of Pecans

**DINNER:** Lobster with a Mixed Green Salad

**Figure 3.4:** Summary of the Ten Metabolic Hormones

| HORMONE | FOODS AND FACTORS THAT CAN DISTURB THE HORMONE | FOODS AND FACTORS THAT CAN BALANCE THE HORMONE | SIGNS AND SYMPTOMS THAT YOU HAVE TOO MUCH | SIGNS AND SYMPTOMS THAT YOU HAVE TOO LITTLE | DISEASES AND CONDITIONS ASSOCIATED WITH UNBALANCED LEVELS |
|---|---|---|---|---|---|
| INSULIN | Refined carbs, sweets, sugar, soda, alcohol, hydrogenated fats, starchy vegetables (potatoes), some food additives, certain diabetes medications, stress, consuming too many calories, lack of exercise | Protein, natural fats, slow-digesting carbs (fiber-rich vegetables), whole grains, regular exercise, eating on a regular schedule, following a balanced diet, weight loss | Obesity, depression, skin tags (benign growth of the skin), acne, dark patches in the armpits, irregular periods, fatigue, low sex drive | Blurred vision, excessive thirst, dizziness, rapid breathing, increased urination, excessive weight loss | Diabetes, pre-diabetes, gestational diabetes (diabetes in pregnancy), heart disease, elevated blood pressure, elevated cholesterol, fatigue, fasting sugar higher than 70 mg/dL, irregular periods, infertility, polycystic ovary syndrome (PCOS) |
| GLUCAGON | Consuming too many calories, eating frequent meals, high insulin secretions | Natural fats, adequate protein, slow digesting carbs | Excessive weight loss | Obesity | Pancreatic tumors |
| LEPTIN | Refined carbs, large late-night dinners, alcohol, candy, soda, sugar, hydrogenated fats, lack of adequate or deep sleep, obesity, stress | Omega-3 fatty acids (found in seafood), adequate protein (organic eggs, poultry, and seafood), nuts, slow digesting carbs | Obesity | Constant hunger, depression | Anorexia nervosa, diabetes, insulin resistance, elevated cholesterol, high blood pressure, stroke, skin tags |
| THYROID HORMONE | Low-fat diets, low-carb/high-protein diets, too much iodized salt, polyunsaturated oils, some artificial sweeteners, fluoride in toothpaste, certain drugs (amiodorone and lithium) | Red meat ( beef and lamb) in moderation, seafood (herring and salmon) in moderation, mono-unsaturated fats (olive oil and avocados), selenium-rich food (whole grains, brewer's yeast), vegetables, fruits | Emotional instability, rapid weight loss, bulging eyes, irritability, nervousness, mania, irregular heartbeats, dangerous arrhythmias, excessive sweating, diarrhea | Weight gain, swelling all over the body, morning fatigue, intolerance to heat or cold, dry hair, hair loss, dry skin, slow-growing nails, muscle pain, constipation depression, excessive fatigue, irregular periods, infertility | Overactive thyroid (hyperthyroidism), sluggish thyroid (hypothyroidism) |

| HORMONE | FOODS AND FACTORS THAT CAN DISTURB THE HORMONE | FOODS AND FACTORS THAT CAN BALANCE THE HORMONE | SIGNS AND SYMPTOMS THAT YOU HAVE TOO MUCH | SIGNS AND SYMPTOMS THAT YOU HAVE TOO LITTLE | DISEASES AND CONDITIONS ASSOCIATED WITH UNBALANCED LEVELS |
|---|---|---|---|---|---|
| HGH | Aging, lack of exercise, caffeine, lack of sleep, vinegar, shallow sleep, high body fat, stress, too much dietary fat, pesticides, vegetarian diets | Anaerobic exercise, weight loss, a diet with the right amounts of natural fat and protein | Before puberty: very tall stature<br><br>After puberty: Signs and symptoms are rarely seen except in certain conditions such as acromegaly (too much HGH from tumors) and HGH abuse by athletes. These symptoms include thickening of the bones in the jaw, hands, and feet; male breast enlargement; and excessive muscle development | Before puberty: short stature or hunching over due to spine kyphosis, small muscles<br><br>After puberty: weight gain, droopy eyelids, sagging cheeks, droopy skin in the arms, stretch marks in the abdomen, wrinkles, low energy, double chin, fatigue even after getting a good night's sleep, lack of inner peace, outbursts of panic and anxiety, decreased muscle mass, decreased sex drive, lack of dreams | Before puberty: gigantism, and dwarfism<br><br>After puberty: acromegaly (excess secretions from pituitary tumors), HGH deficiency |
| CORTISOL | Alcohol, sugar, caffeine, too much salt, low-fat diets, lack of sleep, skipping meals, stress, excessive fears | A balanced diet, high-fiber foods, a diet low in sugar, food rich in vitamin C (citrus fruits, tomatoes, and strawberries), food rich in phosphatidyl-serine (beans, chicken, mackerel, green leafy vegetables), getting adequate sleep, relaxation | Belly fat (the "spare tire"), depression, insomnia, irregular periods, reduced sex drive, weight gain | Cravings for salt, chronic diarrhea, weakness, unnatural dark skin in certain parts, paleness, excessive or unintentional weight loss | Insulin resistance, diabetes, Cushing's syndrome (excess secretions of cortisol), adrenal insufficiency |

| HORMONE | FOODS AND FACTORS THAT CAN DISTURB THE HORMONE | FOODS AND FACTORS THAT CAN BALANCE THE HORMONE | SIGNS AND SYMPTOMS THAT YOU HAVE TOO MUCH | SIGNS AND SYMPTOMS THAT YOU HAVE TOO LITTLE | DISEASES AND CONDITIONS ASSOCIATED WITH UNBALANCED LEVELS |
|---|---|---|---|---|---|
| DHEA | Aging, sugar, refined carbs, a diet high in trans fats, soy | Eating adequate amounts of natural fat (especially saturated fat found in butter), food rich in magnesium (beans, seeds, and whole grains) | Acne | Weight gain, lack of sex drive | DHEA excess resulting from tumors or too much supplementation and DHEA deficiency |
| ESTROGEN<br><br>PROGES-TERONE | Aging, caffeine, refined carbs, trans fats, alcohol, too much sugar, fat-free dairy, soy, environmental toxins, stress, contraceptive pills | Eating adequate amounts of natural fats, whole milk, fruits, fiber-rich vegetables, and organic animal products; green tea; pomegranate | In women: tender breasts, anxiety, cyclical headaches or migraines, irregular bleeding, water retention, weight gain<br><br>In men: enlarged male breasts, feminization, frequent urination from an enlarged prostate<br><br>In women: unopposed estrogen, which can lead to irregular periods, depression, and weight gain<br><br>In men: too much progesterone rarely occurs | In women: droopy breasts, fatigue, depression, decreased sex drive, hot flashes, night sweats, vaginal itching and dryness, decreased vaginal lubrication, recurrent urinary tract infections<br><br>In men: a deficiency of estrogen rarely occurs<br><br>In women: breast cysts, heavy menstrual bleeding<br><br>In men: nervous behavior, anxiety, enlarged prostate | In women: menopause, polycystic ovary syndrome, infertility, endometriosis, heavy bleeding, fibroids, breast and uterine cancer, melasma (pigmentation of the face), heart disease, stroke.<br><br>In men: excess estrogen can lead to: an enlarged prostate, decreased sperm count, lowered testosterone<br><br>Progesterone deficiency |

| HORMONE | FOODS AND FACTORS THAT CAN DISTURB THE HORMONE | FOODS AND FACTORS THAT CAN BALANCE THE HORMONE | SIGNS AND SYMPTOMS THAT YOU HAVE TOO MUCH | SIGNS AND SYMPTOMS THAT YOU HAVE TOO LITTLE | DISEASES AND CONDITIONS ASSOCIATED WITH UNBALANCED LEVELS |
|---|---|---|---|---|---|
| TESTOSTERONE | Aging, refined carbs, sweets, alcohol, low-fat diet, low-protein diet, soy, licorice, stress, smoking, drugs, a diet high in hydrogenated fats or trans fats, lack of sexual activity | Eating adequate amounts of natural fat (including saturated fat), protein, foods rich in zinc (oysters, Dungeness carbs, dark meat in poultry, nuts) | Athletes abusing steroids or hormone replacements<br><br>In men: acne, frequent urination from an enlarged prostate, baldness (hair loss), excessive muscle development<br><br>In women: loss of hair, development of masculine traits, deepening of the voice | In men: weight gain, aging appearance, decreased sex drive, erection problems, fatigue, depression, decreased muscle mass, wrinkles, loss of self confidence, indecisiveness<br><br>In women: depression, excessive anxiety and fears, hysterical reactions, absent sex drive, absent orgasms, decreased clitoris and nipple sensitivity, painful intercourse, vaginal pruritus (itching), hair recession at the sides of the forehead, aging appearance, atrophied muscles | In men: testosterone deficiency or male andropause<br><br>In women: testosterone deficiency |

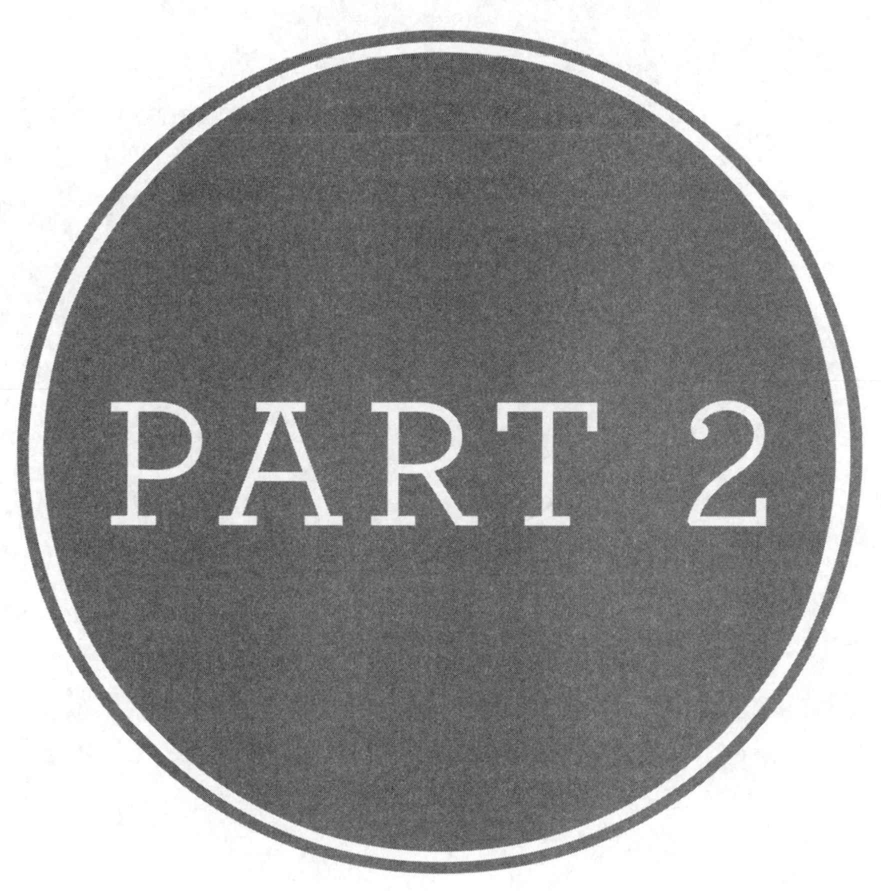

# PART 2

CHAPTER 4

# The Nutrients Your Body Needs

## Can We Regain Our Health?

I'm an optimist. The way I see it, the earlier you start, the better off you are. You need a balanced diet to get all the nutrients your body requires. A Ferrari needs premium fuel, not regular fuel. The same goes for your body. It needs organic real food, not fake fat-free food, so don't even try giving me a pathetic excuse like, "But if I eat fat, Doctor, I'll gain weight." That's so 1980s. You want to have a perfect 10 body, don't you? Eating natural fats will get you a perfect 10 physique and fantastic health. That's right, the kinds of fats present in omelets, avocados, olives, and even butter and cheese.

I realize that when I tell you to follow a high-fat/low-carb diet and go against the conventional wisdom, it will create controversy. But I won't be swayed from my goal to help you achieve perfect 10 health.

Let's look at a different scenario. When you follow a balanced diet with fewer carbs—especially refined carbs—you're less likely to get heart disease or age prematurely. If sugar levels in your bloodstream remain low, insulin levels are also stabilized. In turn, glucagon, leptin, cortisol, and sex hormones follow. Wow! That simultaneously improves your health and speeds up fat loss. It gets even better—disease is less likely to develop when your insulin level is near rock bottom. Amazing, isn't it?

While no one can tell you exactly the amount of fat you should eat, I can tell you this: *it definitely shouldn't be low in fat.* The road to health is a balanced diet in all the macronutrients. A healthy approach is neither a low-fat nor a low-carb diet; instead, it's about balance.

In this chapter, I will introduce to you the nutrients your body needs to function properly. Your body requires 6 essential nutrient classes for growth, maintenance, and repair of its tissues. These classes are carbohydrates, protein, fat, vitamins, minerals, and water. Carbohydrates, protein, and fat are the macronutrients. Vitamins, minerals, and water are the micronutrients.

## The Formula for a Healthy Diet Is Balance

A healthy diet balances all the macronutrients in a very specific way, and this balance is the cornerstone of the Perfect 10 Diet. The Perfect 10 Diet balance is 40 percent carbohydrates, 20 percent protein, and about 40 percent fat (Fig. 4.1). Low-fat diets, or diets with less than 30 percent fat, tend to be high in carbohydrates and sugar, and they cause the body to overproduce insulin. This causes the body to store fat and gain weight. On the other hand, diets that tend to be high in protein, like popular low-carb programs, force your body to use protein as a source of energy. They trick your body by not allowing sugar at all or mimicking starvation. As a result, you lose weight as your insulin levels are stabilized. But protein is not a clean source of energy for your body to use as its main source of fuel, and it can cause a variety of health problems.

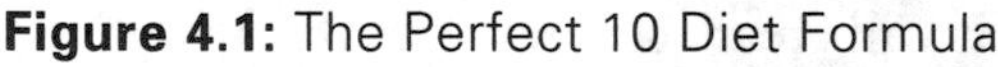

**Figure 4.1:** The Perfect 10 Diet Formula

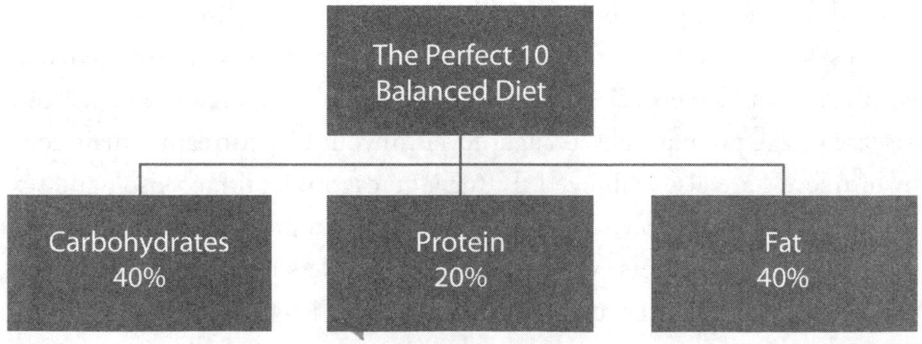

The Perfect 10 Diet is the only diet that promotes nutritional balance, with a 40/20/40 ratio that will keep your sugar level stable and your metabolic system working efficiently. Balance is a key step in promoting perfect 10 health. Why? Your body can use both fat and carbs as a clean source of energy. A diet that includes an appropriate amount of natural fat will help you feel more satisfied with less food, and it will allow your body to slowly absorb the sugar into the bloodstream. That will lead to decreased insulin secretions. Decreased insulin levels equal weight loss. And let's not forget that decreased insulin levels also lower your chances of developing disease.

Eating natural fat is a key step toward successful and sustained weight loss. By eating 40 percent carbs, you also get enough nutrients to support your hormones with vitamins and minerals. You also get enough fiber. By definition, fiber is the indigestible parts of fruits, seeds, vegetables, and whole grains. But for me, it's nothing short of a miracle nutrient. By eating fiber-rich foods, you not only decrease food cravings, but you also reduce your chances of developing heart disease, stroke, high blood pressure, and diabetes. In women, fiber helps balance excess estrogen.

### The Macronutrients

- Carbohydrates
- Protein
- Fat

## Carbohydrates

Most of the carbohydrates you'll consume on the Perfect 10 Diet are slow-digesting carbs. Many people are unaware that vegetables, fruits, and legumes are carbohydrates, too—it's not all bread, rice, and pasta. Vegetables, fruits, legumes, and whole grains are the good carbs. The bad carbs are refined, like white rice, pasta, and all forms of sugar (including maltose, dextrose, and sucrose); they are nutritionally void and create exaggerated insulin secretions. The challenge for most is to reduce their intake of unhealthy carbs from sugar, refined carbohydrates, and fat-free foods filled with high-fructose corn syrup, and to increase their intake of high-fiber carbs. The Perfect 10 Diet will make this easy for you to do.

## What Are Carbohydrates?

Carbohydrates are molecules made of carbon, hydrogen, and oxygen that are used as a source of energy by the body. They can be simple (glucose) or complex (many glucose molecules attached together), and it's best when we consume carbohydrates that occur naturally. Plant sources are the complex carbs that contain the wonder nutrient, fiber.

## What Are the Good Carbs?

The good carbs are those that are absorbed slowly in the bloodstream and don't impact your blood sugar or insulin in any dramatic way. They are found in most fiber-rich vegetables, fruits, and whole grains. Good carbs balance insulin, boost glucagon, support thyroid health, and optimize the production of sex hormones and DHEA. All these hormones are essential for you to be fit, radiant, and healthy. Your body needs these good carbs, but we eat far too few of them. A healthy diet must include 5 to 9 servings of fruits and vegetables a day. So are you on the right dietary track?

I am extremely disturbed when some of my patients say they avoid eating whole fruits because they're not recommended on their low-carb diets. On the other hand, someone on a low-fat diet might drink a gallon of orange juice, believing it's a healthy option for vitamin C and antioxidants. But, in reality, he or she is taking in massive amounts of sugar, throwing off insulin secretions. Again, it's about balance.

## What Are the Bad Carbs?

Believe me, sugar is the devil. It's here to ruin you. If you don't eliminate it from your diet, you will never achieve the perfect 10 physique you dream of. The same goes for refined carbs. Want to be a fit man? Well, you have to avoid those fat-free muffins and low-fat cakes. "Anti-nutrients" like these are prohibited on the Perfect 10 Diet, and they should be completely eliminated from your life. You take in bad carbs every time you drink a soda or a beer, or eat products made with refined white flour or high-fructose corn syrup-laden low-fat products. To your body, this junk food is no different from pure table sugar. When you eat these things, your bloodstream is flooded with sugar, which causes an instant spike in insulin levels. After this spike, your blood sugar level will crash, and you'll be overcome with hunger. That crash is the strange feeling of tiredness or sleepiness you probably feel after a big meal of pasta or pancakes. This leads to a vicious cycle, because subsequently you'll crave more sugar to fix that crash.

Sugar is like crack, but without its appetite-suppressing qualities. You'll eat a single cookie, and before you know it, you won't be able to resist having one more, and then another, and another. An important part of any recovery for addiction is taking one meal at a time. Don't torture yourself with thoughts like, "I can never eat cookies again" or "I can't have pasta or pizza." Instead, set mini goals for yourself, like I'll treat myself to a cookie every now and then. Almost everything, including a scoop of ice cream from Häagen-Dazs, is all right in moderation. You'll feel motivated, instead of deprived. If you find yourself tempted to have more, just envision the damaging effects of sugar on your organs, mood, hormones, overall appearance, and sex life.

Okay, that's enough melodrama. My point is that sugar is a treat, and you must pretty much eliminate it from your diet if you truly want to have a perfect 10 physique.

It's important to know that sugar is everywhere, and it hides behind many different names. See Figure 4.2 for examples.

**Figure 4.2:** Various Names for Sugar

- Beet sugar
- Brown sugar
- Corn syrup
- Dextrose
- Galactose
- Glucose
- Grape sugar
- High-fructose corn syrup
- Honey
- Malt
- Maltose
- Maple syrup
- Molasses
- Raw sugar
- Rice syrup
- Sucrose
- Syrup

**Figure 4.3:** Top 20 Sources of Carbohydrates in the American Diet*

| | | |
|---|---|---|
| 1. Potatoes (mashed or baked) | 8. Pizza | 15. Pancakes |
| 2. White bread | 9. Pasta | 16. Table sugar |
| 3. Cold breakfast cereal | 10. Muffins | 17. Jam |
| 4. Dark bread | 11. Fruit punch | 18. Fruit juice |
| 5. Orange juice | 12. Soft drinks | 19. French fries |
| 6. Bananas | 13. Apples | 20. Candy |
| 7. White rice | 14. Skim milk | |

Dr. Simin Liu, Harvard University School of Public Health
* This data represents the findings of the Harvard Nurses' Health Study (2002).

You can see in Figure 4.3 that the American diet is fraught with bad carbohydrates. You've got to replace many of those bad carbs with more natural fats. Eat avocados and eggs instead of cereal for breakfast, and olives or avocados instead of cookies for snacks.

## Which Are Better—Complex or Simple Carbs?

I'd rather you ask whether carbs contain fiber or not, since the classification of complex and simple carbohydrates is incorrect. The science that resulted in the classifications was based on the idea that the sugars in complex carbs break down slowly in the body, while the sugar in simple carbs breaks down rapidly. The glycemic index, a wonderful tool devised by Dr. David Jenkins, can help you understand this more clearly.

## The Glycemic Index (GI)

Dr. Jenkins illustrated that many of the so-called "complex" carbohydrates, such as white bread, are more hostile than pure sugar inside the body. A diet based on white bread, white rice, cereals, soda, and low-fat products is loaded with sugar. Interestingly, some root vegetables that lack fiber, such as potatoes and pumpkins, also raise glucose levels in the bloodstream faster than pure table sugar. That's because the carbs or starches present in potatoes act like sugar. The rapid rise in blood sugar you experience after eating a baked potato is the same as you'd experience after eating a doughnut! A potato has fewer calories, of course, but it leads to a high insulin level, which can make you hungry.

Most versions of the glycemic index assign sugar with the number 100 and compare other foods on an ascending or descending scale from that point (Fig. 4.4). Foods that are low on the glycemic index are usually high in fiber and have been shown to promote satiety by allowing the gradual release of sugar into the bloodstream (and they don't make you feel hungry) (Fig. 4.5). On the other hand, foods that are high on the glycemic index, like potatoes, lack fiber and have been shown to promote weight gain by increasing insulin secretion.

Unless the consumer understands the differences in carbs (the glycemic index offers an easy way to do this), he or she will not understand that a low-fat diet increases the risk of heart disease, obesity, and diabetes. But portion size counts too. Americans are eating more high-glycemic foods and taking in very little fat to delay the absorption of sugar into the bloodstream. In other words, eating some mashed potatoes with some sour cream once in a while may not harm you, but if you eat a lot of mashed potatoes with no fat at all and don't

**Figure 4.4:** Glycemic Index of Various Foods

| HIGH GLYCEMIC CARBOHYDRATES | (SUGAR = 100) |
|---|---|
| Croissant | 100 |
| Fat-free muffin | 130 |
| French toast | 90 |
| French baguette bread | 100 |
| Honey Nut Cheerios | 85 |
| Special K cereal | 90 |
| Pancakes | 100 |
| Potatoes (baked) | 160 |
| Pretzels | 100 |
| Waffles | 100 |
| White bread | 100 |
| White rice | 100 |
| | |
| LOW-GLYCEMIC CARBOHYDRATES | |
| Most fiber-rich vegetables | <20 |
| Most whole grains | <35 |
| Most fruit | <20 to 70 |

burn the sugar, you are guaranteed to gain weight. Why? You'll produce too much insulin and inhibit glucagon, the hormone that melts the fat.

Eating processed foods, like most breakfast cereals (it gets worse when you add fat-free milk), will raise your blood sugar level faster than if you eat pure sugar. People who eat low-fat muffins for breakfast are bound to gain more weight than people who eat eggs with cheese simply because they are taking in only sugar, which leads to increased insulin secretions.

**Figure 4.5:** Blood Glucose Levels in Relation to Low and High Glycemic Index Food

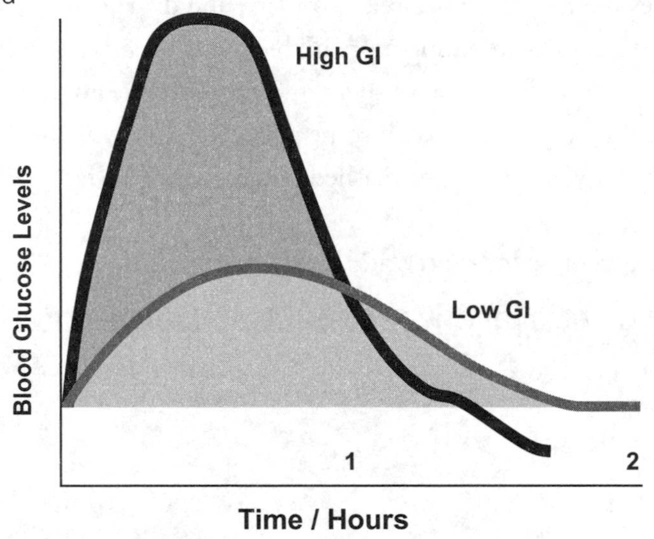


The amount of carbohydrate in the reference and test food must be the same.

## Vegetables

Eat your vegetables to have a perfect 10 physique. It sounds like a cliché, but it works. If you're the kind of person who says, "But I hate vegetables, Doctor," get real. Vegetables should constitute the base of every meal you eat. They provide your body with large amounts of vitamins, minerals, and fiber. It's the fiber in vegetables that makes them so nutritious, as it slows the absorption of nutrients in the bloodstream. The fiber in vegetables will also lower your risk of heart disease.

You can have your vegetables raw, mildly steamed, stir-fried, or juiced. Again, vegetables that are low in fiber (such as white potatoes) act like pure sugar in your body, so they should be greatly limited or avoided until you lose weight. It's easy to see why obesity is so rampant these days, when the only vegetable eaten by many is potatoes—either baked or as French fries. Other starchy vegetables, such as carrots (especially cooked) and beets can also cause unhealthy surges in blood sugar if they're eaten in large quantities and without a portion of protein or fat to delay their absorption. Fiber-rich vegetables are always preferable, and should always be your first choice on the Perfect 10 Diet.

When you eat low-fiber vegetables, such as potatoes, carrots, or beets, do so in moderation. These starchy vegetables should only be eaten by people who exercise regularly, since they can lead to weight gain. The bright colors of vegetables indicate that they are full of antioxidants, which mitigate free radical damage. Veggies like spinach and kale contain vitamin K, which contributes to heart health.

Cruciferous vegetables, such as broccoli and cauliflower, help neutralize dangerous estrogen metabolites in men and women. I must provide a word of caution, however; if you suffer from a sluggish thyroid, be aware that certain vegetables (broccoli, Brussels sprouts, cabbage, cauliflower, kale, turnips, rutabaga, spinach, and watercress), when eaten raw and in large quantities, can block the uptake of iodine. That can aggravate your condition. If you do have a sluggish thyroid, these healthy vegetables should be eaten lightly cooked. If you had your thyroid removed and are already on thyroid medications, you don't have to be concerned about this issue at all. For folks who don't have a thyroid problem, eating these vegetables is actually a good thing.

As you eliminate refined carbs from your diet and increase your fiber-rich vegetable intake, your taste buds will get used to the naturally sweet tastes of cauliflower, eggplant, and zucchini. As a matter of fact, it may feel strange to go back to eating pasta, pizza, or sweets.

## Fruit

Fruit is an extremely healthy addition to your diet. On the Perfect 10 Diet, it's also an amazingly convenient snack food. It's packed with goodness and available in different shapes, sizes, and flavors. Fruit is generally high in vitamins, minerals, enzymes, water, and fiber. The fiber in fruit helps slow the digestion process, keeping you full longer so you don't experience energy crashes. Fruit also contains a sugar called fructose, which is good for energy. Many people on low-carb diets avoid fruit because of carbs, but eating fruit can optimize many of the hormones discussed on the Perfect 10 Diet.

Fructose, which is naturally present in fruit, does not negatively affect insulin levels like glucose. Nevertheless, consuming excessive amounts of fructose (like a glass of a fruit juice) in your bloodstream can be as harmful as eating pure sugar, which your body will store as fat if it isn't quickly burned off. A fruit juice concentrate can contain as much sugar as a can of soda, and a fresh-squeezed glass of juice (which, stripped of its fiber, no longer slows the delivery of sugar to the blood) can have even more. For this reason, you can eat whole fruits, but you should eliminate fruit juices from your diet. Don't drink your calories. Chewing takes longer and ultimately provides more satisfaction.

Which fruits should you eat? I love cantaloupe, cherries, and all kinds of berries on the Perfect 10 Diet. They're great for weight loss since they are very low in sugar and calories.

Oranges are high in vitamin C and can help balance cortisol, making them a great stress-relieving food. Do you like grapes? Wonderful! They're rich in resveratrol, which is good for your heart. Ladies, if you want to show off your killer legs in a pair of Jimmy Choos or Manolo Blahniks, how about eating plums regularly? They are rich in vitamin K—much more so than any other fruit—which helps reduce the appearance of spider and varicose veins.

All fruits are good for you, but you should limit tropical fruits like mangoes and bananas if you're having a hard time losing weight. For those of you with a sluggish thyroid, strawberries should also be limited as they can interfere with the thyroid hormone production.

Are you really hungry? How about enjoying a piece of cheese with your favorite fruit, or top a piece of fruit with a few teaspoons of unsweetened whipped cream. It will fill you up nicely. The fat from the cheese or the whipped cream will delay the absorption of fructose into your bloodstream and will leave you feeling full and satisfied.

The most nutritious part of many fruits are the skins, which are rich in antioxidants, so don't peel them. You should eliminate dried fruits from your diet, since they no longer contain the water that helps fill you up.

## Legumes

Legumes should be part of a healthy diet. Try to eat them 3 to 4 times a week. They're a good source of carbs and also contain small amounts of protein. In fact, legumes are bona fide belly flatteners. The list includes black beans, black-eyed peas, garbanzo beans, kidney beans, navy beans, pinto beans, and lentils. They're high in soluble fiber, so they're low on the glycemic index and do not impact your blood sugar or insulin levels in any negative way.

Legumes are also a great source of antioxidants, the antidote to free radicals. Antioxidants prevent heart disease and cancer. In fact, recent research indicates that eating legumes can prevent colon adenomas and colon cancer. I encourage you to include many Middle Eastern dishes made with legumes, such as hummus and tahini, in your diet. Legumes are also great as healthy snacks or appetizers.

There is one exception. Soybeans, which are mostly genetically modified, are the only legumes that I want you to avoid. It's estimated that 85 percent of American soy crops are genetically modified to enhance resistance to spoilage. In Europe, such genetic engineering is banned. Until we know more about the possible health risks associated with genetically modified soy, steer clear of it.

## Grains

Fear not. You don't have to give up whole-wheat bread or pasta on the Perfect 10 Diet to have a perfect 10 body. It's just the *refined* grains that you have to avoid. Whole grains are good carbs that do not negatively impact insulin levels, and they can be eaten in moderation. A breakfast of non-instant oatmeal is a perfectly acceptable choice as part of a healthy diet. It's full of vitamins, minerals, and soluble fiber, and it can lower your cholesterol level.

When it comes to bread, I prefer that you choose rye or pumpernickel, since they contain the highest amount of fiber and the lowest amount of sugar. The way to pick healthy bread is to look for the highest fiber content. Whole grains contain minerals, such as magnesium, potassium, phosphorus, copper, and manganese. But buyer beware: many whole-grain breads have added sugar or molasses, so read the labels carefully before dropping a loaf of bread into your shopping cart.

For all grain-based products, make sure you read all ingredients carefully. Many cereals that claim to be made with whole grains also contain added sugar, high-fructose corn syrup, or even partially hydrogenated fats. All these added ingredients have a negative impact on hormones, and that's bad. When it comes to rice, choose wild over brown rice for its higher fiber content. When it comes to pasta, go for whole-wheat pasta. Cook it al dente (for a short time, so it's a bit underdone) to slow the digestive process.

## You Need Fiber in Your Diet

Fiber is the roughage, or the indigestible part, of fruits, vegetables, and whole grains. It's nothing short of a miracle nutrient. Fiber delays your digestive tract's efforts to get at the sugars and starches in carbohydrates, which makes you feel full and satisfied. You should eat about 40 to 50 grams of fiber a day.

Fiber is classified as either soluble or insoluble, depending on how it reacts with water. Soluble fibers, such as pectin, gum, and mucilage, break down in water and form a gel in the intestines. Insoluble fibers, such as cellulose and hemicellulose, do not dissolve and sweep through the intestines like a broom.

Soluble fiber is found in apples, barley, and peas, and it has been shown to promote healthy sugar levels. Insoluble fiber, which is found in cauliflower and beans, improves bowel function and removes toxins from the colon. High-fiber diets help manage hunger and eliminate calories from foods by leading them out of the body via the stool. As a result, it's easier for you to lose weight.

## Eating the Right Kinds of Carbs Can Make a Big Difference

It is a clinically proven fact that in order to lose weight, you must consume fewer calories than you burn. This can be accomplished by eating fiber-rich foods. Fiber is Mother Nature's natural appetite reducer. By eating 40 to 50 grams of fiber a day, you will lose weight and reduce your risk for heart disease, diabetes, and a host of other related conditions. Always remember: the right carbs do not come in boxes that state they are low in fat or fat-free.

**Figure 4.6:** Top Fiber Foods

| Food | Portion | Fiber (g) |
|---|---|---|
| **VEGETABLES** | | |
| Artichoke | 1 medium | 3 |
| Broccoli | ½ cup | 2.4 |
| Brussels sprouts | ½ cup | 3 |
| Sweet potatoes | ½ cup | 4 |
| Zucchini | ½ cup | 5 |
| **FRUITS** | | |
| Avocados | 1 medium | 6.9 |
| Apple | 1 medium | 4 |
| Kiwi | 1 medium | 2.7 |
| Strawberries | ½ cup | 3 |
| **LEGUMES** | | |
| Black beans | ½ cup | 6 |
| Butter beans | ½ cup | 7 |
| Kidney beans | ½ cup | 7 |
| Lentils | ½ cup | 5.1 |
| **WHOLE GRAINS** | | |
| Oatmeal | ½ cup | 4.4 |
| Rye bread | 1 slice | 5 |
| Whole-wheat bread | 1 slice | 3 |

## *Joanne's Story in Her Own Words*

I've been overweight since I was a teenager. I've followed practically every low-fat diet on the planet and have lost weight on them—only to gain it all back, and then some. I counted calories and watched portions for years with no success.

By age 42, I gave up on losing weight and ballooned up to 180 pounds. I recently started on cholesterol and blood pressure drugs. I heard about the Perfect 10 Diet from a friend, and after a consultation with Dr. Michael Aziz, all my beliefs changed. I was shocked to learn that the low-fat products I consumed were causing me to gain weight. How could this make sense, with all the "healthy" signs on fat-free salad dressings and cereals?

I started reading the labels and realized I was eating pure sugar. I started to eat more fiber-rich vegetables as side dishes with each meal instead of pasta and baked potatoes. I started to eat eggs with cheese for breakfast instead of my favorite cereal when I realized it contained partially hydrogenated fat in addition to high-fructose corn syrup. I gave up the orange juice I drank every morning when I realized the enormous amount of sugar I was consuming on a daily basis. I snacked on nuts and avocados instead of baked potato chips and fat-free rice cakes.

My appetite switch has been turned off, and my body is so "cleansed" of sugar that when I do decide to indulge, I experience immediate consequences (like a yeast infection or a drop in energy). The truth is that I had become insulin resistant, which is why I gained weight, and I didn't even know it. I lost 30 pounds in one year, and my insulin level dropped from 45 to 5. I am totally off all my cholesterol and blood pressure drugs. I am amazed at the transformation. I look and feel great—a perfect 10.

I finally feel sexy again 24/7.

## A Typical Day on the Perfect 10 Diet

**BREAKFAST:** Turkey Breast on Whole-Wheat Toast and 1 Apple
**OPTIONAL MIDMORNING SNACK:** 1 Cup Chick Peas
**LUNCH:** Grilled Tilapia with Baked Tomatoes and a Side Salad
**OPTIONAL MIDAFTERNOON SNACK:** ½ Cup Cherries
**DINNER:** Natural Granola and 1 Glass of Milk

## *Julie's Story in Her Own Words*

I am 37 years old, and my weight has risen steadily since my marriage 12 years ago. After my third child was born, I exercised less, and my weight reached 200 pounds. I have been on many different popular low-fat diets over the years, but they never worked. I would lose weight on prepackaged meals with popular diet programs and low-fat shakes, but I always regained the weight.

I have also tried low-carb diets, but I hated giving up fruit, and I didn't think eating bacon was a healthy thing to do. The Perfect 10 Diet, a rich diet that is completely different from any low-fat or low-carb diets I've ever tried, allowed me to eat more vegetables with each meal, as well as fruits. It's very balanced, and it does not make me feel deprived of the carbs I love, like whole-grain bread and fruits. All I had to give up was sugar, fruit juices, and refined carbohydrates.

As a matter of fact, I really don't feel like I've given up anything now, because when I indulge in those foods, I get a strange taste in my mouth. The Perfect 10 Diet allows me to eat more fats from butter, coconut, and avocados, foods I avoided for years because I believed they were bad for my cholesterol. Who could ask for anything more? I've lost 70 pounds on the Perfect 10 Diet in 16 months, and my fasting insulin level has dropped from 40 to 4. Nothing tastes as good as being thin feels.

## A Typical Day on the Perfect 10 Diet

**BREAKFAST:** Mushroom Omelet with 2 Chicken Sausages and 1 Orange

**OPTIONAL MIDMORNING SNACK:** Unsalted Sunflower Seeds

**LUNCH:** Grilled Duck Breast with Dill, Mushrooms, and a Side Salad

**OPTIONAL MIDAFTERNOON SNACK:** Mixed Fruit Salad

**DINNER:** Cheese Fondue with 2 Whole-Wheat Crackers

## Protein

### Why Do We Need Protein?

Protein comes from the Greek word *proteus*, which means "of first importance." That's exactly what it is. Protein is the basic building block of all tissues and organs and is involved in almost all chemical reactions in the body. Protein is also needed to relay messages between cells and transport nutrients. Foods that are rich in animal protein include fish, fowl, eggs, and red meat. Animal protein is essential to optimize glucagon and growth hormone production, and this helps melt fat.

The trick with protein is to eat it in the right amounts, which on the Perfect 10 Diet means roughly 20 percent of your daily food intake. Why? A diet that's low in protein can lead to weight gain by disturbing hormone production. On the other hand, a diet that is too high in protein can cause gout. It's all about balance.

The weight-loss benefits of low-carb diets have been observed for over 150 years. But they really took off in the last 20 years. The Atkins and Protein Power diets have helped millions lose weight, but come on! You must be from a carnivorous tribe or another planet if you think eating protein all day long is a healthy thing to do. These high-protein and very low-carb diets will ultimately take a toll on your health.

Sure, you'll lose weight on extreme protein diets because you'll eliminate sugar and bad carbs and balance your insulin. But what about the downsides? First, you may experience constipation and acidic breath if you use protein and fat as your main source of energy. Hmm. That's not sexy. Okay, so now you're probably thinking, "*Who cares about constipation or bad breath? I'll take a laxative and brush my teeth more often. I just want to be thin.*" Well, you could do that, but high-protein diets can eventually make you suffer from kidney stones, gout, and osteoporosis.

As I also mentioned earlier, high-protein/low-carb diets are bad for your thyroid, since excess protein prevents the conversion of thyroid hormone to its active form. A sluggish thyroid means dry skin, hair loss, depression, and, eventually, a slow metabolism.

Unlike the Perfect 10 Diet that can make you look younger by boosting HGH levels, high-protein/low-carb diets can make you age faster by depressing HGH levels. You see, these types of diets are also way too high in fat, and this simply shuts down your growth hormone or HGH production, the fountain of youth hormone. Eating excessive amounts of fat (50 or 60 percent of your caloric intake) is an enemy to HGH secretion. In turn, you'll develop early wrinkles, bags under the eyes, a double chin, sagging skin, and a sluggish metabolism. Additionally, these diets are too low in fiber, which can lead to a higher estrogen level in women. An imbalance in the estrogen-progesterone ratio can lead to many problems, such as headaches and irregular periods.

So what do you think of these diets now? Do you still want to follow a high-protein/low-carb diet ? You see, it's not only about getting thin and having immediate results. You need to preserve your health first before you can become a perfect 10 on the inside and the outside.

## How Much Protein Can I Eat?

I recommend that protein should be about 20 percent of your total daily food intake *if* you exercise regularly (exercise is a core part of the Perfect 10 Diet to boost growth hormone production). As a matter of fact, most people need only 15 percent protein in their daily diet.

However, there are exceptions on the Perfect 10 Diet. For individuals who are involved in heavy anaerobic activities, such as body builders and others who are involved in weight lifting, the Perfect 10 Diet can be adjusted to include more protein.

If you are a guy who is doing a lot of anaerobic activity and wants to build big muscles, you should consume 25 or even 30 percent of your daily caloric intake from protein. This amount won't harm your thyroid or your health, because all the excess protein will be used to build muscles. The rest of your macronutrients should come from carbs and fat. A good equation would be 40 percent carbohydrates, 25 percent protein, and 35 percent fat, because getting 20 percent of your calories from protein may not be enough.

In other words, your protein requirement on the Perfect 10 Diet depends on you—your physical build and your activity level. That's what a flexible, versatile diet like the Perfect 10 Diet is all about. It's custom-tailored because everybody's activity level is different, and it can vary from time to time, depending on your exercise routine. If you're a body builder, this diet is perfect, and if you're a sedentary senior citizen, this diet is also perfect.

The Perfect 10 Diet has two optional snacks in case you work out regularly and want to focus on building muscle.

There are multiple formulas to determine your body's protein requirements, and they can be complicated. I like to use a simple and practical formula: if you're sedentary, eat protein in 1 to 2 of your 3 daily meals. If you are involved in some exercise or anaerobic training, such as working out 2 to 3 times a week, eat protein in 2 to 3 meals. If you are involved in heavy weight lifting, eat protein in all your 3 meals and maybe in one of your snacks. Isn't that easy? Most people require 50 to 160 grams of protein daily, and the rest should come from carbs and fat. Remember, your protein requirement on the Perfect 10 Diet depends on your activity level. Twenty percent of total calories is the average requirement needed for most people on the Perfect 10 Diet in combination with a moderate exercise program.

## Protein Sources

The protein sources I recommend are based on the protein itself rather than the amount of fat or cholesterol the food may contain. This is because saturated fat and cholesterol-rich foods have no relationship to heart disease. While no protein sources are strictly prohibited, I do believe that some are healthier than others. When you eat animal protein, it would be wise to eat food closer to the bottom of the food chain, such as poultry, rather than beef. Why? Environmental toxins can accumulate in large, long-lived animals. And you know what toxins do to your endocrine system and hormones: they mess them up.

## The Most Favorable Protein Sources

The most favorable protein sources are eggs, poultry (including duck and goose), fish and other seafood, mushrooms, and liver. These protein sources can improve your health and support your hormones.

### EGGS

Eggs are perfectly fine food. I'm talking about real eggs here, not vegetable oil–based, fabricated foods like Egg Beaters. Back in the old days, eggs were considered healthy. Unfortunately, some faulty research that came out in the 1980s gave eggs a bad rap. Recent research indicates there is no harm in eating eggs—even on a daily basis—since most cholesterol is produced *inside* our bodies. In fact, if you eat cholesterol-rich foods like eggs, your body will use the ingested dietary cholesterol to repair tissues and make essential sex hormones (estrogen, progesterone, and testosterone) that keep you young, healthy, radiant, and fit.

The medical establishment is still encouraging us to avoid egg yolks for fear of heart disease, but this is inaccurate advice. When you eat eggs, you are better off eating the yolks than the whites, since the yolks contain healthy vitamins and the good omega-3 fatty acids that prevent heart disease. One large egg yolk also contains 245 IU (international units) of vitamin A, 18 IU of vitamin D, and lutein, which is essential for healthy eyes. Eggs also contain chromium, which enhances insulin function.

Today, most chickens are given hormones and antibiotics. They are fed corn, which makes the amount of omega-6 fatty acids in their eggs higher than the healthy omega-3 fatty acids. For this reason, it is vastly superior if you can buy eggs produced from pasture-fed or free-range chickens. Eggs from pasture-fed chickens contain more omega-3 fatty acids and vitamins, since their diet includes green plants and insects. Eggs from pasture-fed chickens can be bought from organic food stores, local farmers, and online. Organic eggs (which don't have quite the nutritional content of pasture-fed eggs since the chickens' diet is artificial) are readily available in most supermarkets.

Eat your eggs any way you like. Boil a bunch of eggs every few days and place them in your refrigerator to eat as a healthy snack or for a quick healthy breakfast. If you're having an omelet, cook your eggs in butter (yes, butter) rather than in polyunsaturated vegetable oils to prevent the cholesterol oxidation that occurs when these oils are heated, which leads to the formation of cell-damaging free radicals. On the Perfect 10 Diet, you can eat eggs on a daily basis and rest assured that you are making a very healthy, as well as a sound, choice.

### POULTRY

Poultry is an excellent source of protein. Many body builders swear that they build more muscles by eating lean chicken and turkey. This may be the effects of good quality protein on HGH production and testosterone.

Poultry also contains vitamins and minerals, such as phosphorus and copper, essential for good health. Poultry (especially the dark meat) contains zinc, which is essential to support the production of female and male sex hormones (estrogen, progesterone, and testosterone). Zinc also improves skin complexion. Again, I recommend that you eat pasture-fed or free-range birds. You can buy pasture-fed chicken from organic foods stores, local farmers, and online. Organic poultry is readily available in most supermarkets. (A list of suppliers is also provided at the end of this book.) Eating poultry regularly seems to have an inverse relationship to colon cancer compared to the consumption of red meat. On the Perfect 10 Diet, I encourage you to eat chicken, turkey, pheasant, and duck. Rest assured that poultry, whether it's lean like chicken or fatty like duck, will positively impact your health. Enjoy your poultry cooked any way you like, except deep-fried.

### FISH

Fish is an excellent source of protein and fat. It contains healthy omega-3 fatty acids, which play a role in the prevention of cardiovascular disease and the optimization of sex hormones. Studies confirm that people who eat fish regularly are less likely to suffer strokes, since fish, like aspirin, prolongs bleeding time.

Eating fish regularly has also been shown to be inversely related to the development of colon and other types of cancer, including stomach and esophageal. Epidemiologic studies that show this advantage make fish a very favorable protein choice on the Perfect 10 Diet. Eating fish regularly has been shown to control the levels of leptin, the satiety hormone. That can lead to weight loss.

When it comes to fish, stay with ocean-caught fish rather than farm-raised fish or fish from lakes in order to avoid ingesting mercury and other contaminants that can throw your metabolism off balance. Don't throw away fish heads, either, as they are nutrient rich. Instead, use them to make fish broth. Fish broth is a staple of the Japanese diet, which is rich in the minerals and iodine that are essential for thyroid health.

**Figure 4.7:** Omega-3 Content per 6-Ounce Serving

| | |
|---|---|
| Mackerel | 3.5 |
| Ocean-farmed Atlantic salmon | 2.9 |
| Wild Pacific salmon* | 1.8 |
| Swordfish | 0.9 |
| Bluefin tuna | 0.3 |
| Flounder | 0.3 |
| Tilapia | 0.2 |

USDA Nutrient Database for Standard Reference, Release 19 (2005)
EPA & DHA* Average of 5 species

## DOES FARM-RAISED FISH CONTAIN HEALTHY OMEGA-3 FATTY ACIDS?

Both wild and farm-raised fish contain healthy omega-3 fatty acids. However, some farm-raised salmon are also fed dyes to give their flesh the orange tint of wild salmon. Farm-raised fish are fed soy. Choose fish that is labeled wild or frozen, meaning it was ocean-caught, and stay away from fish without labels or that's labeled "fresh," which means it was probably farm raised. You can easily find wild fish in your local supermarket. (A list of wild fish suppliers is provided at the end of this book.)

## SHELLFISH

The term "shellfish" applies to 2 different kinds of animals: crustaceans and mollusks. Crustaceans include crabs, crayfish, lobster, and shrimp. Mollusks include clams, oysters, mussels, scallops, octopus, and squid. All shellfish provide the body with high-quality protein and contain healthy minerals and vitamins. Shellfish also contain healthy omega-3 fatty acids (although in lesser amounts than other fish).

Oysters are high in zinc, which plays a role in fertility by preserving the male and female sex hormones (estrogen, progesterone, and testosterone). It's no wonder that oysters are considered to be an aphrodisiac in many cultures. Oysters also contain vanadium, which helps improve sugar control.

## SEAFOOD AND THYROID HEALTH

On the Perfect 10 Diet, seafood is an excellent protein choice that you can benefit from daily. Seafood is great for thyroid health. However, if you have an underactive thyroid, eat seafood no more than 3 times a week. Eating too much seafood can adversely affect thyroid function, as shown in a Japanese study. In the study, 50 percent of patients with an underactive thyroid who stopped eating seafood had an increase in thyroid hormone levels in a matter of a few weeks. This is related to the dangers of having too much iodine in your food. It's true—too much of a good thing can be bad, but finding the right balance optimizes your thyroid hormone production.

## YOU RECOMMEND SEAFOOD AS A FAVORITE PROTEIN, BUT WHAT ABOUT MERCURY?

Mercury is very harmful to the developing brains of unborn babies and young children. That's why young children and women who are pregnant, who are planning to become pregnant, or who are nursing are advised to be cautious when eating fish. For those people, the United States government recommends no more than 12 ounces per week of a variety of seafood to limit their risk. The Environmental Protection Agency (EPA) suggests more stringent guidelines, limiting fish to 1 serving per week (6 ounces of cooked fish for women and 2 ounces for young children).

For the rest of us, the benefits of eating fish regularly outweigh any risks. You can reduce your exposure to mercury by eating fish known to have low mercury levels. Just stick to eating small fish and avoid large ones, such as swordfish, shark, and king mackerel.

Fish is a very healthy addition to your diet. Fish will provide you with the essential fatty acids (omega-3) that help prevent heart disease, cancer, and Alzheimer's disease.

## DOES CANNED TUNA CONTAIN A LOT OF MERCURY?

That depends on what kind of canned tuna you buy. The species used in canned tuna tend to be smaller than the long-lived, larger species sold at the fish counter. Choose chunk light, as it tends to contain less mercury than solid white or chunk white. Albacore "white" tuna has more mercury;

**Figure 4.8:** Seafood: What to Enjoy and What to Avoid to Limit Mercury Exposure

| SEAFOOD TO ENJOY | | SEAFOOD TO AVOID |
|---|---|---|
| Abalone | Scallops | Bass (freshwater) |
| Crawfish | Sea bass | Bluefish |
| Crab | Shrimp | Catfish |
| Haddock | Sole | Cod |
| Halibut | Spiny lobster | Great Lakes salmon |
| Mahimahi | Squid | Lake trout |
| Marlin | Tilapia | Maine lobster |
| Octopus | Tuna (small species like skipjack) | Mackerel |
| Pacific salmon (wild) | Wahoo | Ocean perch |
| Red snapper | Yellowtail | Shark |
| Sardines | | Striped bass |
| | | Sturgeon |
| | | Swordfish |
| | | Tilefish |
| | | Tuna (fresh and frozen) |

those who are at risk should consume no more than 6 ounces per week. Some consumer groups have recommended that pregnant women should not eat any tuna at all.

## MUSHROOMS

Mushrooms are neither vegetables nor plants. They are classified in a separate biological kingdom that is more closely related to animals. In fact, their flesh, especially when cooked, resembles animal tissue more than plants. Mushrooms offer important health benefits, such as lowered cholesterol, enhanced immunity, and protection from cancer. Mushrooms contain a respectable amount of protein and trace vitamins and minerals.

The mushrooms sold in your local supermarket are probably white or brown button mushrooms and the large portobello variety. Popular Asian varieties also sold in supermarkets include shiitake, oysters, and maitake. On the Perfect 10 Diet, you can eat mushrooms as a side dish, appetizer, or as a healthy snack.

#### LEGUMES

Legumes, which are more commonly known as beans, are good sources of protein and carbs. Legumes also contain calcium, which is essential for bone health. They can be eaten fresh or dried. On the Perfect 10 Diet, have bean soups or add beans to your salads. All legumes are allowed on the Perfect 10 Diet except genetically modified soy.

#### LIVER

Do you like French cuisine? How about foie gras? Liver is shunned by many, as some doctors claim it contains toxins and cholesterol. However, toxins and pesticides are generally found in animal fat, rather than organ meats. The cholesterol found in liver is also used to make sex hormones and repair tissues. Maintaining a good level of sex hormones means staying younger longer. Liver is also a good source of iron and other minerals our bodies need. Liver is very high in vitamin A, which is essential for healthy skin and vision. Some scientists have voiced concerns that the high vitamin A content might be toxic or could lead to vitamin overdose, but that's untrue. High doses of synthetic vitamin A are toxic, but the natural vitamin A found in food is not, unless it's consumed in excess of 100,000 IU per day. You can certainly enjoy a liver dish—even on a daily basis—without worry. Don't miss out on this nutrient-dense food. Liver is also a good source of niacin, which can lower cholesterol.

### Moderately Favorable Sources of Protein

These protein sources should be included in your diet in moderation. Again, these choices are related to the protein source itself, rather than the amount of fat. This list includes lamb, pork, beef, and soy.

#### LAMB, PORK, AND BEEF

Lamb, pork, and beef are healthy protein choices. Rich in vitamin $B_{12}$, meat can help reduce cortisol, the stress hormone linked to belly fat. When you eat red meat, always stick with organic sources. You can find buffalo burgers in most supermarkets and many restaurants. Pasture-fed red meat is easily found in stores that carry a range of organic products, such as Whole Foods and Trader Joe's. It's important to note that not all beef is the same. Meat from grass-fed cows is better for your health than meat from farm-raised cows.

Farm-raised cows are often treated inhumanely, caged in confined spaces, injected with the growth hormone rBST to increase milk production, and slaughtered once they stop producing milk. Farm-raised cows are also fed corn and injected with other artificial hormones to promote weight gain. As a result, farm-raised cows have higher levels of fat, and that fat contains toxins and environmental pollutants that are harmful to your health and endocrine glands. I must add that the artificial hormones given to the cows interfere with weight loss and can even cause cancer. Farm-raised cows may also be fed meat from other cows. In some instances, this has led to mad cow disease, which is deadly to humans.

Farm-raised cows and pigs are slaughtered brutally—stunned with electric shocks and left to bleed to death while dangling by their feet. It's a treatment no animal should ever endure. Don't think that inhumane methods of overcrowding, artificial feeds, artificial hormones, and antibiotics do not affect your health—they do. Please take action, and stop inhumane farming practices by boycotting these products.

Regardless of their source—organic or not—the link between these protein choices and colon cancer has been raised in medical literature. It is worth noting that this statement can be controversial at times, since, for example, Mormons suffer lower rates of colon cancer even though their diet includes red meat. It gets more confusing since we know now that fiber is not protective against this disease. However, many large epidemiologic studies have found that eating red meat in abundance has been linked to the development of this type of cancer. This relationship is caused by the protein itself, not the fat. For this reason, limit the amount of red meat you eat to once a month or so. The relationship between red meat and colon cancer was associated with grilled or well-done preparations in particular. This may be related to the heterocyclic amines that form when meat is grilled at high temperatures.

For this reason, organic red meat is only a moderately favorable source on the Perfect 10 Diet. When you eat organic red meat, make sure it's boiled, steamed, or stir-fried. If you must have grilled meat, make sure it's prepared rare or medium, and never well done. There is one exception: people with a sluggish thyroid can benefit from eating organic red meat on the rare side more often than once every 3 weeks on the Perfect 10 Diet. Why? It's rich in iron, which accelerates the conversion of thyroid hormone to its active form.

## SOY

For years we have heard from the "experts" about the benefits of soy and what a super food it is. But soy is only a moderately favorable source on the Perfect 10 Diet—as long as it is not genetically modified (non-GMO). Soy is part of the legume family. In forms like tofu, tempeh, or soy milk, we are told that soy will help lower cholesterol, protect bones, help symptoms of menopause, and even protect against cancer. Many of these statements are simply not true. The role that soy plays in cancer prevention is still unproven, as the research is contradictory.

Eating soy in excess can be dangerous, since soy crops have a large level of insecticides. Soy contains isoflavones. Isoflavones are serious endocrine disrupters. In other words, if you like to eat a small amount of soy products, such as tofu or edamame, that's okay. But when you eat a lot of soy, your body does not know what to do with the three or four times the amount of isoflavones.

The relationship between soy and thyroid health is complicated. Some studies found that children who were fed soy formulas developed a sluggish thyroid. However, in adults, this does not appear to be the case. After all, the Japanese eat soy and do not have an increased incidence of thyroid disease. But in Asia, they don't eat anywhere near as much soy as we do, so the issue is still unclear.

Soy crops tend to be high in phytates, which are acids that block the body's intake of essential minerals such as calcium, magnesium, iron, and zinc. Some studies on testosterone levels indicated that men who eat soy frequently tend to have lower testosterone levels than men who eat animal products. Soy is considered one of those gender-bender foods. Soy contains more natural estrogen than any other food. For this reason, women with a certain type of breast cancer should completely avoid soy, since it can lead to progression of the disease.

## Unfavorable Protein Sources

Some protein sources can upset your hormone balance and should never be eaten. Proteins to keep off your diet include soy protein isolate and all preserved meats.

### SOY PROTEIN ISOLATE

Modern technology has made it possible to extract soy protein isolate from soy, and it is now found in many low-carb protein shakes, low-carb chocolate bars, soy cheese, faux meats, and some brands of soy milk. These poisonous products have been boosted by the low-carb mania that swept the nation in the last two decades. This food is highly processed. Soy protein isolate is manufactured with added chemicals and then spray-dried at high temperatures to become a protein powder. Nitrites, which are potent cancer promoters, are formed in the process; as a result, the protein is denatured and contaminated. MSG, a neurotoxin, is added to mask its beany taste. If you are used to snacking on popular low-carb snacks and shakes made with this overprocessed soy, it's time for you to stop.

### PRESERVED MEATS

Preserved meats include bacon, Canadian bacon, sausage, hot dogs, and cold cuts. Cured meats are extremely high in sodium, which is bad for your blood pressure. The meat fillers used in some cured meats may contain allergy-triggering components.

So move over, cold cuts and bacon. Preserved meats have no place at any time or in any amount on the Perfect 10 Diet. The same goes for smoked meats, if you want to stay healthy. This type of meat preservation was invented before refrigeration to keep meats free from the harmful effects of unhealthy microorganisms.

Exactly what constitutes "smoked" or "cured" meat can be somewhat confusing. One would assume that if something is smoked, it has been exposed to smoke. Wrong. Commercially available food products that are smoked have most likely not been touched by real smoke at all. Rather, a chemical liquid smoke is used to flavor the meat. Liquid smoke contains hundreds of dangerous chemicals, some of which are known carcinogens.

In cured meats, nitrites are injected via a special process, and that's bad in every way to your hormones and health.

I've explained earlier that low-carb diets help you balance insulin, and that's why you lose weight. That's great, but wait a minute—that improvement is temporary. Low-carb diets eventually damage the same hormone they initially help balance, just like low-fat diets. According to a 2002 study published in the journal *Diabetes Care*, researchers found that a diet of hot dogs, bologna, and bacon (often the choices on low-carb diets) increased the risk of type 2 diabetes by about 48 percent in men. The project, which began in 1986, followed 40,000 men aged 40 to 75 who were healthy and free of diabetes or cancer for a period of 12 years. By the end of the study, it became clear that processed meats were an independent risk factor for diabetes, and get a load of this—the American Diabetes Association (ADA) has voiced its support of low-carb diets for the management of diabetes. The endorsement was part of the ADA's 2008 Clinical Practice Recommendations, which are intended to guide diabetes health-care providers. This endorsement leaves me speechless.

With or without an official endorsement, the Atkins, Zone, and South Beach diets are now more popular than ever. Beware: this greatness is like the Titanic; it won't get you very far, as it's destined to sink. If you're on one of these diets, get off it immediately, before it's too late. Eating processed meats is associated with increased total mortality, according to several studies. One large study that was published in the *Archives of Internal Medicines* in March 2009 showed increases in total mortality, cancer, and cardiovascular disease. Some of the types of cancer linked to processed meats include esophagus, stomach, colon, and prostate. This may be caused by nitrites in processed meats, which are converted in the stomach to carcinogenic nitrosamines. Unlike low-carb diets, which can shorten your life and increase your risk for cancer, the Perfect 10 Diet can extend your life and prevent cancer.

Don't be tempted to try these diets because they correctly condemn sugar and make you lose a few pounds. Be smart.

## What about Other Sources of Animal Protein and Organs?

In different parts of the world, other animal protein sources are eaten. There is no information in medical literature about these different protein sources. However, they certainly do not contain any dangerous fats or deadly trans fats you must avoid. Rabbit, frog legs, and snails (escargots), which are common in French cuisine, are indeed healthy choices, and you can probably treat yourself to these protein sources without any undue fear for your health. In fact, protein can be used to make hormones. For those of you who like exotic cuisines, I have included a rabbit recipe at the end of this book. Ostrich, another delicacy, is very low in calories and quite healthy.

Cow brain, which is high in fat, should be completely avoided on the Perfect 10 Diet. The risk of bovine spongiform encephalopathy (mad cow disease), a fatal disease, is too great, however rare it may be.

## Is It Healthy to Be a Strict Vegetarian?

That's an easy question to answer: no. Vegetarian diets are often high in carbohydrates, which can lead to exaggerated insulin secretions. A high insulin level equals getting fat.

A vegetarian diet is also too low in fat. The greatest advantage of a diet with adequate fat intake is what it does to your sex hormones. A cholesterol-rich diet yields more sex hormones than a vegetarian diet. For guys, a body of research indicates that a diet with 40 percent of its calories from fat yields more testosterone than one with 30 percent of its calories from fat. The latest research clearly supports my diet plan. Strict vegetarians can develop a sluggish thyroid since their diet may be too low in protein, and an underactive thyroid equals weight gain. A diet low in protein may not support HGH production, the hormone that keeps you young and fit.

If you are a guy trying to build muscles, let me ask you this: do you really think you can sculpt a body and build muscles by eating bread and rice? Why do you think all the drinks at your gym are protein-based? Protein boosts HGH and helps you build muscles.

I know we are constantly told that vegetarians live longer than people who eat meat, but this is a myth. Vitamin $B_{12}$, which is present in animal products, is an important vitamin that is needed to lower homocysteine, a marker of heart disease.

## What about Excessive Levels of Cholesterol in Some of the Protein Choices You Recommend?

Despite what we're constantly told by the medical establishment, recent solid research indicates no relationship between cholesterol in food and blood serum levels. Most of the cholesterol is produced by our bodies. The cholesterol you ingest is used to make sex hormones and repair tissues.

As a matter of fact, when you eat cholesterol-rich food, your body shuts down its own production of cholesterol. The myth of cholesterol in food and its relationship to heart disease can be best debunked by looking at the Japanese diet. The Japanese eat more cholesterol (from shellfish and other organ meats) than the rest of the world, but the average lifespan of the Japanese is among the longest in the world. There is simply no link between cholesterol in food and the onset of heart disease. Please don't believe what you hear on the cereal commercials.

## Isn't Your Recommendation of Fatty Meat over Leaner Meat Contradictory to Mainstream Advice?

Animal fat has nothing to do with heart disease. It's the manufactured fats, not the natural fats, that contribute to heart disease. I know we've all been brainwashed into thinking white-meat poultry is healthier than dark-meat poultry, or that veal is healthier than duck. It's simply not true. There are no studies that prove white meat is healthier than dark meat or that chicken is safer for your heart than duck.

As a matter of fact, I advise my patients not to throw away the skin, fat, and bones from "organic" animal products. Instead, place them in boiling hot water to make a healthy broth. Animal broth from poultry, lamb, and beef contains calcium, magnesium, and potassium. Calcium is essential for healthy bones. The gelatin-rich goodness of real animal stock is beneficial in improving digestive disorders, including hyperacidity, colitis, and Crohn's disease. Although gelatin is not a complete protein source, it allows the body to utilize proteins from other foods.

## Eating the Right Types of Protein on the Perfect 10 Diet Is Not Negotiable

Take a moment to think about every low-fat diet you've tried. Chances are you were told to eat more lean meats (soy, pork, and veal), egg substitutes, or egg whites. You were told to avoid whole eggs, liver, shrimp, and lobster. And you listened. Then came the low-carb craze, which advised you to eat ham, bacon, and sausage, and you also listened. But on the Perfect 10 Diet, eating the right types of protein can mean the difference between life and death. You have a choice and I hope I've made it clear what types of protein are good for your health so you can start to implement these changes immediately.

### *Carmen's Story in Her Own Words*

I am 40 years old. I'm 5 feet, 6 inches, and I've been overweight since I injured my back in a car accident many years ago. Several years ago, I gave up on low-fat diets and followed one of the popular low-carb programs. I was rather nervous about eating ham and bacon for breakfast, but I continued to do so since the diet seemed to work, and I lost a lot of weight. Ham, sausage, and bacon with eggs or egg whites with smoked salmon were my daily routine.

One day, I experienced severe back pain. I thought it was related to my old injury, but it turned out to be kidney stones. My urologist analyzed the stones and attributed them to my high-protein/low-carb diet.

I consulted Dr. Aziz after hearing him on a popular New York radio station. When I first met Dr. Aziz, I weighed 190 pounds. The Perfect 10 Diet principles were completely new and different from anything I had ever heard or tried before.

On the Perfect 10 Diet, I ate much less protein than I had on the low-carb diet, but I still lost weight. I began to understand that my diet needed to be balanced. I gave up eating protein snacks and started to eat more vegetables and fruits. I ate avocados or eggs with fruit instead of bacon and sausage. I gave up low-carb protein shakes and low-carb chocolate bars when I realized both contained soy protein isolate. Now I only eat unprocessed food. I read the labels and all the fine print on every food I buy so I'm not fooled into buying products loaded with chemicals and trans fats. I also started swimming to improve my back and my overall fitness level. I've lost 60 pounds in just a little more than a year, and I've never felt better. Today, I'm 4 sizes smaller. The Perfect 10 Diet is truly miracle bliss.

## A Typical Day on the Perfect 10 Diet

**BREAKFAST:** 3 Pieces of Wild Salmon with 2 Teaspoons of Cream Cheese and 1 Apricot
**OPTIONAL MIDMORNING SNACK:** 1 or 2 Boiled Eggs
**LUNCH:** Grilled Shrimp with Steamed Asparagus
**OPTIONAL MIDAFTERNOON SNACK:** ½ Cantaloupe
**DINNER:** Squash Soup

## *John's Story in His Own Words*

For years, I only consumed the leanest meat, and drank only fat-free milk. I worked hard to keep up with the advice of the experts of the day, and I ate copious amounts of bread, pasta, and cereals.

Halfway through my 40s, reality began to bite. Despite my so-called "healthy" diet and daily exercise, my blood pressure went up. I also noticed it was becoming increasingly hard for me to maintain the lean look I had always prided myself on. I was tired, sluggish, and I felt hungry at all times. I heard about the Perfect 10 Diet from a friend and went to see Dr. Aziz, who diagnosed me with reactive hypoglycemia. My testosterone level was very low, and my fasting insulin level stood at a whopping 40—which was way too high. It was not until I gave up my low-fat diet that I began to feel much better.

I switched to full-fat salad dressing and full-fat cheese. I began to eat shellfish, liver, and duck, which I had avoided for years. My blood pressure improved. My testosterone inched upwards, and I felt more energized. I felt less hungry as my fasting insulin level dropped to rock-bottom levels. I lost a lot of weight. Now, as I'm approaching my 50s, I feel healthier and leaner than ever before.

### A Typical Day on the Perfect 10 Diet

**BREAKFAST:** Few Strawberries with Cottage Cheese
**OPTIONAL MIDMORNING SNACK:** Celery with Guacamole
**LUNCH:** Orange Duck
**OPTIONAL MIDAFTERNOON SNACK:** Fruit Cup
**DINNER:** Stir-Fried Scallops with Mushrooms

## Fat

It's essential to incorporate "natural" fat in the right amounts into your diet to stabilize insulin levels and other hormones. How much fat should you eat? On the Perfect 10 Diet, 40 percent of your diet should come from fat, but don't overdo it. Too much fat (say, 50 percent) is bad for growth hormone, or HGH, since excess fat, again, is its enemy. At 40 percent or a little less, you will feel less hungry and more energetic and dynamic, and you'll lose weight.

However, incorporating fat back into your diet does not mean turning to manufactured vegetable oils or tub margarines, which are promoted as cholesterol-free. Yes, your blood cholesterol levels may be deceptively lower, but you're more likely to suffer from heart disease and cancer.

On the Perfect 10 Diet, you'll increase your intake of healthy natural fat. The buzzword here is "natural." At the same time, you'll eliminate refined carbs in order to rebalance your diet. You'll eat more nuts instead of cookies or potato chips, and more olives instead of pretzels. This will dramatically reduce your insulin secretions, balance your glucagon, and ultimately lead to weight loss.

Remember, the Perfect 10 Diet focuses on *balancing* nutrients rather than promoting one over another. That word that you've learned to hate, *fat*, you must learn to love. By eating more "good" fat and fewer "bad" carbohydrates, you will lose weight while improving your health. Fat is an essential macronutrient that must be appropriately included in your diet to achieve optimal, perfect 10 health.

A lack of natural fat in your diet can only lead to disease. Fat promotes the building blocks of brain cells in children, promotes nerve cell growth, and assists with the absorption of fat-soluble vitamins K, E, D, and A. Fat provides you with more energy and stamina, and you'll be less likely to overeat. Fat is often blamed as a cause of obesity because it provides almost twice the calories of carbohydrates and protein per gram, but it's just not true. Actually, fat spares the protein from being used for energy, so you're able to build chiseled muscles.

## Three Kinds of Fat

- Saturated
- Monounsaturated
- Polyunsaturated

Fat is made up of collections of molecules called triglycerides. The classification of fat as saturated or unsaturated is based on its chemical structure.

All fat is made of chains of carbon and hydrogen atoms, with oxygen atoms attached at the end. If all the carbon atoms are bound to the most hydrogen atoms they can possibly hold, the fat is considered saturated. If the carbon atoms are missing hydrogen connections, the fat is considered unsaturated. Unsaturated fat is further divided into monounsaturated (with one extra hydrogen bond missing) and polyunsaturated (with more than one bond missing). Saturated fats, such as butter, are solid at room temperature and below. Monounsaturated fats, such as olive oil, are liquid at room temperature but solid when placed in the refrigerator. Polyunsaturated oils, such as corn and soybean, are liquid at both room temperature and when refrigerated. The human body manufactures both saturated and monounsaturated fats when we gain weight to store energy and for cellular repair. It is a basic metabolic process for survival.

## 1. Saturated Fat (Excellent)

Saturated fat is found in coconut and palm oils, dairy products, and in animal products to some degree. Probably the single greatest nutritional myth of past decades has been that saturated fat is unhealthy. A huge body of research published in respected medical journals shows the exact opposite is true. Sadly, the majority of people never hear about it.

Eating foods rich in saturated fat, such as eggs and butter, boosts the production (and thereby the effects) of hormones whose structures are built upon cholesterol. These are the steroid hormones, which include the female and male sex hormones estrogen, progesterone, and testosterone. Sex hormones keep you looking young, enhance sex drive, and prevent wrinkles and osteoporosis.

Saturated fat is also needed for the production of adrenal sex hormones like DHEA. DHEA is a hormone that prevents autoimmune diseases. It has been linked to longevity and also enhances your sex drive. Imagine the harm you're doing to yourself when you deprive your body of these good fats. As you incorporate saturated fat back into your diet, don't be ashamed or surprised if your sexual partner starts to complain about your high sex drive. That's a sign of good sex hormones levels.

Saturated fat is also needed for the proper functioning of your cells. Saturated fat improves the body's proper absorption and conversion of essential fatty acids like omega-3 fatty acids. Saturated fat is also needed for calcium to be deposited into the bones.

I know you might be thinking, "Great, Doc, you'll help me balance my hormones, but in doing so, you'll pave the way to a heart attack." I have news for you: There is no relationship between saturated fat and heart disease. After all, the epidemic of heart disease didn't start in this country until margarine and vegetable shortening—which contain trans fats, not saturated fats—were added to our diet in the last century. Before that, lard and butter were widely used, and heart disease was rare. In fact, I will go on to say that many research studies and observations indicate that saturated fat may even *protect* against heart disease. Yep, you read that right. Saturated fat can prevent heart disease. This information is not new. It's been witnessed in many cultures for decades, but the food industry makes sure you never hear about it.

## The Masai of Kenya

In the 1960s, researcher Dr. George Mann noted that the Masai of Kenya, who have one of the richest diets in animal fats in the world, do not have any incidence of heart disease. The Masai are known to drink a gallon of milk a day and eat massive amounts of meat, but they are strong and lean. Autopsies performed on Masai cadavers revealed no incidence of atherosclerosis, despite their high animal fat intake.

## The Samburus

Another East African tribe, the Samburus, eat even more animal fat than the Masai—a whopping 400 grams of fat daily. You'd expect that they would have astronomical rates of heart disease and stroke, but researchers have found the exact opposite to be true. As a group, the Samburus have incredibly low blood cholesterol levels and a notable absence of heart disease.

## The Fulani of Nigeria

The Fulani of Nigeria also have a diet high in animal fat and a low incidence of heart disease. Interestingly, once these people migrated to Western countries and adopted a modern diet high in refined carbohydrates, partially hydrogenated vegetable oils, and the like, their risk of heart disease increased dramatically.

## The French

The so-called French paradox describes the relative low incidence of atherosclerosis and heart disease in the French despite the high amounts of saturated fat in their diet. The French are famous for their love of high-fat appetizers, butter-based dishes, and a finale of cheese for dessert, yet they have a longer lifespan than many other people in the world. As you can see, the French paradox isn't a paradox at all. Their low risk for heart disease is related to the fact that saturated fats do not oxidize when they're heated. On the other hand, the polyunsaturated oils we consume in massive amounts in this country are likely to damage cholesterol by creating free radicals and causing plaque ruptures in the arteries. More heart attacks are related to plaque ruptures than stenosis.

Saturated fat is classified as small chain, medium chain, and long chain, depending upon the length of the fat molecule. When you eat small- and medium-chain saturated fats in butter and coconut, your body uses most of the fat for energy rather than storing it. For this reason, eating butter and coconut do not impact your cholesterol level in any negative way. Plant sources of saturated fat, such as coconut and palm kernel oil, have been used in cooking for hundreds of years. They are very stable when heated and do not oxidize easily. In addition, they do not contain any dangerous trans fats or added chemicals when extracted.

## Coconut

Coconut was used extensively by the food industry in the United States before it was replaced with hydrogenated fats (thanks to the edible oil industry and its lobbyists). Coconut is the preferred cooking fat in many Asian countries, including Thailand and Sri Lanka. In fact, coconut makes up nearly 50 percent of the calories in the Sri Lankan diet (Sri Lankans eat an average of about 120 coconuts per person per year). Given that coconut is 90 percent saturated fat, you'd expect heart disease to be rampant. Yet the incidence of heart disease in Sri Lanka, according to the WHO, is the lowest in the world: 1 in 1,000. Thailand, where coconuts are also a huge part of the daily diet, also has a very low incidence of heart disease.

Coconut is mostly made of a medium-chain triglyceride called lauric acid, a saturated fat that the body cannot make or store. It is used for energy and actually can speed up your metabolism. This can help your body burn calories more efficiently and can contribute to weight loss. However, research on weight loss is contradictory on the topic. Some studies have shown fat loss, and others failed to show any weight change. But there is one thing for sure: coconut is a safe and healthy fat.

In addition, the lauric acid present in coconut changes in the body into monolaurin, which has antimicrobial properties. The antimicrobial activity helps the body fight infection from bacteria to viruses, including herpes and HIV. Some of the research that denounced coconut in the past was done on a hydrogenated variety, and the data from that research is flawed. Adding coconut to your diet can, in fact, help you lower your cholesterol. Eating fresh or unprocessed coconut is always a boon to your health. Coconut is a favorite fat on the Perfect 10 Diet; it's excellent for cooking.

You can buy coconut milk in most health-food stores. Warm it for to 2 to 3 minutes on the stove and add the fruit of your choice for a delightful and filling treat. (You can mix coconut milk with a little water if it happens to be too rich for your taste.) You can also drink coconut water after exercise since it contains the right mix of minerals.

## Palm Oil

Palm oil is also a great healthy addition to your diet. Like coconut oil, it's a medium-chain triglyceride that does not affect your cholesterol in a negative way. Palm oil has been used for centuries in both Africa and Asia. It is a good source of beta-carotene and vitamin E, which are beneficial in maintaining membrane fluidity and function. This can reduce the risk of stroke.

In addition, new study findings have demonstrated that palm oil has beneficial effects on blood lipids. It is extremely stable when heated and is excellent for cooking. Although I discourage frying in general, if you must deep-fry foods, use palm oil, because it has a high burning point.

Coconut and palm oils are truly healthy fats. Both are extracted without the use of harsh chemicals and do not contain any deadly trans fats. Coconut and palm oils have high smoke points and resist oxidation when heated. At present, scientific evidence demonstrates that both coconut and palm oils are healthy choices. Yet both coconut and palm oil continue to be condemned by many medical authorities. Coconut and palm oil are not readily available at most grocery chains, but you can find both in organic and health-food stores.

## Cocoa Butter (Found in Chocolate)

Cocoa butter is a saturated fat found in cocoa beans and is used for making chocolate. It has a melting point just below the body temperature, and that's why chocolate melts in your mouth. Cocoa butter is neutral to cholesterol, but it continues to be condemned by the American Heart Association as an atherogenic fat!

Trying to lose some weight? Eat some dark chocolate made with cocoa butter. It will help you feel full. Chocolate is made out of the cocoa butter and the cacao beans. The beans lost their name cacao in translation and became cocoa. On the Perfect 10 Diet, look for organic dark chocolate that is at least 70 percent cocoa. The higher the percentage of cocoa found in chocolate, the better it is for your cardiovascular health. Just be vigilant about the chocolate's sugar content.

Cornell University scientists discovered that cocoa has nearly twice the antioxidants of red wine, and up to three times the antioxidants found in green tea. In fact, raw cocoa has the highest antioxidant value of all natural foods in the world. I'm sure you have heard some of the research emerging every day about the benefits of eating dark chocolate. Cocoa contains flavinoids, which have anti-platelet properties that prevent blood clotting. Scientists continue to find many benefits of chocolate.

However, it's important to note that chocolate loses its flavinoids when it is processed, so don't be a kid in a candy store; look specifically for organic super dark brands with little or no added sugar. A Dutch study found that eating dark chocolate can cut the risk of cardiovascular disease by 21 percent and can add years to life expectancy. Hallelujah. Anecdotally, chocolate is even said to be an aphrodisiac because of its tryptophan, which has an effect on mood.

Unfortunately, much of the chocolate sold in the United States has a lot of added sugar, is processed, or is made with partially hydrogenated oils, and not with cocoa butter. That's not the kind of chocolate you buy on the Perfect 10 Diet. Milk chocolate does not offer the same benefits as dark chocolate, so watch how much of it you eat. White chocolate is similar to milk chocolate, but without the cocoa base. Without any real cocoa bean content, white chocolate is not really chocolate at all. Organic dark chocolate made with reduced sugar and real cocoa butter is a favorite on the Perfect 10 Diet. It's easy on insulin, and does not contain trans fats to mess up your leptin levels. To cut down on calories, try some berries dipped in some warm chocolate instead of eating a big chocolate bar. It is a delicious dessert or snack that is quite rich and healthy.

## Butter

Want to be a sex goddess or a real macho man? How about going back to eating rich and creamy butter! Yes, butter; it is good for your sex hormones. And I think you would agree it is better to be a perfect 10 bombshell with good sex hormone levels than have a bomb explode in your arteries from all these fake fats such as I Can't Believe It's Not Butter. Butter has fewer calories and is more stable for cooking than refined vegetable oils. Butter, which is mostly made up of medium- and short-chain fatty acids, contains many healthful compounds, including lecithin, which assists the body in breaking down cholesterol. It's also a rich source of vitamins A and C and the mineral selenium. Butter protects against free radical damage, which can weaken and destroy artery walls.

It's hard for most people to believe that eating butter can decrease their cholesterol levels, but lipoprotein (a), another subdivision of bad cholesterol, LDL, is lowered when you eat butter. Butter is also rich in conjugated linoleic acid, which has cancer-fighting properties. Butter contains a short-chain saturated fat called butyric acid, which is quite unique to it, and it has anti-fungal properties.

Despite reliable scientific evidence that butter is healthy, it continues to be condemned by the medical authorities as atherogenic. But what about the French? Wouldn't you like to share their paradox? The French, for the most part, do not have the obesity problem we have in the United States. Butter is rich in conjugated linoleic acid, which has fat-burning properties. Chanel and Gaultier are expensive, but you can have the perfect 10 body to fit in their clothes if you copy the French. Butter does not interfere with cellular communications or cause abnormal hormonal secretions like margarine. The notion that eating butter can promote heart disease is nothing but nonsense. Remember, a balanced diet should contain some beneficial saturated fat, such as that found in butter. Use butter for all your cooking and spread a little on whole-grain bread for a delicious, rich, and filling breakfast.

## Ghee

Gee, ghee, you're so wonderful. Ghee, a clarified form of butter that has been used for cooking in many African and Asian countries for centuries, is similar to butter in its health benefits, and it's good for your sex hormones. Ghee is resistant to bacteria and rancidity because its milk solids and water have been removed, and it is excellent for cooking since it doesn't burn at high temperatures. Like butter, ghee does not interfere with cellular communications, so it does not interfere with hormone secretion. You can find ghee in most health-food stores.

## Dairy

Got milk? You probably do, since we consume a lot of it in the United States. But researchers at Harvard found that adults do not need to consume *any* dairy to achieve optimal health. This directly contradicts widespread advertising campaigns on the part of the dairy industry that promote heavy milk consumption to the tune of 3 servings a day. As a matter of fact, some research has linked heavy dairy consumption to acne, asthma, allergies, and ovarian and prostate cancers. Excessive amounts of dairy in your diet can make it too high in protein which can negatively affect thyroid health.

You might be thinking, "But milk is natural, Doctor. How can it be bad?" Yes, milk is natural, but cows' milk, by design, grows a 75-pound calf into a 1,750-pound cow over the course of 2 years. We're humans, for heaven's sake, not cows. Do you really think that you can drink 3 servings of dairy daily and have a perfect 10 physique?

Behind the milk hype is the multibillion-dollar dairy industry, which has convinced most doctors, consumers, and government agencies that milk is essential for bone health. That's simply not true. As a matter of fact, in the countries with the highest rates of osteoporosis—such as the United States—milk is consumed in abundance. Do adults need to drink milk? Nope.

But maybe you're thinking, "Oh, but I love milk." I wouldn't ask you to give up milk or dairy products. As a matter of fact, having some dairy in moderation (like 1 serving a day or less for those with no underlying health-related issues, such as lactose intolerance) does have benefits. Dairy provides a good source of carbs, protein, and fat.

When it comes to the fat in dairy, most people believe that whole milk is unhealthy, so they drink skim milk (1or 2 percent). That's dead wrong. The natural fat present in milk is good for your health. Ironically, when you choose fat-free dairy such as yogurt, you're choosing a type of dairy that is lacking in nutrition and has added sugar. A serving of fat-free milk can possibly lead to more insulin secretions than a glass of whole milk.

The danger does not stop here: researchers at Harvard University found that women who consume 2 servings of fat-free dairy per day are more likely to be infertile. Ovulation decreases by 28 percent. Removing fat from milk radically changes its balance, which can lead to a disturbance in sex hormone production. If you are a woman trying to conceive, make the switch to whole milk now.

The health conscious often shun whole milk for fear of excess calories, but new research suggests that adults who favor full-fat dairy gain less weight over time. These new findings indicate that the fat in dairy plays a role in weight control, while low-fat dairy does not. Fat in dairy products contains conjugated linoleic acid (CLA), which promotes weight loss. CLA is a potent cancer inhibitor that plays a role in the prevention of heart disease. Dairy products contain a certain type of fat that can raise high-density lipoprotein (C-HDL) levels, and that "good cholesterol" is protective at higher levels. All these healthy ingredients (including vitamins) are eliminated when the fat is removed.

I discussed earlier how raw milk has more nutrients than pasteurized milk. However, raw milk is very hard, if not impossible, to find, and it's actually outlawed in many U.S. cities. Don't worry. I won't ask you to move to a farm, or raise a cow in your own backyard. The Perfect 10 Diet is about practicality. Instead, choose organic whole pasteurized milk, as it contains no pesticides, antibiotics, or hormones, such as rBST. Organic milk is readily available in your local supermarket.

The same goes for goat milk, which you can purchase at health-food stores. Goat milk is less allergenic than cow milk.

If you are lactose intolerant, you may find that it's easier to tolerate fermented dairy products. The healthy bacteria used to make cheese and yogurt changes the lactose in milk, which is hard for many people to digest, into a sugar called galactose. Raw cheese, which has a higher nutritional value than pasteurized cheese, can be easily found in health-food stores.

Kefir, a cousin of yogurt with roots going back more than 2,000 years, is another healthy addition to your diet. Pour kefir over granola for breakfast or blend it with a few berries to make a smoothie as a snack, or have as is. Delicious. But remember, when I recommend dairy in small amounts, that doesn't mean 3 servings a day.

Unsaturated fat is further divided into monounsaturated and polyunsaturated fat.

## 2. Monounsaturated (Healthy When Natural, but Dangerous When Manufactured)

Monounsaturated fat is mostly found in olive oil, avocados, nuts, and animal fat.

### ANIMAL FAT

Believe it or not, animal fat is placed in the saturated fat category by incorrect practice. Animal fat is mostly monounsaturated. For this reason, animal fat has a positive influence on cholesterol—just like olive oil. Animal fat has other health benefits, too, including antimicrobial activity. The stearic acid found in animal fat is the best fuel for the heart muscle. Incidentally, the saturated fat that is found in animal products also aids in mineral absorption.

It's hard for most people to believe that animal fat is healthy, but humans have eaten animal fat for thousands of years. Animal fat is used for cooking in many Asian and African cultures, where there is a low incidence of heart disease. It has no relationship to colon cancer, either. It is an innocent bystander that is wrongly blamed when we eat too much red meat.

### POULTRY FAT

The percentage of saturation of poultry fat depends on what the birds are fed. Poultry fat is rich in antimicrobial compounds, which are excellent against cold and viral infections. (Chicken soup has been known for generations to be an excellent remedy for colds and the flu.) Goose and duck fat are sold in fancy food shops.

### LARD FAT

This is the fat rendered from pigs. It is about 40 percent saturated and 60 percent unsaturated. It is used for cooking in many parts of China and several European countries. Like poultry fat, lard fat also contains antimicrobial compounds.

### TALLOW FAT

This fat from ruminant animals, such as cattle, sheep, or lamb, has been used for cooking by many cultures for centuries. It does not oxidize or form free radicals when heated, so it's excellent for cooking.

## Should I Avoid Animal Fat If I've Already Had a Heart Attack?

Numerous studies on dietary patterns and the risk of heart disease have found that animal fat consumption is no different in people *with* heart disease and those without it. Unfortunately, the big pharmaceutical companies and other proponents of the cholesterol theory have ensured that many of these studies refuting their hypothesis never get publicized. As a result, we're convinced that we should avoid animal fat.

Don't get me wrong. Am I telling you to be a cave dweller and start to eat animal fat? Absolutely not. There have been dramatic changes in the fatty composition of meats in the last century due to changes in the diets of animals. Today, animal fat has fewer omega-3 fatty acids, and more toxins, pesticides, and artificial hormones (gender benders). All these things are bad for your body and endocrine glands and can lead to serious hormonal disruption. You should trim the fat from the meats you consume, but my point remains that animal fat from organic sources will not harm you. You can certainly use animal fat from organic sources for cooking if you prefer it over butter, and rest assured that your food will be tastier and contain fewer calories than if you cooked it with refined vegetable oils like corn or soybean.

Other examples of monounsaturated fat include olive oil, avocados, and nuts. These healthy fats have been shown to have beneficial effects on cholesterol by lowering the bad cholesterol, low-density lipoprotein (LDL) and raising the good, high-density lipoprotein (HDL).

## Avocados

Want to enjoy Tex-Mex cuisine? Sure, but skip the tortillas, of course. And don't let the fat content of an avocado (30 grams) scare you—that's what makes it a top weight-loss food on the Perfect 10 Diet. It's heart-healthy and rich in monounsaturated fats, which can increase satiety by stabilizing insulin. Avocados are great support for both male and female sex hormones, and they are high in fiber and low in sugar. They're virtually a perfect food.

Include avocados in your diet as a snack or vegetable side dish. Want to treat yourself to a delicious snack? Mix half an avocado with some lime, sea salt, and pepper and serve it with some raw vegetables. It will fill you up nicely.

## Olive Oil

Move over, Adonis and Venus, for the Perfect 10 Diet followers. The secret of the Greek and Roman gods has been revealed. Like avocados, olive oil satisfies your appetite and helps you make sex hormones. Good sex hormone levels equal looking younger longer. But that's hardly its only positive feature. Olive oil, which is used extensively in Greece, Italy, and Spain, has many antioxidant properties. It's one of the main reasons the Mediterranean diet promotes superior heart health.

The greener the oil is, the better. Extra-virgin olive oil is the oil that comes from the first press of the olive; it contains more nutrients than oils extracted by other means. Stay away from "light" olive oil, as it is bleached with peroxide, and solvents are used in the process. If you find the flavor of extra-virgin olive oil to be too strong, you can mix it with a little almond or macadamia nut oil.

Cooking with extra-virgin olive oil is preferable to cooking with refined polyunsaturated oils. But reserve it for light cooking since it can oxidize at high temperatures. I want you to dress your salads with olive oil instead of using commercially produced salad dressings, which often contain added sugar and are bad for your insulin.

## Nuts/Nut Butters

Nuts are mostly made from oleic acid, which has been shown to have a positive influence on cardiovascular health. On the Perfect 10 Diet, I want you to include nuts in your diet as a healthy snack, but be sure to always place a serving in a cup. Doing so will prevent you from overeating. If you eat too many nuts, you may hinder your weight-loss efforts because of their high caloric content. Several large studies have shown that people who eat nuts more than 4 times a week lowered their risk for heart disease by 40 to 50 percent. Macadamia nuts contain selenium, which research indicates may prevent cancer. Buy nuts only in airtight jars or packages, and not from open bins, as they could be rancid.

I also encourage you to buy macadamia butter and almond butter from health-food stores. Macadamia or almond butter paired with whole-grain bread make an excellent healthy breakfast that's rich in good fats and leaves you full and hunger-free for hours.

Peanuts are legumes, not nuts, so they're not included in this category. Eat peanuts in limited amounts since they contain higher quantities of omega-6 fatty acids, which can undermine your health if eaten to excess.

## Nut Oils

Nut oils include almond, macadamia, walnut, and other nut varieties. Although these monounsaturated fats are quite stable, they can still oxidize when heated. Nut oils should always be purchased cold pressed (meaning that they were extracted without the use of high heat or any chemicals).

Nut oils are ideal for light cooking and over salads. They should be stored in a sealed tin or dark bottle kept in a dark place to protect them from air and light (both of which can hasten oxidation). It's not necessary to freeze or refrigerate these oils unless they are used infrequently.

## Canola Oil (Manufactured)

Canola oil is extracted from the poisonous rapeseed tree; its name stands for "Canada oil." It is refined or manufactured. Canola oil is genetically modified and contains erucic acid, a toxic fatty acid removed by mechanical and solvent extraction. The oil is marketed as a good source of omega-3 fatty acids, but most of the omega-3s are lost during the refinement process.

Canola oil, at times, is partially hydrogenated to make it more stable. What does this mean for the Perfect 10 Diet followers? Needless to say, you should pass it up. If you must use canola oil, buy the organic, expeller-pressed, non-hydrogenated variety available at health-food stores. The presence of any trans fats in your diet will hinder your weight-loss efforts and harm you.

### Peanut Oil

Peanut oil is a monounsaturated fat. Peanuts of lesser quality that are not used to make peanut butter are used to make peanut oil. It can be allergenic to some people, and solvents are used in its extraction process. It contains an excess of omega-6 fatty acids, which have been linked to disease development. (Remember, a disturbance in the omega-6 to omega-3 ratio is behind many of our modern-day illnesses.) It is best to avoid peanut oil or use it sparingly on the Perfect 10 Diet.

### 3. Polyunsaturated Oils (Essential When Natural)

Polyunsaturated oils are missing several hydrogen atoms. These oils are essential to our health since our bodies cannot manufacture them. Polyunsaturated oils are needed for hormone production and to regulate bodily activities. There are two types of polyunsaturated oils: omega-3 fatty acids, which are present in fish, eggs, and flaxseed oil, and omega-6 fatty acids, which are present in seeds and their oils.

### Omega-3 Fatty Acids

Eggs, nuts, and cold-water fish, such as salmon and mackerel, contain the healthy polyunsaturated omega-3 fatty acids, which have been shown to have a positive effect on cholesterol and prevent inflammation, a hallmark for atherosclerosis. For this reason, adding fish to your diet will help prevent heart disease.

Quick tip: Supplementing your diet with omega-3 fatty acids pills can curb your appetite and can make you feel full hours after a meal, since it helps control insulin and leptin. Omega-3 fatty acids also support your sex hormones and play a role in cancer prevention, male fertility, bone health, and mood disorders, including depression.

Omega-3 fatty acids have anti-inflammatory benefits and may reduce the symptoms of Crohn's disease. These fatty acids are also found in eggs, nuts, and flaxseed oil, which comes in dark bottles to prevent oxidation and must be refrigerated. It can be used on salads and cooked food, but it should never be heated or used for cooking. Have a teaspoon of flaxseed oil 2 to 3 times a week.

### Omega-6 Fatty Acids

You've heard me saying over and over again that too many omega-6 fatty acids are bad, but you may become deficient if you exclude these fats completely. Omega-6 fatty acids should be included in your diet, but only in moderation. They are found in corn, peanuts, and seeds, such as sunflower seeds.

How do you get the right amounts? How about munching on a few sunflower seeds every now and then? Omega-6 fatty acids are also found in evening primrose and borage oils, which can ease arthritis and premenstrual symptoms.

You get the right amount of omega-6 fatty acids on the Perfect 10 Diet by eating real food and seeds, just like your grandparents did. Omega-6 is also present in the vegetable oils extracted from seeds, such as unrefined safflower and sunflower oils, which you can purchase at health-food stores.

You can consume these oils, without heating them, in small amounts on salads, as long they are not refined or hydrogenated. However, consuming them to excess can pose a risk to your health. Again, you will find these oils in dark bottles to prevent their oxidation.

## Killer Fats (Manufactured Fats)

### Refined Polyunsaturated Vegetable and Hydrogenated Oils

These fats are the same polyunsaturated oils (corn, cottonseed, safflower, sunflower, and soybean) in a refined form that continue to be bizarrely promoted by the medical organizations, including the American Heart Association! These oils are also promoted by low-fat diet gurus and some low-carb diets, and they're heavily used by the fast-food industry. Sorry to disappoint you, folks, but McDonald's and other fast-food fried menu choices are not on the Perfect 10 Diet menu. I'm sure you don't need a doctor to tell you that. These oils are bad for your thyroid health. Furthermore, research indicates that a diet high in refined vegetable oils can lead to the development of both heart disease and cancer.

The process of making these oils includes the use of chemicals. Once extracted, these oils are mixed with nickel oxide and then heated. Emulsifiers are squeezed into the mixture and cleaned to remove the unpleasant odor. Artificial flavors and colors are added to make it taste pleasant, and then it's placed on store shelves in clear bottles exposed to light. Refined polyunsaturated oils are sometimes hydrogenated to prolong shelf life and resist the repeated heating needed in the fast-food industry to make crispy French fries. As discussed, hydrogenated fats are bad for many of the hormones discussed on the Perfect 10 Diet, including insulin, leptin, and sex hormones. Most low-fat and many low-carb processed products contain these deadly fats.

## Don't Trust the FDA Food Labels on Trans Fats

Don't trust labels that say "0g trans fats." I'm not kidding. Just about every single boxed or bagged food you find on a supermarket shelf contains some amount of hydrogenated or trans fats, but it can still bear a label that states it's trans-fat free. Trans fats are found in many brands of chocolate, salad dressings, some flat breads, granola bars, cakes, cookies, crackers, potato chips, some brands of ice cream, packaged meals, low-fat products, low-carb products, frozen dinners and entrées…and even your beloved pet's food. I'm an animal lover, so please be vigilant about excluding trans fats from your pet's diet, too. Trans fats are everywhere—fast-food restaurants, popular coffee chains, doughnut shops, and even your own kitchen.

How did this happen? We can thank the food industry lobbyists for this modern-day tragedy. Processed foods use hydrogenated fats extensively to prolong their shelf life. You simply cannot make snacks like cookies or doughnuts that can sit on shelves for months, or even years, using butter. The food industry would lose money. Butter melts at room temperature, which means that the end product will be greasy and will have a short shelf life. Partially hydrogenated fats fit the bill for food manufacturers—they're cheap and can be added to products without any greasy taste or texture.

Partially hydrogenated fat remains solid at high temperatures, and foods made with them can sit in boxes without melting for a long time. It's pure poison, but 70 percent of all processed foods in supermarkets contain partially hydrogenated fat. When you eat trans fats in any amount, they incorporate in your cells and interfere with cellular communications. The good news is that you can purge your cells of trans fats and replace them with natural fats. With time, your cells will respond to insulin and other hormones.

But in order to be a savvy consumer and exclude these types of dangerous fats, you have to be a clever detective. That means reading the fine print for all ingredients in any processed food rather than just reading the food industry claims printed on the box. Don't be fooled by the "0g trans fats" on the label. As a matter of fact, that should be a red flag.

Let me explain. Let's say you want to cheat on the Perfect 10 Diet one day and buy a box of cookies from your local supermarket. The label clearly states, "This product contains 0 trans fats," but a closer look reveals the cookies are made with partially hydrogenated oil or vegetable shortening (Fig. 4.9). Confusing? You bet.

You see, according to the FDA, food products can be labeled as being trans-fats free even when they contain as much as ½ gram of trans fats per serving. That's ridiculous. One cookie may not contain any trans fats, according to the FDA, but eat 2 cookies and you just consumed 1 gram of trans fats, which can mess up your hormones and clog your arteries. Do the math, because who eats just 2 cookies?

The American Heart Association recommends on its website to limit trans fats to 1 percent of your total calories, but research indicates that there is *no* safe limit. On the Perfect 10 Diet, the number is "*zero*." If you're going to include any processed food in your diet, read the list of ingredients on the box for the presence of any partially hydrogenated oils, instead of just looking for trans fats information on the label.

**Figure 4.9:** Look for the Presence of Vegetable Shortening or Partially Hydrogenated Oils Rather than the Presence of Trans Fats on Labels

**Nutrition Facts**

Serving Size 1 cup (200g)
Servings per container 2

| Amount per serving | |
|---|---|
| Calories 220 | Calories from Fat 100 |
| | % Daily Value* |
| Total Fat 12g | 18% |
| Saturated Fat 3g | 15% |
| Trans Fat 2g | |
| Cholesterol 30 mg | 10% |
| Sodium 235 mg | 10% |
| Total Carbohydrate 16g | 5% |
| Dietary Fiber 5g | 20% |
| Sugars 4g | |
| Protein 6g | |
| Vitamin A | |
| Vitamin C | |
| Calcium | |

* Percent Daily Values are based on a 2,000 calorie diet. Your Daily Values may be higher or lower depending on your calorie needs:

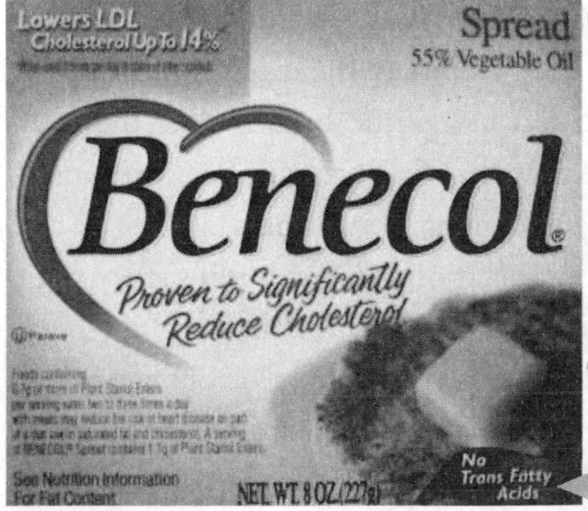


No Trans Fatty Acids

**Nutrition Facts**

Serv. Size 1 Tasp. (14g)
Servings 16
**Calories** 70
Fal Cal. 70

| Amount/Serving | %DV* | Amount/Serving | %DV* |
|---|---|---|---|
| Total Fat 8g | 12% | Cholest. 0mg | 0% |
| Sat. Fat 1g | 5% | Sodium 110mg | 5% |
| Polyunsat. Fat 2g | | Total Carb. Og | 0% |
| Monounsat. Fat 4g | | Protein 0g | |
| Vitamin A 10% | | Vitamin E 20% | |

* Percent Daily Values (DV) are based on a 2,000 calorie diet.

Not a significant source of dietary fiber, sugars, vitamin C, calcium and iron.

**Ingredients:** Liquid Canola Oil, Water, Plant Stanol Ester Partially Hydrogenated Soybean Oil, Salt, Emulsifiers (Vegetable Mono- and Diglycerides, Soy Lesithin, Polyglycerol Esters of Fatty Acids), Hydrogenated Soybean Oil, Potassium Sorbate, Citric Acid and Calcium Disodium EDTA to Preserve Freshness, Artificial Flavor, dl-□-Tocopheryl Acetate, Vitamin A Palmitate Colored with Beta Carotene.

Shutterstock

## Where Else Can You Find Hydrogenated and Trans Fats?

Sometimes the terms "hydrogenated" and "partially hydrogenated" are used interchangeably. Both are horrible for your health. In order to be a perfect 10, you must be vigilant about completely excluding trans fats from your diet. For instance, to save money, many restaurants use a butter blend that is really margarine. Never order your bread or toast pre-buttered; instead, ask for real butter packets and put it on the toast yourself.

Thought you got rid of trans fats simply by looking for the presence of partially hydrogenated oils and hydrogenated oils? Think again. Soybean oil is the most commonly used oil in commercial products. It may contain trans fats up to 50 percent of the time, even with no hydrogenation. You should avoid all food products containing soybean oil, and that's not easy. Soybean oil is present in most commercial mayonnaise brands, salad dressings, many brands of nonhydrogenated margarine, and mixed vegetable oils.

The misguided public frequently buys fat-free and low-fat processed products that contain partially hydrogenated or soybean oil in the belief that they're making a healthy choice for themselves and their families. Don't be fooled. It's really disturbing to see that we have turned to toxic, processed foods, such as low-fat salad dressings, low-calorie frozen dinners, and imitation butter in the belief that we're making healthy choices.

At present, the American Heart Association has apologized for its previous support of dangerous hydrogenated margarine, but it now advises us to use nonhydrogenated margarine brands instead. These types of margarine came with brand names such as Smart Balance. Smart Balance has fewer trans fats than hydrogenated margarine brands. But the well-informed Perfect 10 Diet followers know that that type of margarine *unbalances* your hormones, and ultimately endangers your health.

It's nice that the American Heart Association is sorry, but it's still wrong. Nonhydrogenated margarine poses a risk to your health, since it's made with refined vegetable oils, contains excessive amounts of omega-6 fatty acids, and may contain trans fats—even with no hydrogenation. There should be *no* margarine in your diet, period.

Here is a sample of the amount of trans fats in various foods with partially hydrogenated fat or soybean oil:

| | Grams of Trans Fats |
|---|---|
| Croissant cooked in vegetable oil | 4.0 |
| Popular fast-food restaurant large fries | 7.0 |
| Glazed doughnut | 4.0 |
| Packaged buttermilk biscuit | 3.0 |
| Low-fat frozen entrée | 3.0 |
| 5 crackers | 1.5 |
| 2 teaspoons of powdered non-dairy creamer | 1.0 |
| 2 frozen waffles | 2.0 |
| Hamburger roll | 1.0 |
| Mayonnaise made with soybean oil | Trace |
| Powdered milk | Trace |
| Salad dressing made with soybean oil | Trace |

## Which Fats Are Best to Cook With?

Saturated fats, such as butter, ghee, and coconut, are best to cook with since they are extremely stable at high temperatures and do not oxidize, create free radicals, or interfere with hormone production. Monounsaturated oils, such as extra-virgin olive oil, can also be used, but at much lower temperatures. Refined polyunsaturated oils should never be used for cooking, since they create free radicals when heated.

## Eating the Right Kind of Fats Is Key for Successful Weight Loss and Good Health

Only by eating the right kind of fats can you lose weight, stabilize your insulin and other hormones, and prevent disease. The natural fat I favor on the Perfect 10 Diet can turn off your hunger hormones for hours. That's pretty amazing, but if you're still thinking, "Why is everybody else saying the exact opposite?" then, my friends, remember that our dietary recommendations were written by politicians, not scientists.

**Figure 4.10:** Classifications of Fats and Oils by Long-Chain Fatty Acids C14-22

| (Mostly) Saturated | (Mostly) Mono-unsaturated | (Mostly) Polyunsaturated | | | |
|---|---|---|---|---|---|
| | ω 9 Oleic | ω 6 Linoleic | ω 6 y-Linolenic | ω 3 a-Linolenic | ω 3 EPA & DHA |
| Cocoa butter<br>Dairy fats<br>Nutmeg<br>Butter<br>Palm<br>Tallow<br>(Stearines) | Canola*<br>Chicken fat<br>Duck fat<br>Goose fat<br>Lard**<br>Macadamia<br>Olive<br>Peanut<br>Safflower (hybrid)<br>Sunflower (hybrid)<br>Turkey fat | Corn**<br>Cotton*<br>Soy*<br>Safflower** (regular)<br>Sunflower** (regular)<br>↓<br>Hydro-genation or partial hydro-genation<br>↓<br>Trans fats, shortenings/ margarines | Black currant<br>Borage<br>Primrose | Flaxseed (Linseed) | Fish** |

Why Greek names and numbers? The end of the fatty acid farthest from the acid is called the omega end. The chemical structure counted from the omega end denotes whether a fatty acid belongs to the omega-6, omega-3, or other omega family.

*Usually partially hydrogenated **Sometimes partially hydrogenated

"Know Your Fats: The Complete Primer for Understanding the Nutrition of Fats, Oils and Cholesterol," Mary G. Enig, PhD

## *Jim's Story in His Own Words*

I am 60 years old, and I recently suffered a heart attack. I never followed any particular diet. After my diagnosis, I was advised by both my cardiologist and nutritionist to follow a low-fat/low-cholesterol diet. I started to eat cereal for breakfast every day, and my wife started to cook with tub margarine and other refined vegetable oils. I avoided eggs, shrimp, and cheese. My wife and I started to buy only low-fat products, like salad dressings and crackers. My cardiologist recently increased the dosage of my cholesterol-lowering drug since my triglyceride levels went up, and he also placed me on a second blood pressure pill. My weight has gone up, particularly since I haven't been able to exercise much since my heart attack.

I learned about the Perfect 10 Diet after seeing Dr. Aziz on TV. I was shocked to learn that a low-fat diet could actually increase my chances of getting another heart attack. My biggest surprise came when I learned that the refined vegetable oils my wife was using for cooking were the heart-clogging fats, instead of the saturated fats I'd been avoiding. I checked most of the low-fat products that I regularly ate only to find out that most contained partially hydrogenated oil, sugar, and high-fructose corn syrup. I am very angry about the deceptive and misleading information promoted by the food industry.

After learning about the dangers of trans fats, my wife threw out all the mixed vegetable oils and liquid margarine she used for cooking. I started to eat organic vegetables, and I began to use only extra-virgin olive oil on my salads. My cholesterol came down to very low levels. I am 6 feet, 2 inches tall and weighed 240 pounds before I started the Perfect 10 Diet, and now I've lost 50 pounds. My fasting insulin level also dropped from 44 to 4 in just 2 months. My triglyceride levels dropped. I feel better, and more energetic.

## A Typical Day on the Perfect 10 Diet

**BREAKFAST:** Whole-Wheat Croissant with Butter
**OPTIONAL MIDMORNING SNACK:** ½ Cup Berries
**LUNCH:** Belgian Steamed Mussels and Cauliflower Puree
**OPTIONAL MIDAFTERNOON SNACK:** Vegetable Juice
**DINNER:** Seafood Bisque Soup

## *Diane's Story*

Diane is a 42-year-old teacher who consulted me for relief from muscular aches and fatigue. Diane is 5 feet, 6 inches tall and weighed 150 pounds. Her cholesterol was elevated, and she had been taking a lipid-lowering drug for 3 years. Diane followed a low-fat diet and rarely ate cholesterol-rich foods like shellfish; she confessed that her only weakness was milk chocolate, which she ate regularly. Diane also loved pasta and cooked only with margarine.

I diagnosed Diane with rhabdomyolysis, a condition of muscle damage that can occur in people who take cholesterol-lowering drugs. Her insulin was also high, and her female sex hormones were simply nonexistent. Her muscle pain was caused by the rhabdomyolysis, and the fatigue was related to very low sex hormone levels.

I advised Diane to stop taking cholesterol-lowering drugs until I obtained a blood test to confirm my diagnosis. Once the diagnosis was confirmed, I ordered an advanced lipid profile for Diane. The analysis of her cholesterol subdivisions indicated that the problem was related to massive carbohydrate and trans fat consumption.

It amazed Diane to learn that her cholesterol was elevated because of her low-fat food choices. I put Diane on the Perfect 10 Diet, advising her to eat more natural fats and to avoid all refined carbohydrates, sugar, and margarine. She certainly could continue to eat chocolate, but she had to limit it to dark brands with reduced sugar that contained no partially hydrogenated fat. Diane lost 14 pounds in 3 weeks on the Perfect 10 Diet, and her cholesterol level normalized without the need for drugs. In no time, her sex hormones also improved when she got off the cholesterol-lowering drug.

## A Typical Day on the Perfect 10 Diet

**BREAKFAST:** Yogurt Smoothie with Mixed Berries
**OPTIONAL MIDMORNING SNACK:** Raw Veggies
**LUNCH:** Whole-Wheat Pasta with Shrimp
**OPTIONAL MIDAFTERNOON SNACK:** Mixed Nuts
**DINNER:** Squash Soup and a Side Salad

# The Micronutrients

Now let's talk about the micronutrients your body needs to function properly. These are vitamins, minerals, and water.

## Vitamins

Vitamins and minerals are the essential compounds that act as cofactors for many of your bodily functions. A diet high in refined carbohydrates is often deficient in vitamins and minerals. Vitamins help fight the free radical formation caused by smoking and consuming sugar and polyunsaturated oils. Multiple vitamin deficiencies can lead to the early development of heart disease and hormonal disturbances.

## Minerals

Minerals are classified according to the percentage of the body's total weight they comprise. Minerals that make up 0.01 percent or more are known as macrominerals, while those that make up less are called trace minerals.

Among the macrominerals is calcium. Each day, the standard American diet supplies only 1/3 of the calcium your body needs. That's too low. Calcium is essential for healthy bones, teeth, and skin. It also regulates blood pressure.

Where can you get the calcium you need without consuming lots of dairy products? Good news: calcium is found in dark green leafy vegetables, broccoli, salmon, sardines, and almonds. I also advise you to take calcium supplements.

There are ten officially recognized trace minerals that your body needs for optimal health, including boron and chromium. All play a vital role in our health.

## Are We Getting Enough Nutrients?

No. That's because most vegetables these days are grown in depleted soil. We have to eat nearly ten times the amount of fruits and vegetables our grandparents ate in order to get the same nutritional value they had.

I recommend you eat organic food as much as possible to mitigate the pesticide issue, and consider taking a whole-food vitamin pill that provides your daily requirements of basic vitamins and minerals. I don't recommend synthetic vitamins because they can be dangerous to your health.

## Water

Is it *that* important? Yes, it is. The mineral activity of cortisol and sex hormones are improved by drinking lots of water, as the process is reliant on both water and salt. Choose mineral water bottled in glass bottles or filtered tap water. Why filtered? The fluoride in tap water is bad for your thyroid, and the chlorine in tap water can promote cholesterol oxidation. Oxidized cholesterol promotes heart disease.

Although bottled water in plastic bottles is convenient and portable, bisphenol A (BPA) is a key component used in the manufacture of a wide variety of plastic bottles. Studies have found that BPA (a gender bender) is a particularly dangerous toxin since it can interact with the body's endocrine system. Over the last decade, extensive research has exposed BPA as a powerful hormone disrupter that can damage reproductive organs. Animal lab studies have shown that exposure to BPA during pregnancy can lead to developmental abnormalities, reduced survival, and delayed puberty. That's why you should always use glass bottles. Filtered tap water should only be stored in glass bottles or BPA-free containers.

How much water you need to drink depends on your body size and activity level. Eight glasses may be fine for a small-framed or an inactive person. A larger or more active person needs at least 11 or even 12 glasses a day. To make sure you're getting this much, drink 1 to 2 glasses of water right before each meal or snack.

Drinking water has many benefits beyond filling your stomach. It allows your cells to receive nutrients. Thirst is often mistaken for hunger, and that's why drinking enough water is so important. If you feel hungry, have a glass of water or two and wait a few minutes. If you're still hungry, have a snack or a meal. There are other advantages to drinking water, too—it may reduce the risk of bladder cancer.

I recommend that you keep a bottle of water with you at all times. It's especially important to drink more water when you're exercising since you need extra hydration during your workout.

Of course, drinking plain water is pretty boring. How about adding a lemon or orange wedge for a little flavor? It's also worth noting that contrary to common belief, decaffeinated beverages do count toward the recommended amount of water you should drink on a daily basis. You can even lose weight just by adding ice to your water—your body will burn as many as 80 calories just warming itself up.

CHAPTER 5

# The Key Principles of the Perfect 10 Diet

Now that we've dispelled some really big dietary myths, you're ready to begin the Perfect 10 Diet. The following is a questionnaire I developed to help you get started. Answer yes or no to the following questions:

- Is your diet properly balanced in terms of the amounts of carbs, protein, and fat you consume?
- Do you eat at least 5 servings of fruits and vegetables every day?
- Does your diet supply ample amounts of fat to absorb fat-soluble vitamins?
- Does your diet include food groups that provide essential fatty acids, such as seeds, eggs, and fish?
- Do you eat sufficient amounts of high-quality protein to sustain your physiological functions every day?
- Do you eat green foods every day?
- Do you avoid processed foods?
- Do you eat different colored vegetables every day?
- Do you avoid sugar and refined carbs?
- Are you vigilant about excluding trans fats from your diet?

If you answered yes to all the questions, you are already on the right track. If you answered no to any question, the Perfect 10 Diet will help get you on the road to health.

## The Perfect 10 Diet Formula

The Perfect 10 Diet is all about nutritional balance—40 percent carbohydrates, 40 percent fat, and 20 percent protein. When you balance your macronutrient intake this way, you stabilize your blood sugar levels and offer your body the best sources of energy. While you can certainly lose weight on a low-fat diet by reducing calories, you pose a risk to your health by raising your insulin levels and becoming fat deficient. That's not a good scenario.

For this reason, I want you to eat more natural fats and eliminate bad carbs to lose weight and achieve perfect 10 hormones and health. Rest assured that you will not be hungry on the Perfect 10 Diet, as you will be eating real, whole foods that will provide you with the satiety you can only get from natural fats.

As you begin to incorporate natural fats into your diet, you will lose weight. I am talking about eating more fish, nuts, avocados, and chocolate made with real cocoa butter. That shouldn't be too hard to take, but you will have to eliminate sugar in all forms including soda, fruit juices, candy, ice cream, low-fat foods, fat-free foods, and all refined carbs. You'll lose weight as your hormones improve and become balanced.

## The New USDA Food Pyramid

Unlike the ever-changing food pyramid designed by the USDA (Fig. 5.1), the Perfect 10 Diet food pyramid is as solid as the great pyramid of Egypt. It may get old, but it is here to stay. I want you to start fresh, with a pyramid that will truly make you a perfect 10.

To help you get used to this new way of eating, I've put together the Perfect 10 Diet food pyramid. You will notice that this pyramid is the exact opposite of the original USDA food pyramid you remember from your childhood, which had carbohydrates at the base and fat at its apex. Natural fats are at the base of the Perfect 10 Diet food pyramid, and refined carbs are at its apex. It's the right way to balance hormones and lose weight.

The Perfect 10 Diet food pyramid also differs from the newer USDA food pyramid. The new USDA food pyramid recommends that half your grains should be whole grains. Does that mean the other half should be refined? That's awfully confusing. The current USDA food pyramid also places all protein in the same category. Do red meat, fish, and beans have equal health benefits? I don't think so. As I previously mentioned, red meat is not a healthy food choice on a daily basis because of its relationship to cancer. Red meat, pork, and lamb should only be consumed once every 3 weeks.

Finally, 3 servings of fat-free dairy daily are considered a sound, healthy choice. The recommendations to consume 3 servings of fat-free dairy on a daily basis have also not been proven to achieve optimal health. An abundance of fat-free dairy in your diet can lead to exaggerated insulin secretions. Their newer food pyramid, just like the previous one, is riddled with so many errors and inconsistencies that it's functionally worthless.

**Figure 5.1:** The New USDA Food Pyramid



| CATEGORY | Grains | Vegetables | Fruits | Milk | Meat and Beans | Recommended nutrient intakes at 12-calorie levels can be found on ***mypyramid.gov.*** |
|---|---|---|---|---|---|---|
| RECOMMENDATION | Half of all grains consumed should be whole grains. | Vary the types of vegetables you eat. | Eat a variety of fruits. Go easy on juices. | Eat low-fat or fat-free dairy products. | Eat lean cuts, seafood, and beans. Avoid frying. | |
| DAILY AMOUNT *Based on a 2,000 calorie diet.* | 6 oz. | 2.5 cups | 2 cups | 3 cups | 5.5 oz. | |

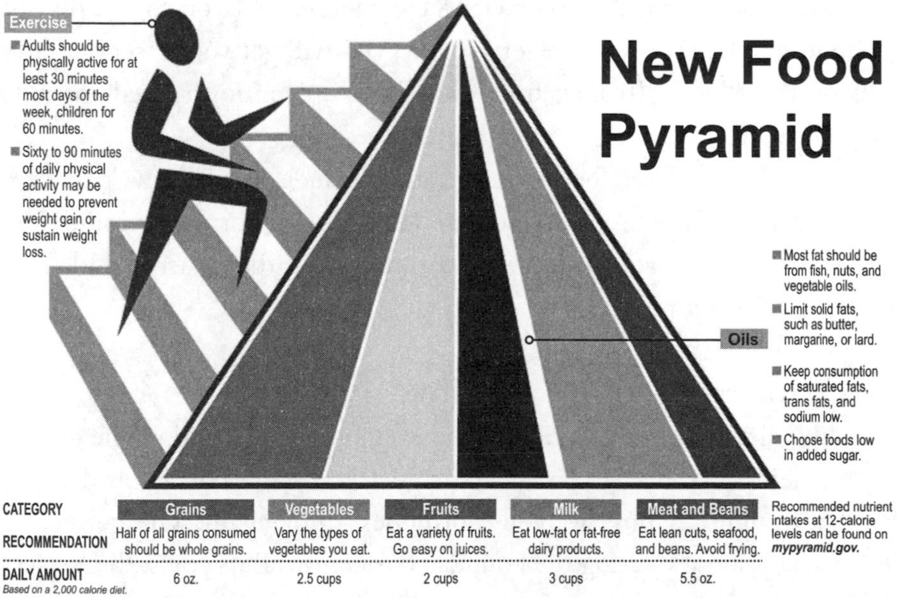

USDA website

## The Perfect 10 Diet Food Pyramid

The Perfect 10 Diet food pyramid (Fig. 5.2) will guide you to make healthy food choices as you embark on a new eating plan for life. The base of your diet should always be an abundance of fiber-rich vegetables at each meal, rather than refined carbohydrates.

Natural fat should constitute a large percentage of your daily calories. They are about 40 percent of the calories you'll consume on the Perfect 10 Diet, or a bit less.

Fruit should also be part of your diet.

Your protein sources should come primarily from poultry, fish, and other seafood, and you should eat nuts and legumes at least 3 to 4 times a week.

Calcium supplementation is preferred over heavy dairy consumption at all times. If you do consume dairy, do so in small amounts.

You may eat whole grains, but in moderation rather than in abundance. Refined carbohydrates, like pasta, cereals, candy, and sweets, should be completely eliminated from your diet, since they are synonymous with sugar.

Red meat, pork, and lamb appear at the apex of the pyramid; they are to be eaten sparingly because of their link to cancer. Once every 3 weeks is plenty.

Contrary to what the current USDA guidelines tell you to do, do not consume any manufactured vegetable oils; you will get your essential fatty acids on the Perfect 10 Diet from munching on sunflower seeds or nuts here and there.

The Perfect 10 Diet food pyramid also includes exercise as part of a healthy lifestyle. Exercise is essential to boost growth hormone production, which can keep you young, lean, and fit. And your diet must include 8 to 10 glasses of water per day.

## The Three Stages of the Perfect 10 Diet

A healthy diet must include fiber-rich vegetables, fruits, and whole grains. But no diet can be perfect unless all its goals are achieved. If you thought this diet would only improve your hormones, think again. The Perfect 10 Diet is really about melting the pounds. To achieve all its goals, the Perfect 10 Diet is divided into three easy stages, specifically designed to help people

**Figure 5.2:** The Perfect 10 Diet Food Pyramid

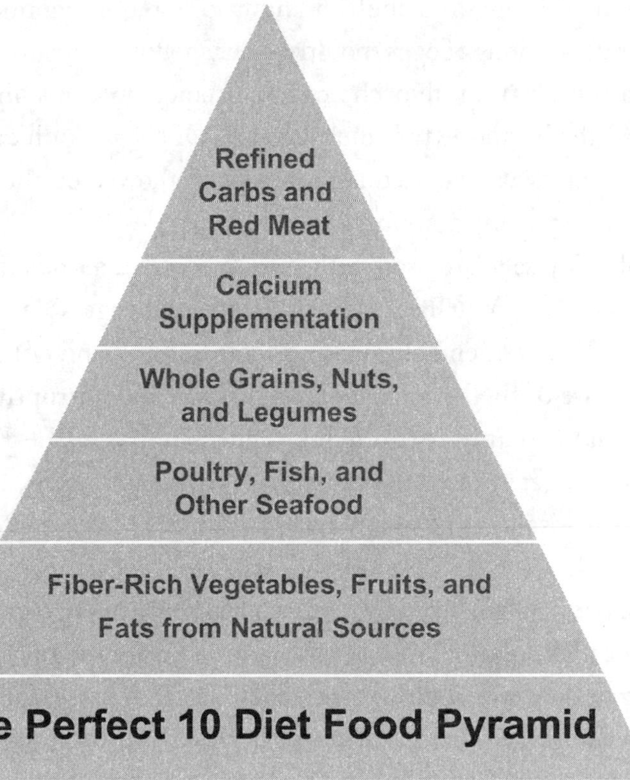


with different goals. Stages One and Two are for those of you who desire to lose weight and melt the pounds. Stage Three is optimal for those who just want to eat healthy and fight disease for life.

## Stage One (Initiation)

Stage One of the Perfect 10 Diet will last three weeks, and most people will lose an average of 10 to 14 pounds during this time. That's a lot of weight in a short period of time, but don't be alarmed with your initial results. Some of the weight loss in this stage is water. Later on, your weight will go down at a slower pace. During this stage, you'll eat 3 meals a day, and you'll also have the option to eat 1 to 2 snacks a day on the days you work out or if you're hungry.

Stage One is relatively short because it is not sustainable over the long term. It is only designed to jump-start your weight loss and give you an idea about your own metabolism and calorie requirements. You will have normal size portions of eggs, poultry, fish, shellfish, mushrooms, and beans. These are healthy protein choices to balance your insulin and optimize glucagon, the hormone that melts the fat. Of course, unlike low-carb diets, no processed meats like bacon or sausage are allowed on the Perfect 10 Diet at any time or in any amounts.

You'll enjoy salads tossed with nuts (pecans, almonds, and walnuts are all good choices). You'll eat plenty of fiber-rich vegetables with each meal. However, I recommend eliminating beets, carrots, and potatoes during this stage because of their starchy nature; they are very disruptive for insulin.

Fruits are certainly permitted and encouraged on the Perfect 10 Diet. I love low-sugar fruits such as berries, kiwis, honeydew, and cantaloupe, and the fructose present in any types of fruit will not negatively affect your insulin level.

You'll also drink plenty of water from glass bottles if you can. Unsweetened lemonade and decaffeinated beverages are also acceptable.

Being fit does take a little work, so let's get to what you have to give up in this short stage. You must cut your calories if you want to lose weight.

It is back to a Paleolithic diet on Stage One of the Perfect 10 Diet. Since your body needs protein and fat to function optimally, you must focus on cutting out carbs. The only carbs you need to cut back on without any risks to your health in this short stage are whole grains. This means you won't eat any cereal, bread of any kind, rice, or pasta during the 3-week period of Stage One. If you are the kind of person who says, "Wait a minute, Doc. I can't give up bread," or "Mama mia, I'm Italian, what are you saying to me?" Don't worry; you'll have bread and pasta in no time at all. You can safely eliminate whole grains. After all, grains weren't a part of the human diet for most of our history. Agriculture didn't exist for 99.9 percent of our human existence. The Perfect 10 Diet is not about deprivations. It's about freedom and variety. Give it a shot, and you will be amazed with the results. Of course, there was no dairy in Paleolithic time. But I won't make you wait 2 million years or even 3 weeks; I will let you have some dairy. Of course, no alcohol of any kind or any amount is allowed during Stage One of the Perfect 10 Diet.

Although Stage One may be the strictest stage of the Perfect 10 Diet, I guarantee you won't be hungry or feel deprived during this time.

## Stage Two (Ongoing Weight Loss)

Stage Two of the Perfect 10 Diet builds on Stage One's principles. Stage Two of the Perfect 10 Diet is similar to the human diet after the advent of agriculture. You will be getting more calories than in Stage One, but you'll get an even better indication about your body's metabolism and calorie requirements.

Vegetables, fruits, eggs, poultry, seafood, and nuts are still encouraged. You still eat 3 meals, and you'll also have the option of eating 1 to 2 snacks a day if you're still hungry.

Bread and pasta are also back—the whole-grain kind, of course. Whole grains are added back in small amounts during this longer stage to prevent the feelings of deprivation that frequently occur with dieting. Add 1 to 3 servings of whole grains to your daily diet, such as a bowl of oatmeal, a slice of high-fiber bread, a scoop of brown rice, or even a portion of whole-wheat pasta. Whole grains make a comeback in this stage because deprivation leaves us with a desire to overeat what is prohibited, which can lead to eventual diet failure. Whole grains can still support your hormones and fill you up nicely.

If you find that your weight plateaus during this stage, simply cut down on whole grains or increase your exercise routine. Stage Two of the Perfect 10 Diet is specifically designed to make your weight loss easy, painless, and without a lot of sacrifice.

If you like to drink, alcohol is allowed in very limited amounts during this longer stage (1 or 2 drinks a week at the most is okay). Most people should continue to lose weight if they correctly follow the principles of the Perfect 10 Diet.

How long should you stay in Stage Two of the Perfect 10 Diet? That all depends on you and factors like your initial body weight, desired ultimate goal weight, metabolism, hormone levels, activity level, exercise routine, and your dedication to following the Perfect 10 Diet principles on a daily basis. You can stay in Stage Two as long as it takes you to reach your ultimate desired weight. It may take a few days or a few years to get to the end of this stage, but either is perfectly okay.

## Stage Three (Life Maintenance)

You can feel free to start your diet transformation with Stage Three of the Perfect 10 Diet right from the start if you just want to improve your health, balance hormones, and fight disease and are not interested in losing weight. Stage Three is our modern diet but with lots of discipline. Stage Three is similar to Stage Two but with a little more freedom now that you've lost the excess weight. It's designed to set you on a healthy course for the rest of your life.

During Stage Three, you'll still eat 3 meals a day, and will have the option to eat 1 to 2 additional snacks per day if you're hungry. You can eat more whole grains than you could in Stage Two (up to 4 servings a day). Potatoes are also acceptable now that you've lost the weight, but if you consume potatoes or other starchy vegetables, cut back on the whole grains. It is okay to treat yourself to sweets once in a while as long as you don't overdo it.

Stage Three is our modern diet with its unhealthy challenges. So how do you deal with sweets or pizza on the Perfect 10 Diet? It takes a lot of discipline, since the Perfect 10 Diet is not a calorie-focused diet. Let me give you a couple examples. If you're really craving regular pizza, have a thin-crust pie loaded with lots of vegetables to limit the refined carbs. If you are going to eat ice cream, have one scoop only, and make sure it's the full-fat, not the fat-free variety. The fat-free variety contains too much sugar and you will end up having three scoops instead of one. Sugar is a treat, not a nutrient. Don't go for the sugar-free treats either as they contain artificial sweeteners, which are worse than sugar. If you do eat anything sweet or starchy, hit the gym immediately so the trickle effect of sugar won't damage your hormones. Frequent misbehaving is not a good thing if you want to be truly a perfect 10. Stage Three is also great for diabetics, people with thyroid disease, women in menopause, men with low testosterone, body builders, and anyone who wants to be in perfect 10 health but is not looking to lose weight.

The greatest thing about the Perfect 10 Diet is its versatility. You can always go back to Stage One at any time if your weight starts to go up. Let's say you went on a vacation and you've fallen off track; go right back to Stage One. This means no grains. Learning how to "go off plan" is an important part of the Perfect 10 Diet. That's when the Perfect 10 Diet becomes your way of life.

**Figure 5.3:** The Three Stages of the Perfect 10 Diet

### *Stage One*

Duration: 3 Weeks

This stage is the Paleolithic diet (vegetables, fruits, poultry, seafood, beans, nuts and seeds).

### *Stage Two*

Duration: Flexible

This stage is the human diet following the advent of agriculture (vegetables, fruits, poultry, seafood, beans, nuts and seeds, and whole grains).

### *Stage Three*

Duration: Life

This stage is our modern diet with some modifications (vegetables, fruits, poultry, seafood, beans, nuts and seeds, and more whole grains). If you eat sweets or refined carbs, do so sparingly.

Dairy should be kept to a minimum at all times. Alcohol should be enjoyed only in moderation in Stages Two and Three.

CHAPTER 6

# Getting Started on the Perfect 10 Diet

Now that you understand how natural fats help you lose weight, and how a diet of nutrient-dense whole foods is absolutely critical for maintaining good hormone levels, you're ready to get started on the Perfect 10 Diet by putting all this knowledge into practice.

## The Three Stages of the Perfect 10 Diet

- Stage One: You will eat 3 meals a day. No grains or alcohol are allowed.
- Stage Two: You will eat 3 meals a day, and now you can add 1 to 3 servings of whole grains to your diet. If you must drink alcohol, do so in small amounts.
- Stage Three: You will eat 3 meals a day. You can increase your whole-grain consumption to 3 or 4 servings a day. If you must eat sweets, do so sparingly.

At Stage Two and Three, cut grains out completely if you start to gain weight.

## Carbohydrates

The Perfect 10 Diet allows you to eat liberal amounts of carbohydrates, up to 40 percent of your daily food intake. Remember, the Perfect 10 Diet is not a low-carb diet, rather, it is a balanced diet with respect to all macronutrients. By eating enough of the right carbs, you'll get plenty of fiber.

In Stage One of the Perfect 10 Diet, your carbohydrates will come from vegetables, beans, and fruits. In Stages Two and Three, your carbohydrates will also come from whole grains, such as wild or brown rice, whole-wheat pasta, and whole-grain bread.

## Vegetables to Enjoy

- Asparagus
- Artichokes
- Arugula
- Bamboo shoots
- Bell peppers (orange, green, red, and yellow)
- Broccoli
- Brussels sprouts
- Cabbage
- Celery
- Chard
- Chives
- Cilantro
- Cucumbers
- Endive
- Eggplant
- Greens (chard, collard, mustard, and turnip)
- Hot peppers
- Kale
- Lettuce (all varieties)
- Leeks
- Okra
- Onions
- Parsley
- Radicchio
- Radishes
- Rutabaga
- Scallions
- Spinach
- Sprouts (all varieties)
- String beans
- Turnips
- Zucchini

## Vegetables to Limit

The vegetables to limit on the Perfect 10 Diet lack fiber and are starchy in nature. Consumption of these vegetables leads to rapid sugar absorption, which can raise insulin levels and mess up other hormones if eaten in large amounts.

- Carrots (consume only small amounts, and make sure they're raw—once they're cooked, they climb up the glycemic index)
- Sweet potatoes

## Vegetables to Avoid

- Potatoes
- Beets

## Fruits to Enjoy

- Apples
- Avocados
- Bananas
- Blackberries
- Blueberries
- Cantaloupe
- Cherries
- Cranberries
- Grapes
- Honeydew
- Kiwi
- Mangos
- Oranges
- Pears
- Pineapples
- Raspberries
- Strawberries
- Tomatoes

## Fruits to Avoid

- All fruit juices (except tomato)
- Dried fruits

## Legumes to Enjoy

- All legumes (except genetically modified soy)

## When Can I Start to Eat Grains on the Perfect 10 Diet?

Despite what you've been told about the benefits of grains, they did not become part of the human diet until relatively recent times. Bread, rice, and pasta are certainly allowed on the Perfect 10 Diet. However, you can only consume the whole-grain variety, and even that doesn't begin until Stage Two. Whole grains should be limited to 1 to 3 servings a day in Stage Two, and the amount of grains your body can sustain will also depend on your activity level. If your weight loss in Stage Two of the

Perfect 10 Diet plateaus, scale back the amount of grains from 3 to 2 or from 2 to 1 serving per day.

You can eat 4 servings of grains a day during Stage Three of the Perfect 10 Diet if you're very active or not interested in weight loss. However, the risks always outweigh the benefits, as you may start to regain weight you've worked hard to lose. I'd rather see you eat more fiber-rich vegetables than bread or rice with each meal. If you do, you're less likely to put the pounds back on.

## Acceptable Grains

- Barley
- Bread (rye, pumpernickel, and whole grain)
- Corn (small amounts)
- Oatmeal (non-instant)
- Rice (brown and wild*)
- Whole-grain cereals with no added sugar or chemicals
- Whole-wheat pasta

**Wild rice is preferred over brown rice because it has more fiber.*

## You Recommend One to Three Servings of Grains in Stage Two. How Many Can I Really Eat?

I don't advise you to increase grain consumption in Stage Two of the Perfect 10 Diet beyond 1 serving a day during the first month. If you follow this direction, you'll begin to get a handle on your own body's metabolism. If you find yourself losing too much weight, you can add an additional serving or 2 of grains per week. If your weight plateaus, limit grains from 3 to 2 or from 2 to 1 serving. You are the only one who can gauge what your body needs depending on the pace of your weight loss and your activity level.

## Grains to Avoid

- All refined grains (white bread, white rice, and white pasta)
- All pastries made with white flour
- Low-fat and fat-free products containing added sugar or high-fructose corn syrup

## Protein

It's important that you get enough protein, which should be roughly 20 percent of daily food intake for most of us. If you're very athletic and involved in anaerobic activities like weight lifting, you can eat a little more than that. If you're not very active, 15 percent should be plenty.

Remember, the Perfect 10 Diet is flexible and versatile, and designed to meet your needs. Most people will need about 50 to 160 grams of protein daily for optimal health. You should divide this amount equally throughout the day to stabilize your blood sugar levels. Eating too much or too little protein can be detrimental to your hormones and overall health.

### Protein to Enjoy

- All shellfish
- Fish (halibut, herring, tuna, sardines, and wild salmon)
- Legumes (except soy)
- Liver
- Mushrooms
- Ostrich
- Poultry, including chicken, Cornish game hen, duck, turkey, goose, and pheasant
- Rabbit

### Protein Sources to Eat Sparingly

- Buffalo burgers
- Organic red meat, pork, and lamb (eat moderately or sparingly, as their frequent consumption has been related to colon cancer)
- Soy (tofu, tempeh)

### Protein Sources to Avoid

- Canned tuna in soybean oil (contains trans fats)
- Cow brain (linked to mad cow disease)
- Nitrite-containing products, including hot dogs, bacon, Canadian bacon, ham, and sausage (avoid completely for the strong link to colon cancer)

- Soy protein isolate (chemically treated with nitrites)
- Soy burgers made with soy protein isolate

### Putting Natural Fat Back into Your Diet

Learning new ways of eating can be challenging now that supermarket shelves are filled with low-fat sugary cereals and fat-free foods, and margarine containers that have heart-healthy logos plastered all over them. However, this is the food you must eliminate from the Perfect 10 Diet since it is processed, filled with sugar, and contains deadly trans fats. Eating this junk will wreak havoc on your metabolic system, and it'll make you gain weight in no time at all.

Start by shopping for vegetables instead of processed foods. Make it a habit to shop in health-food stores, and buy raw nuts and nut butters, such as macadamia or almond butter, to use instead of jam or jellies made with high-fructose corn syrup.

Eating nuts regularly can prevent heart disease. Buy avocados instead of cookies. Remember, you can eat even saturated fats on the Perfect 10 Diet, such as butter, full-fat raw cheese, and coconut.

Start dressing salads with extra-virgin olive oil instead of low-fat dressings made with high-fructose corn syrup. Toss nuts into your salads instead of white-flour croutons. Eat fish and other seafood at least 3 to 4 times a week. Don't stop there—treat yourself to a piece of dark chocolate made with real cocoa butter once in a while.

## Fats

### Dairy to Enjoy

A splash of cream or organic whole (cow or goat) milk in decaffeinated beverages is acceptable on the Perfect 10 Diet. But limit dairy at all times if you can.

- Cheese
    - Cheddar cheese
    - Cottage cheese

    - Goat cheese
    - Farmer cheese
    - Feta cheese
    - Mozzarella cheese
    - Parmesan cheese
    - Ricotta cheese
    - Swiss cheese
- Kefir
- Yogurt

## Nuts to Enjoy

These nuts should be eaten raw and unsalted, and not roasted. It is also acceptable to eat nut butters that are extracted organically, without chemicals.

- Almonds
- Brazil nuts
- Cashews*
- Hazelnuts
- Macadamias
- Pecans
- Walnuts

**I have placed cashews in the nuts category, but they are fruits.*

## Oils to Enjoy

- Almond oil (cold on salads)
- Avocado oil (cold on salads)
- Macadamia oil (also useful for cooking)
- Extra-virgin olive oil (use for light cooking and to dress salads)
- Unrefined cold-pressed polyunsaturated oils, such as safflower and sunflower, in small amounts (use to dress salads; do not heat)

## Fats to Enjoy

- Butter
- Coconut
- Ghee (clarified butter) (use for cooking if you don't like the taste of butter)
- Palm oil

## Fats to Avoid

- All refined vegetable oils (corn, safflower, sunflower, soybean, and mixed vegetable oil)
- Animal fat from nonorganic sources (may contain toxins, hormones, and pesticides)
- Nonhydrogenated margarine
- Partially hydrogenated oils and fats (fast-food oils and margarine brands like I Can't Believe It's Not Butter)
- Vegetable shortening

## What about Desserts on the Perfect 10 Diet?

If you believe desserts are off-limits on the Perfect 10 Diet, think again. The Perfect 10 Diet is crème de la crème of all diets because it allows many delicious, rich desserts. But most desserts are high in sugar, which makes them tough on insulin and many hormones. Desserts that are off-limits are anything made with white flour and sugar, including fat-free cakes and low-fat muffins. Remember, folks, there is no candy on the Perfect 10 Diet—not if you want to be eye candy. I only allow healthy desserts on the Perfect 10 Diet. Almonds or berries dipped in reduced-sugar chocolate make a rich, delicious dessert. Fresh fruit with full-fat yogurt is another great option. If you throw fresh fruit and yogurt or kefir in the blender with ice, you'll probably never miss ice cream. A banana mixed with cocoa powder is also a great choice. These desserts are not only good for your health, but they'll satisfy your sweet tooth without wreaking havoc inside your body. Healthy desserts will also keep you from feeling deprived, so you'll be better able to stick to the Perfect 10 Diet at all times.

## Which Sweeteners Are Best?

You've already read that sugar is bad, so you might be thinking that artificial sweeteners are okay on the Perfect 10 Diet. Actually, they're worse. There are many sweeteners on the market. The list includes saccharin (Sweet'N Low), aspartame (Equal), and sucralose (Splenda). It's important to note that all these sweeteners are manmade. Aspartame has been linked to cancer in animal studies. Splenda has been linked as a trigger for migraines, and to a sluggish thyroid. Artificial sweeteners are not natural to our bodies, and they're loaded with chemicals. The long-term effects on our health are unknown, so avoid them.

On the Perfect 10 Diet, I prefer stevia and agave. Stevia, which is sweeter than sugar, is extracted from the *Stevia rebaudiana* leaf, a shrub found in South America. Indians have safely consumed it for hundreds of years. I carry stevia packets to use in my tea when I'm away from home. Unfortunately, stevia is not widely available in supermarkets since the FDA banned its sale in 1991 because of some safety issues. Just a few years ago, this ban was lifted, and the study used to support the ban was later found to be flawed. Look for stevia at GNC and Whole Foods stores.

I also like agave on the Perfect 10 Diet, which is extracted from a Mexican cactus. It is natural and has a low glycemic index, which makes it a safe sweetener for diabetics, and it has a minimal impact on insulin. If you must use sweeteners at high temperatures, use agave.

## Sweeteners to Avoid

- High-fructose corn syrup
- Honey*
- Maple syrup*
- Molasses
- Sugar

**Although these sweeteners are natural, the body treats them exactly the same way as sugar, so they should be avoided.*

## Beverages on the Perfect 10 Diet

The list of acceptable beverages on the Perfect 10 Diet is quite extensive, but several should be completely avoided. I will go over them all—the good, the bad, and the ugly.

### What about Soda?

All sodas should be avoided on the Perfect 10 Diet. Recent research indicates that drinking more than one soda a day—even if it's diet—is associated with a cluster of risk factors linked to the development of diabetes and heart disease. Soda can throw off your insulin and sex hormones, since just 1 can contains as much as 10 teaspoons of sugar.

That's not all. Some research has linked consumption of soda to pancreatic cancer, and both regular and diet sodas contain a preservative called benzoate to maintain freshness. Benzoate interacts with vitamin C and breaks down to benzene, a major carcinogen that has been linked to leukemia. Although the amount of benzoate present in soda is quite small, it's something to consider when you contemplate the massive amounts of soda you'll consume over a lifetime.

Regular soda contains massive amounts of high-fructose corn syrup, and diet sodas have aspartame. Both perpetuate sugar cravings and lead to weight gain.

### What about Milk Substitutes, Such as Soy, Rice, and Almond Milk?

Many people who are lactose intolerant turn to vegetarian milk substitutes such as soy and rice milk. We are told that these are healthy alternatives to whole milk. I'm not a fan of either of them. Rice milk is made out of white rice, and it can contain more than 30 grams of sugar in a single serving.

On the other hand, soy milk contains little sugar, but it contains excessive amounts of polyunsaturated oils that are also bad for your health. If you are lactose intolerant and want to have a milk substitute, I prefer unsweetened almond milk, which you can find in organic and whole-food stores. Almond milk is made from raw almonds soaked in water. It has very little sugar and is a perfectly healthy choice.

## What about Coffee and Tea on the Perfect 10 Diet?

A daily trip to Dunkin' Donuts or Starbucks for a grande or a venti latte will not get you a perfect 10 physique. You need to kick the caffeine habit. On the Perfect 10 Diet, I'd rather see you stick to decaffeinated beverages at all times, but if you can't kick the caffeine habit, at least cut down to 1 cup a day.

Excess caffeine promotes excess insulin secretion, which can lead to hunger. I know you might be saying, "But coffee has no calories, so how can it be bad?" Caffeine stimulates your nervous system so you feel a little on edge. In turn, your adrenals pump the stress hormones epinephrine and norepinephrine and lead your liver to release some sugar into the bloodstream. Next, insulin is secreted to lower the sugar. Pretty soon you feel the need for a second cup of coffee, a cigarette, or a piece of candy or a chocolate bar.

Coffee has a negative effect on both growth hormone and testosterone. Too much caffeine can lead to a disturbance in testosterone levels in men—including making it break down to estrogen, the female sex hormone. You can also become addicted to doses of daily caffeine. Heavy caffeine users may develop withdrawal symptoms, such as headaches, drowsiness, difficulty concentrating, and irritability. When you are irritable, you are more likely to have sugar cravings.

Is addiction to caffeine a serious problem? Probably not, unless some of the withdrawal symptoms are disrupting your life. However, caffeine can increase a woman's risk of miscarriage, and that's why pregnant women are advised to avoid coffee.

Tea, on the other hand, may have an edge over coffee. I love green tea. Green tea contains less caffeine than coffee, and contains epigallcatechin gallate (EGCG), one of the strongest and most studied antioxidants. EGCG has shown impressive activity against many types of cancer. It appears to protect the heart and arteries from oxidative damage, and, applied topically, it can reverse precancerous skin lesions. One cup of unsweetened green tea a day is fine, or you can consume even more of decaffeinated varieties.

## What about Energy Drinks?

Energy drinks are not permitted on the Perfect 10 Diet. The excess caffeine in energy drinks is addictive, and they're loaded with sugar. Energy drinks lose effectiveness over time, and they set you up for a rebound as soon as you discontinue them.

## What about Alcohol on the Perfect 10 Diet?

I talked about how bad alcohol is for your hormones in the beginning of the book. Give it up, folks. Of course, this is easier said than done—especially for those of you who are used to drinking every day or every weekend. However, it's necessary, because alcohol jacks up your blood sugar levels, which is bad for your insulin and your physique.

Alcohol is like a double-edged sword: it can be both good and bad. One drink a day can cut your risk of heart disease by 32 percent, but excessive amounts of alcohol can increase both morbidity and mortality. Drinking alcohol to excess can increase your chance of developing liver disease, and there are also reports in the scientific literature about increased risk of breast cancer among women who consume alcohol to excess. If you drink more than 1 or 2 drinks a week, you are more likely to end up with an atrophied, smaller brain as you get older. You're also more likely to have less muscle mass and more fat. You can forget about your sex hormones once you've had too much alcohol. Yeah, you might become less inhibited, but you will have no performance.

Sure you can have more fun after you've had a few cocktails or beers, but being drunk makes you unattractive no matter how charming you may be. And didn't I just mention excess alcohol will make you fat, too? Does this mean I want you to give up alcohol completely on the Perfect 10 Diet? Of course not. Alcohol is allowed in moderation in Stages Two and Three of the Perfect 10 Diet, but when it's consumed in excess, alcohol is poisonous to every system of your body. If you drink a lot of alcohol, you are guaranteed to gain weight. Why? Because alcohol is a sugar that's used for energy before being stored as fat. This means that if you drink a lot of alcohol, you may not be able to lose any weight—even if you are following the rest of the Perfect 10 Diet principles to the core.

For this reason, I recommend that you avoid alcohol completely if you have a hard time losing weight, have a history of alcohol abuse, or suffer from an existing liver disease. If you have no health issues and still wish to drink, I will not discourage you from occasionally enjoying a glass of your favorite alcoholic beverage after a stressful day at work or with dinner occasionally starting in Stage Two.

I do ask that you trade in your favorite booze and beer for organic red wine. Why organic? Because of sulfites. Sulfites are additives used in food and wines to extend their shelf life, and they have been linked to allergic reactions and asthma. Organic red wine also tastes better. Red wine, in particular, can reduce your risk for heart disease because it contains higher levels of flavinoids. Just like grapes, red wine is rich in resveratrol.

Be sure you avoid all calorie-dense mixed drinks made with added sugar and fruit juices. Beer is high in maltose, a highly glycemic sugar. Because of this, your body will treat beer like any other refined carbohydrates and will increase its insulin secretion. You won't have a perfect 10 body if you have a beer belly. If you must drink beer, go for a low-carb brand.

You should also increase your weekly exercise routine by at least one half hour for every shot you consume. That should inspire you to cut back!

## Beverages to Enjoy

- All vegetable juices (except beet and carrot)*
- Caffeinated herbal and green tea (1 cup per day is fine)
- Decaffeinated tea and coffee
- Lemonade sweetened with stevia or agave
- Mineral water
- Organic hot chocolate with no added sugar (small amounts)*
- Organic full-fat dairy beverages*
- Sparkling water**
- Tomato juice*

**If you have any drink with calories, it should count as a snack.*

***Sparkling water is a secondary choice, as it contains high amounts of carbonic acid.*

## Beverages to Limit

- Alcohol
- Coffee

## Beverages to Avoid

- All carbonated beverages (regular and diet)
- All fruit juices (except tomato)
- Hot chocolate with added sugars and hydrogenated oils
- Energy drinks
- Fat-free, 1 percent and 2 percent milk
- Rice milk
- Soy milk

## Condiments, Spices, and Herbs to Use

Spices are a big component of the Perfect 10 Diet. Put cinnamon on your yogurt, or turmeric, sage, and garlic over your entrées. Every time you spice up your food, you upgrade it to first class. Voilà! It's a superfood.

- Basil
- Black pepper
- Cayenne pepper
- Cajun blended seasonings
- Crushed red pepper flakes
- Cumin
- Curry powder
- Dill
- Fennel
- Garlic* (fresh only)
- Homemade mayonnaise (made with olive oil, not soybean oil)
- Lemon
- Lime
- Nutmeg
- Onion
- Oregano
- Paprika
- Sea salt
- Rosemary
- Tarragon
- Turmeric
- Thyme
- Vanilla
- Worcestershire sauce

## What's So Special about Garlic?

Add lots of garlic to your recipes and salads. Okay, maybe no one will want to kiss you after all that garlic, but it's good for you. Garlic has antibacterial and antifungal properties. Researchers have also found that garlic prevents blood clotting, which makes it cardio-protective. Garlic is also being studied for its abilities to reduce your risk for cancer.

## What about Salt?

Salt in small amounts is essential for thyroid health. Most Americans get plenty of salt in their diet. Adding too much salt to your food is bad: it can suppress your thyroid when used in excess. I'd rather see us use sea salt instead of iodized salt. You still need salt, so don't try to give it up altogether. In fact, as you transition to a healthful diet by eating natural foods, you may not be getting enough salt—especially if you live in a hot climate where you perspire a lot and lose salt in the process.

## Condiments to Limit

- Mustard (contains vinegar)*
- Vinegar*

**Fermented products are yeast-friendly. Yeast is bad for hormones.*

## Condiments to Avoid

- All fat-free salad dressings with added sugars, partially hydrogenated oils, or soybean oil
- Barbecue sauce with added high-fructose corn syrup
- Jellies with high-fructose corn syrup
- Ketchup with added high-fructose corn syrup
- Mayonnaise made with soybean oil (contains trace trans fats)

## Is It Better to Eat Organic Food?

I get asked this question a lot. Don't nickel and dime your health. Organic produce is usually more expensive than conventional produce, but nonorganic food contains pesticides and toxins that prevent you from receiving signals from the hormone leptin, which, as you probably recall, is involved in satiety. Pesticides are also toxic to other glands. You should also avoid any genetically modified foods, which are altered to resist spoilage. In several studies, animals who were given foods made with genetically modified crops refused to eat it and had to be force-fed. Guess what? They developed autoimmune diseases, stomach lesions, and cancer. Perhaps you're wondering why the government approved such dangerous food? Here's the answer: close examination reveals that industry manipulation and political collusion, not sound science, were the driving forces.

## Is Fasting Allowed on the Perfect 10 Diet?

Yes. Fasting is great for boosting HGH. Fasting, or abstaining from food, is a powerful tool to cleanse your body and get rid of toxins. When we don't eat, all of our energy goes toward cleaning the house rather than digesting. As a result, your body can get rid of chemical by-products or free radicals. Fasting can last any length of time, from a few hours to a few days.

Fasting on drinking water alone is challenging and may be dangerous, since you can feel dizzy or even faint. I don't recommend it. If you want to try an occasional fast at any stage of the Perfect 10 Diet, start slow. Mix some lime or lemon juice with water and agave to sweeten, and then add some cinnamon. You can also have vegetable juice as long as it's fresh-pressed (and not pasteurized or packaged). It's advisable to read about fasting before starting, and never fast if you're pregnant.

## Should I Eat My Food Raw or Cooked?

Proponents of the raw food movement claim that cooking food drains it of its vitamins and minerals, but people have cooked their food for generations without suffering from nutritionally related diseases.

Cooking food at very high temperatures destroys vitamins, but it also makes the minerals more readily available. For this reason, I'm a firm believer that you can have your food any way you like it—raw or cooked—just as long as it isn't overly cooked or charred.

However, there are some precautions you should take. If you eat raw fish, it must be placed in the freezer for two weeks to kill any parasites. Shellfish should be cooked, especially for the elderly and those with immune deficiencies, such as cancer and HIV. Consumption of raw shellfish can lead to infections such as hepatitis A, which can be deadly in the immunosuppressed.

CHAPTER 7

# Putting the Perfect 10 Diet into Action

Are you ready to have the perfect 10 body of a movie star at a red-carpet event? Sure you can, but you have to star in your most important role—your life—and give your very best performance. Are you ready to accept this role? Are you ready to overcome all the challenges required for this job? Lights! Camera! Action! The Perfect 10 Diet is now on.

## Kitchen Cleaning

The road to good health starts with your kitchen. For this reason, no diet can be successful unless you start with some kitchen cleaning (Fig. 7.1). Educate your family and include them in the process so they don't sabotage your efforts. Open your refrigerator and throw away all the margarine and imitation butters. Get rid of all the fruit juices and soda. Next, go after the condiments, including all jellies, ketchup, barbecue sauces, and fat-free salad dressings that contain high-fructose corn syrup. Throw away your all-purpose white flour, croutons preserved with hydrogenated oil, and breadcrumbs. Artificial sweeteners must go, too. Processed meats? This is the Perfect 10 Diet here, so don't even try to keep those.

Next, get rid of all the refined vegetable oils that contain trans fats, including corn, safflower, and mixed vegetable oil (even if they have an FDA statement on the label that says otherwise).

Next, throw away anything that is labeled low-fat or fat-free, because these products are full of sugar (not to mention chemicals and dyes). The list includes all sugary cereals with added chemicals and dyes.

Don't bother thinking, "But I just bought this cereal, or orange juice—what a waste." Your health is more valuable than all the money in the world. You will be surprised that you were ever able to live on this toxic diet. Don't give it to the Salvation Army either. No human being deserves to be poisoned because he or she is poor.

Now, before you restock your cabinets, make sure you carefully read all the food labels in the supermarket. Avoid buying processed foods at all times. Fill your refrigerator with fresh vegetables, fruits, poultry, and fish. Buy some butter for cooking. Don't forget to get a whole-food supplement pill to take on a daily basis.

**Figure 7.1:** Foods to Remove from Your Kitchen

| | |
|---|---|
| Artificial sweeteners | Margarine |
| Barbecue sauce | Powdered milk |
| Cake | Processed meats |
| Crackers | Refined vegetable oils |
| Fat-free dairy | Soda (regular and diet) |
| Fat-free food | Sugar |
| French fries | Sugary cereals |
| Fruit juices | Vegetable shortening |
| Jam | White bread |
| Jelly | White flour |
| Ketchup | White pasta |

## Taper Your Calories throughout the Day

There is an old proverb that says: "Eat breakfast like a king, lunch like a prince, and dinner like a pauper." Recent studies in 2009 show that if you taper your calories throughout the day, you can lose weight more easily (Fig. 7.2). This eating pattern makes a lot of sense, and that's the mantra of the Perfect 10 Diet, too. You need the most calories in the morning and dinner should be your smallest meal. Tapering your calories throughout the day regulates serotonin, a brain chemical, which plays a role in regulating food intake.

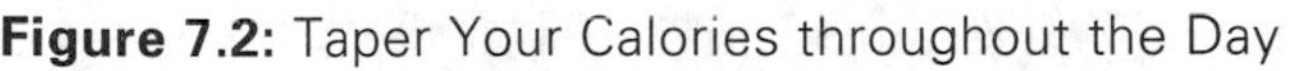

**Figure 7.2:** Taper Your Calories throughout the Day

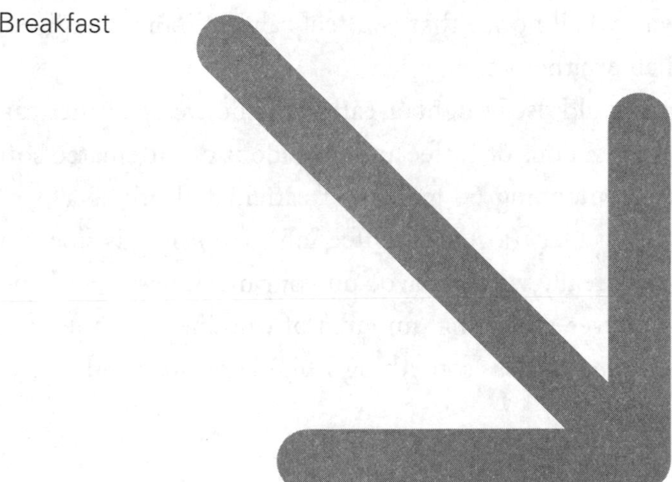


## Breakfast: It's That Important

Start your day right, and eat a big breakfast. One of the major mistakes that dieters make is skipping breakfast, but breakfast is the most important meal of the day. Once we wake up, we begin expending energy at a high rate. We leave for work or run errands, and we need energy for that. Accordingly, it's important that you provide your body with high-quality fuel right from the start.

An ideal breakfast should include protein (eggs) and healthy fats (avocado, butter, or cheese) so your body starts the day with high-quality fuel. A protein breakfast, with or without some fat, will decrease insulin levels and your hunger, as well as the calories you consume. Eating protein and fat for breakfast will delay hunger for 5 to 6 hours.

It's also helpful to have a hot drink (decaffeinated coffee or tea) in the morning to get the digestive processes going after a long night of sleep. Your breakfast certainly should not contain sugar or refined carbs, since this will only prompt your pancreas to make more insulin. That means no Danishes, doughnuts, plain bagels, reduced-fat or fat-free muffins, sugary cereals, or croissants for breakfast. If you eat this junk, you will feel hungry, irritable, and fatigued long before lunch time. If you focus on eating a breakfast free of sugar, you'll notice that you feel calmer, more energized, and more focused than ever before.

A healthy breakfast should also be light on caffeine. The average American drinks approximately 28 gallons of coffee and 32 gallons of caffeinated soft drinks a year. That's a whopping 60 gallons of caffeinated drinks a year! Caffeine in small doses is okay (a cup of coffee in the morning is fine, for example), but too much really wreaks havoc on your metabolism, and you will become reliant on ever-escalating amounts of caffeine simply to feel "up." Breaking the caffeine habit is something I highly recommend.

## What Can I Eat for Breakfast?

My patients often ask this question. My answer to them (and you) is that you may eat anything you like that is good for you, including healthy fats (an avocado, for example), protein (eggs), healthy carbs (a vegetable dish or a fruit salad), and in Stage Two or Three, some whole grains (a small bowl of oatmeal).

Tired of eggs? Try a few slices of turkey or some salmon with some cream cheese. Berries with cottage cheese is another good choice. I encourage my patients to "think out of the box" when it comes to breakfast. Remember, a low-fat cereal with some skim milk is no different from eating pure sugar. It will be detrimental to your health. In the Paleolithic time, humans didn't make distinctions between what kind of food they ate for different meals in the day. If the idea of a salad or leftover vegetables from last night's dinner is unacceptable to you for breakfast, a full-fat yogurt with fruit is a perfectly satisfactory choice.

## Lunch

For lunch, I want you to have some protein, fats, and carbs from fiber-rich vegetables. This balance in macronutrients will slow down digestion time and keep your insulin from quickly peaking.

Lunch should be light or not too high in calories. Either soups or salads are perfect luncheon foods. The following soups are nutritious and contain good carbs: vegetable, black or navy bean, lentil, tomato, and chicken with vegetables. Soups to avoid are starchy or potato based.

For salads, try Greek, Vietnamese, or Thai options. Opt for romaine, endive, or mesclun rather than iceberg lettuce, which has fewer nutrients. Your salad should contain no more than 5 to 6 ingredients to control calories.

Make your own salads at home before leaving for work, or go to a salad bar. Don't pick prepared salads. Some salads appear weight-loss friendly and healthy, but that's deceptive—they could contain added sugar, salt, hydrogenated oils, croutons, or processed deli meats. You have to control what you put in your mouth. Of course, potato and macaroni salads are not on the Perfect 10 Diet. Dressing can add a lot of calories, too, so opt for a teaspoon of extra-virgin olive oil instead. Always stay away from low-fat salad dressings made with sugar or high-fructose corn syrup.

## Dinner

On the Perfect 10 Diet, dinner is the lightest meal of the day. Dinner should be eaten at a reasonable time, like 7:00 or 8:00 p.m. Try to eat dinner at least 2 or 3 hours before going to bed. I want you to enjoy it. I'd love for you to turn off the TV, relax, and really savor your dinner. Set the table, put some music on, and light some candles. Take the time to taste your food and appreciate the close of the day.

For dinner, you should still combine protein, fat, and carbs, but avoid refined and simple carbs altogether. If you're really hungry, it is okay to eat a dinner that is slightly higher in calories than lunch as long as you do not overdo it.

After dinner, you shouldn't eat anything else afterward. Never go to bed on a full stomach. In fact, you should go to bed feeling slightly hungry—

not starving, otherwise hunger pangs will wake you up. Just eat enough that you feel full, but not so full that you can barely move. Also allow at least 11 to 12 hours between dinner and breakfast.

You'll notice on the Perfect 10 Diet menu that the food choices are rich at times, but you don't have to eat a restaurant quality meal every single night. A small turkey or cheese sandwich is fine on the Perfect 10 Diet too. Salads are also an acceptable option for dinner. A rich entrée like chicken with a creamy sauce is allowed, but meals like this can add a lot of calories if you're trying to lose weight. Place sauces on the side, and just use a little to add some taste and help fill you up.

Since the Perfect 10 Diet is an eating plan for life, I know there will be times when you'll want to indulge in rich desserts. If you're still hungry after dinner and are in either of the first two stages of the diet, opt for fruit.

## What Snacks Can I Eat on the Perfect 10 Diet?

Even though you read throughout the book that you can have 1 or 2 snacks a day on the Perfect 10 Diet, they are optional. Why? Frequent snacks are appropriate only if you're hungry or very athletic. I know this goes against the advice of most nutritionists and diet gurus who tell you to eat every 3 hours, but I disagree.

If you need to eat every 3 hours, your metabolism or hormones are not in good shape. Yes, you may lose weight initially if you eat 5 small meals a day, but in no time at all, your weight will plateau. Why? Because even a low-calorie snack increases insulin release, and this inhibits weight loss. Also, HGH is suppressed by frequent meals, and that's not good. By spacing your meals at least 5 hours apart, you take advantage of the feast-fast cycle, which boosts HGH production.

I have designed some days on the Perfect 10 Diet with light meals for those of you who want to snack, but 3 meals a day with a big breakfast should do the job, and you should taper your calories throughout the day. Increasing the amount of time between meals allows proper weight loss to occur. The French, for example, who do not have the obesity problem others have, tend to stick to 3 meals a day, and they rarely snack. The more often you eat, the more likely you will consume more calories and get fat.

Yes, frequent meals are appropriate for people with diabetes or hypoglycemia or for athletes, but for the rest of us, 3 meals are plenty. I started this 3-meal approach years ago, and in time, I felt more energetic, and less hungry. Why? My insulin level stabilized instead of being all over the place every 3 hours. The less often I ate, the less often I became hungry or even thought of food. I snack no more than 3 to 4 times a week, and that's only on the days that I work out. My meals go down in calories throughout the day unless I am really hungry.

Does this mean you should never snack? Of course not. The idea of 3 square meals is just plain boring, and it sounds like being locked in prison. That's where snacks come in. Let's say you are meeting some friends after work or in a gathering that involves food, but it's not dinner time. Hey, have a snack. Really hungry? Had a good workout? Have a snack. Just remember that snacks can be the pitfall of any diet. So forget about snacks that come in packages. They are processed and filled with sugar, and they are detrimental to your health.

Think of healthy choices like:

- banana sprinkled with cocoa powder
- celery with some cream cheese
- coconut milk with some fruit
- dry roasted chick peas
- fruit alone, or with some cheese
- full-fat yogurt topped with fruits
- frosted grapes (grapes frozen for one hour)
- green peas
- olives with some feta cheese
- mashed avocados with some lime juice
- nut butter with some raw vegetables
- nuts (unsalted)
- red radishes
- sliced raw vegetables
- sunflower seeds (unsalted)

## Take Your Measurements

Before you begin the Perfect 10 Diet, use a tape measure to record your vital statistics. Weigh yourself and measure your chest, waist, and hips, and write down those numbers.

Divide your height in inches by 2; the number you get should be close to your ideal waist size. For example, if you're 6 feet tall, that's 72 inches. Divide by 2, and you'll get your target waist size, which is 36. This is just an average; you should shoot for 1 to 2 fewer inches. When you measure yourself again in 3 weeks, you'll be happy and proud of what you did, as the Perfect 10 Diet becomes your diet for life.

## What Should I Expect as I Begin the Perfect 10 Diet?

Everybody is different, and everybody who tries this diet will have a different starting point. Based on my experience, you can expect an average loss of 10 to 14 pounds in the first 3 weeks. You will also experience an increase in your energy level and stamina throughout the day, even though you've reduced your calories. As you continue on the Perfect 10 Diet, your complexion, blood pressure, concentration, hormones, and markers for heart disease, such as cholesterol, should all show a marked improvement.

## Shopping for the Perfect 10 Diet, Stage One

Before you start Stage One of the Perfect 10 Diet, I want you to have all the right food choices at your fingertips. Go to the supermarket and shop in a new way. I love Whole Foods and Trader Joe's, and that's where you should go. Costco is great, too. It has a wide variety of organic food at reasonable prices. Don't live in the city? Go to your local farmer's market—you may find pasture-fed chicken and raw milk.

How much food should you buy? For each day, buy at least five to nine servings of fruits and vegetables. One serving is a cup. One banana, a mango, and an apple count as two servings. Have enough eggs and other rich protein sources to meet your daily protein requirements. If you're shopping for a week, buy a dozen eggs, a pound or two of shrimp, two pieces of wild salmon, and one whole chicken. Always have nuts, organic milk, unsalted butter, olive oil, and cheese handy. Now you're ready to begin the transformation and the extreme makeover of your hormones, body, and health.

**Figure 7.3:** Shopping List for the Perfect 10 Diet, Stage One

VEGETABLES
Asparagus
Artichoke
Broccoli
Cucumber
Eggplant
Endive
Mixed greens
Onions
Parsley
Peppers
Romaine lettuce
Spinach
Scallions
Shallots
Zucchini

FRUITS
Apples
Avocados
Blueberries
Cantaloupe
Cherries
Coconut
Grapefruit
Grapes
Honeydew
Kiwis
Oranges
Mangoes
Peaches
Plums
Pomegranate
Strawberries
Tomatoes
Watermelon

PROTEIN
Beans
Chicken
Clams
Crabs
Duck
Eggs
Fish
Lobsters
Liver
Mushrooms
Oysters
Shrimp
Turkey
Tuna (canned in water or olive oil)

FAT
Butter
Coconut milk
Ghee
Goose fat
Flaxseed oil
Nut butters
Nuts
Olive oil
Palm oil
Safflower oil (nonhydrogenated)

DAIRY
Cheese
Heavy cream
Half and half
Kefir
Milk
Whipped cream (unsweetened)

BEVERAGES
Decaffeinated tea
Green tea
Regular tea
Water (glass bottles)

## Stage One

Welcome your new metabolism. Remember, Stage One will last 3 weeks. Each day, you'll eat 3 meals. You also have the option to have 1 to 2 snacks, but only if you're hungry. Again, Stage One allows no grains. This means that you will not eat any bread, rice, or pasta. Although this may seem hard, you will lose such a significant amount of weight during this stage that you'll be glad you eliminated grains. Remember, no alcohol is allowed.

### A Typical Day on the Perfect 10 Diet, Stage One

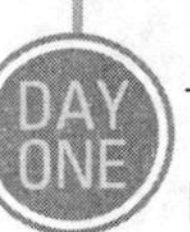


**BREAKFAST:** Fruit Salad and Cottage Cheese
**OPTIONAL MIDMORNING SNACK:** Vegetable Juice
**LUNCH:** Grilled Shrimp and a Side Salad
**OPTIONAL MIDAFTERNOON SNACK:** Lettuce with Guacamole
**DINNER:** Grilled Chicken Breast with Mixed Vegetables

### A Typical Day on the Perfect 10 Diet, Stage One

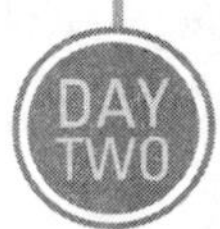


**BREAKFAST:** Full-Fat Yogurt with Sliced Kiwis
**OPTIONAL MIDMORNING SNACK:** A Few Chick Peas
**LUNCH:** Baked Calamari with Mixed Green Vegetables
**OPTIONAL MIDAFTERNOON SNACK:** Celery with 2 Teaspoons Cream Cheese
**DINNER:** Butternut Squash Soup

## A Typical Day on the Perfect 10 Diet, Stage One

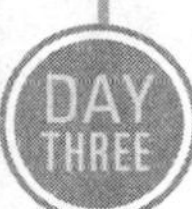


**BREAKFAST:** 3 Boiled Eggs and 2 Slices of Cheese

**OPTIONAL MIDMORNING SNACK:** 2 to 3 Pieces of Turkey

**LUNCH:** Arugula Salad with Extra-Virgin Olive Oil

**OPTIONAL MIDAFTERNOON SNACK:** ½ Cup Fruit with 2 Teaspoons Unsweetened Whipped Cream

**DINNER:** Grilled Tuna with Mixed Greens

## A Typical Day on the Perfect 10 Diet, Stage One

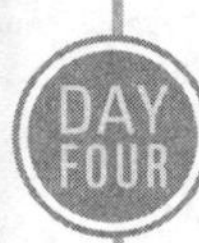


**BREAKFAST:** 1 Cup Mashed Chick Peas on Lettuce

**OPTIONAL MIDMORNING SNACK:** Several Olives with 2 Teaspoons Feta Cheese

**LUNCH:** Chicken Marsala

**OPTIONAL MIDAFTERNOON SNACK:** ½ Cantaloupe

**DINNER:** Grilled Shrimp with Green Peppers and Tomatoes

## A Typical Day on the Perfect 10 Diet, Stage One

**BREAKFAST:** Organic Full-Fat Yogurt with Berries

**OPTIONAL MIDMORNING SNACK:** 1 Orange

**LUNCH:** Grilled Chicken on Watercress

**OPTIONAL MIDAFTERNOON SNACK:** Few Unsalted or Lightly Salted Sunflower Seeds

**DINNER:** Tuna Niçoise Salad

DAY SIX

### A Typical Day on the Perfect 10 Diet, Stage One

**BREAKFAST:** Egg Omelet and 2 Nitrite-Free Turkey Sausages
**OPTIONAL MIDMORNING SNACK:** 1 or 2 Small Bites of Reduced-Sugar Dark Chocolate
**LUNCH:** Red Snapper with Steamed Zucchini
**OPTIONAL MIDAFTERNOON SNACK:** ½ Cup Unsalted Nuts
**DINNER:** Lentil Soup

DAY SEVEN

### A Typical Day on the Perfect 10 Diet, Stage One

**BREAKFAST:** Berries Dipped in Coconut Milk
**OPTIONAL MIDMORNING SNACK:** ½ Cup Red Radishes
**LUNCH:** Tropical Salad (½ Cup Fruit on a Bed of Lettuce, Tomatoes, and Pineapples)
**OPTIONAL MIDAFTERNOON SNACK:** 1 Stir-Fried Portobello Mushroom
**DINNER:** Chicken Shawarma with a Middle Eastern Salad

## Stage Two

Hallelujah. Bread and rice are back. Did you survive your first 3 weeks on the Perfect 10 Diet without whole grains? See, it wasn't that difficult. You can also add whole grains to your daily diet in moderation (1 to 3 servings). Again, the amount of grains you eat will depend upon your metabolism level.

Start with 1 serving of whole grains each day for 4 weeks. As you go along, you will get an idea how much you can really eat. A muscular man who has a physical job may be able to have 2 to 3 servings a day, but a small-framed, sedentary woman may only be able to have 1 serving.

I still encourage you to eat 3 meals daily, with 1 to 2 optional snacks only if you get hungry between meals. If you want to drink alcohol, do so in very small amounts—perhaps a glass of an organic red wine once in a while.

The duration of this stage will depend upon your goal weight, your adherence to the diet, and your exercise level. I don't want you to beat yourself up if you fall off the diet during this longer stage and temporarily go back to your old eating habits. Mistakes happen, and you're only human. Write down your goals, and don't weigh yourself more than once or twice a week. Don't have unrealistic expectations of rapid weight loss. It takes only a few seconds to eat one little cookie, and half an hour on the treadmill to burn off its calories.

For Stage Two, use the same shopping list for Stage One, but now add oatmeal, granola, wild rice, whole-wheat pasta, or a loaf of bread. With one serving a day, a loaf of bread, two boxes of oatmeal, or a box of whole-wheat pasta is enough for a whole week. I've found the following brands to be reputable when it comes to grains:

- Back to Nature
- Bear Naked
- Bob's Red Mill
- Dorset Cereals
- Eden Organic
- Food for Life
- Health Valley
- Lundberg
- Kashi
- Nature's Path
- The Baker
- Whole Foods brands, such as 365
- World of Grains

DAY ONE

## A Typical Day on the Perfect 10 Diet, Stage Two

(A day on the Perfect 10 Diet with 1 serving of grain)

**BREAKFAST:** 1 Cup Slow-Cooked Oatmeal with ½ Glass of Organic Full-Fat Milk

**OPTIONAL MIDMORNING SNACK:** 2 Pieces of Salmon

**LUNCH:** Tuna and Artichoke Salad

**OPTIONAL MIDAFTERNOON SNACK:** ½ Cup Berries

**DINNER:** Athenian Salad (Lettuce, Tomatoes, Scallions, and Feta Cheese)

DAY TWO

## A Typical Day on the Perfect 10 Diet, Stage Two

(A day on the Perfect 10 Diet with 1 serving of grain)

**BREAKFAST:** Vanilla Ricotta Crème

**OPTIONAL MIDMORNING SNACK:** 1 Apple

**LUNCH:** Savory Shrimp and a Side Salad

**OPTIONAL MIDAFTERNOON SNACK:** A Few Olives and 2 Teaspoons Cottage Cheese

**DINNER:** Bean Soup with 1 Slice Rye Bread

DAY THREE

## A Typical Day on the Perfect 10 Diet, Stage Two

(A day on the Perfect 10 Diet with 1 serving of grain)

**BREAKFAST:** A 2-Egg Omelet with 1 Slice Rye Bread

**OPTIONAL MIDMORNING SNACK:** Blueberries Dipped in Reduced-Sugar Dark Organic Chocolate

**LUNCH:** Indian Mulligatawny Soup (Lentil, Curry, and Coconut Milk)

**OPTIONAL MIDAFTERNOON SNACK:** Fruit Salad

**DINNER:** Moroccan Grilled Chicken with Mixed Vegetables

## A Typical Day on the Perfect 10 Diet, Stage Two

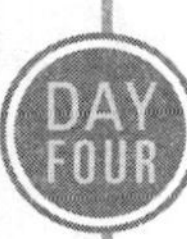

(A day on the Perfect 10 Diet with 2 servings of grains)

**BREAKFAST:** Rye Toast (2 Slices) with Macadamia Butter or Unsalted Butter

**OPTIONAL MIDMORNING SNACK:** ½ Cantaloupe

**LUNCH:** Mediterranean-Style Rabbit

**OPTIONAL MIDAFTERNOON SNACK:** ½ Cup Green Peas

**DINNER:** Chicken Liver with Stir-Fried Mushrooms and Onions

## A Typical Day on the Perfect 10 Diet, Stage Two

(A typical day on the Perfect 10 Diet with 2 servings of grains)

**BREAKFAST:** Tomato Frittata

**OPTIONAL MIDMORNING SNACK:** Fruit and Cheese Platter

**LUNCH:** Asian-Style Chicken, Mixed Vegetables, and 2 Scoops Wild Rice

**OPTIONAL MIDAFTERNOON SNACK:** Strawberry Parfait (½ Cup Strawberries, ½ Cup Yogurt)

**DINNER:** Grilled Tuna on Mixed Greens

## A Typical Day on the Perfect 10 Diet, Stage Two

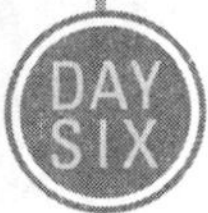

(A day on the Perfect 10 Diet with 3 servings of grains)

**BREAKFAST:** 1 Cup Whole-Grain Cereal or Granola with No Added Sugar, Unsweetened Almond Milk, 1 Teaspoon Chopped Walnuts, Dash of Nutmeg, and 1 Teaspoon Flaxseed Oil

**OPTIONAL MIDMORNING SNACK:** Lettuce with Guacamole Dipping

**LUNCH:** Clams and Shrimp Stir-Fried in Extra-Virgin Olive Oil

**OPTIONAL MIDAFTERNOON SNACK:** 1 Apple with 1 Slice Full-Fat Cheese

**DINNER:** Turkey on Whole-Wheat or Rye Bread (2 Slices) and a Small Side Salad

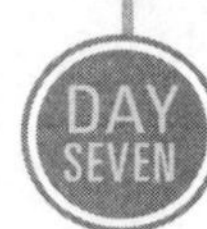


### A Typical Day on the Perfect 10 Diet, Stage Two

(A typical day on the Perfect 10 Diet with 3 servings of grains)

**BREAKFAST:** Vegetable Quiche

**OPTIONAL MIDMORNING SNACK:** ½ Cup Unsalted Nuts of Your Choice

**LUNCH:** Shrimp with 1 Cup Cooked Wild Rice

**OPTIONAL MIDAFTERNOON SNACK:** Fruit Salad

**DINNER:** Tuna on Whole-Wheat Bread (2 Slices) with Lettuce and Tomatoes

## Stage Three

Light the lights, a drum roll, please. It's showtime, and it's time to flaunt it: you've reached your desired weight. Congratulations! My hat's off to you. You've lost the excess weight, and you're ready to start Stage Three. Of course, the final stage of the Perfect 10 Diet can be followed right from the start if you're not looking to lose weight and just want to eat healthy.

You can eat more grains than in Stage Two (up to 4 servings a day). But be careful. Please don't go back to your old eating habits. Remember, you can go back to Stage One at any time if you start to gain weight.

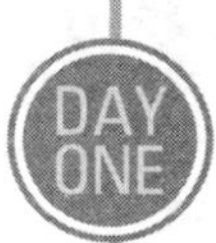


### A Typical Day on the Perfect 10 Diet, Stage Three (Life Maintenance)

(A typical day on the Perfect 10 Diet with 4 servings of grains)

**BREAKFAST:** 1 Cup Natural Whole-Grain Cereal with Almond Milk

**OPTIONAL MIDMORNING SNACK:** 1 Orange

**LUNCH:** Poached Salmon with a Spinach Salad and 1 Scoop Wild Rice

**OPTIONAL MIDAFTERNOON SNACK:** 2 Teaspoons Foie Gras

**DINNER:** Grilled Rosemary Chicken with 2 Scoops Whole-Wheat Pasta

## A Typical Day on the Perfect 10 Diet, Stage Three

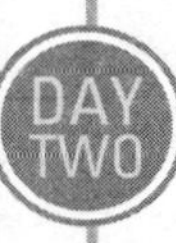


(A typical day on the Perfect 10 Diet with 4 servings of grains)

**BREAKFAST:** 1 Cup Slow-Cooked Oatmeal

**OPTIONAL MIDMORNING SNACK:** Berries in Coconut Milk

**LUNCH:** Duck with Mixed Vegetables and 1 Scoop Wild Rice

**OPTIONAL MIDAFTERNOON SNACK:** A Few Pistachios Dipped in Reduced-Sugar Dark Organic Chocolate

**DINNER:** Tuna, Whole-Wheat Bread (Two Slices), and a Side Salad

## A Typical Day on the Perfect 10 Diet, Stage Three

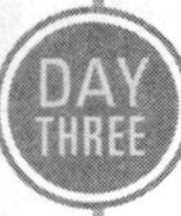


(A typical day on the Perfect 10 Diet with 2 servings of grains and a rich dessert)

**BREAKFAST:** Omelet with Salmon

**OPTIONAL MIDMORNING SNACK:** 1 Bar of Reduced-Sugar Chocolate

**LUNCH:** Shrimp Jambalaya

**OPTIONAL MIDAFTERNOON SNACK:** Mixed Fruit Salad

**DINNER:** Puerto Rican Pigeon Pea Stew with 2 Scoops Brown Rice

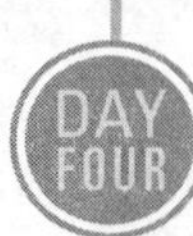


## A Typical Day on the Perfect 10 Diet, Stage Three

(A typical day on the Perfect 10 Diet with 4 servings of grains and some red meat. It's okay to eat red meat once every 3 weeks.)

BREAKFAST: 1 Orange and 2 Slices Multigrain Bread with Butter

OPTIONAL MIDMORNING SNACK: ½ Cup Chick Peas

LUNCH: Lemony Fish with Zucchini in Olive Oil with 2 Scoops Wild Rice

OPTIONAL MIDAFTERNOON SNACK: Sliced Nectarines with 4 Ounces Vanilla Yogurt

DINNER: Marinated Organic London Broil or a Filet Mignon with Grilled Asparagus

## A Typical Day on the Perfect 10 Diet, Stage Three

(A typical day on the Perfect 10 Diet with fewer grains, but with starchy vegetables. You should get some exercise immediately after eating the potatoes so the metabolized sugar won't mess up your hormones.)

BREAKFAST: 2 Slices Multigrain Bread with Macadamia Butter

OPTIONAL MIDMORNING SNACK: 1 Small Latte with Organic Milk

LUNCH: Mediterranean Salad

OPTIONAL MIDAFTERNOON SNACK: ½–1 Cup Herb-Roasted Red Potatoes

DINNER: Fish Poached in Champagne

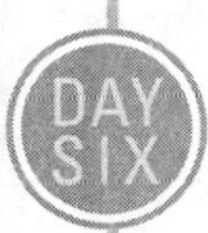


### A Typical Day on the Perfect 10 Diet, Stage Three

(A typical day on the Perfect 10 Diet with a return to Stage One principles, or no grains, if you start to gain weight)

BREAKFAST: 1 Cup Fruit

OPTIONAL MIDMORNING SNACK: ½ Cup Nuts of Your Choice

LUNCH: Baked Shrimp with a Side Salad

OPTIONAL MIDAFTERNOON SNACK: Broccoli Rabe (Cooked in Extra-Virgin Olive Oil)

DINNER: Sashimi (Japanese Fish without the Rice)

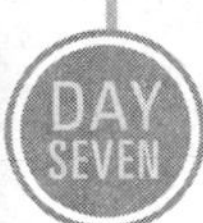


### A Typical Day on the Perfect 10 Diet, Stage Three

(A typical day on the Perfect 10 Diet with 2 servings of grains and an occasional rich dessert)

BREAKFAST: Egg Omelet with 1 Nitrite-Free Turkey Sausage on Rye Toast (2 Slices)

OPTIONAL MIDMORNING SNACK: 1 Pear

LUNCH: Thai Coconut Shrimp

OPTIONAL MIDAFTERNOON SNACK: ½ Slice Cheesecake Made with Agave

DINNER: Baked Chicken Wings with Blue Cheese Dressing

## The Perfect 10 Diet Tips

1. Write down your weight goals and keep a food diary or journal.
2. Set a time frame to lose the weight you can adhere to, and stay disciplined.
3. Always eat organic, natural, nutrient-rich, and unprocessed food.
4. Always eat a big breakfast: it's *that* important.
5. Try not to skip meals, which can lead to overeating.
6. Eat just 3 meals a day, and do not snack every single day.
7. Make exercise part of your daily routine.

8. Always have nuts in your bag. They're a perfect snack if you are hungry.
9. If one of your colleagues is buying lunch, choose and always ask for what you want in advance.
10. Never eat on the go. Take the time to enjoy your food.

## *Martha's Story in Her Own Words*

I used to be rather thin, weighing about 115 pounds when I was 20. After getting married, I stopped caring as much. I was working and trying to start a family. A little at a time, the pounds started to add up. After having 2 babies, I never dropped the extra weight I had gained. Within 5 years, I had gained more than 60 pounds. I tried all the "brand-name" diets out there, but I was never successful. Then, I tried a popular weight-management plan where I got my food delivered, but the food was horrible.

Eventually, I gave up. I felt unhealthy and ugly as I started eating more and more and cared less and less; I was in a downward spiral. Then, I saw Dr. Aziz on TV, and that changed my life. The part that caught my attention was when Dr. Aziz explained how these diets I'd been on had messed up my hormones. It's no wonder I had no control over my appetite. I went to see him, and my views were turned upside down. The Perfect 10 Diet gave me the freedom to eat what I wanted, anyplace, anytime, and with little restrictions. This is exactly what busy people need. I lost 40 pounds, and I am finally on my way to getting my old body back again.

## The Perfect 10 Diet Journal

This convenient journal will assist you in reaching your goals. Use the journal in Stage One every day to keep you motivated. Make several copies and keep them in a folder.

## DAY JOURNAL (STAGE ONE)

Name: ________________ Day ____ of 21 Today's Date: ____________

Breakfast: ________________________________________________

________________________________________________

________________________________________________

Optional Midmorning Snack: ________________________________

________________________________________________

________________________________________________

Lunch: ________________________________________________

________________________________________________

________________________________________________

Optional Midafternoon Snack: ________________________________

________________________________________________

________________________________________________

Dinner: ________________________________________________

________________________________________________

________________________________________________

Exercise: ________________________________________________

________________________________________________

________________________________________________

Water: ________________________________________________

________________________________________________

________________________________________________

How Many Snacks Did I Eat Today? ____________________________

TODAY'S PLAN: ☐ Accomplished ☐ Not Accomplished

## DAY JOURNAL (STAGE TWO)

Name: _______________ Day ____ of 21 Today's Date: ____________

Breakfast: ______________________________________________

______________________________________________

______________________________________________

Optional Midmorning Snack: ______________________________

______________________________________________

______________________________________________

Lunch: ______________________________________________

______________________________________________

______________________________________________

Optional Midafternoon Snack: ____________________________

______________________________________________

______________________________________________

Dinner: ______________________________________________

______________________________________________

______________________________________________

Exercise: ______________________________________________

______________________________________________

Water: ______________________________________________

______________________________________________

______________________________________________

How Many Snacks Did I Eat Today? ____________________

Number of Grain Servings Eaten Today? ________________

Did I Drink Any Alcohol? ____________________________

TODAY'S PLAN: ☐ Accomplished ☐ Not Accomplished

CHAPTER 8

# Being a Savvy Consumer

When you eat the food that your body was designed to recognize, you support your hormones. In turn, you lose weight. But it's so easy to mindlessly consume chemicals. Processed food leaves your body confused about what to do with overloaded chemicals. Too much processed food leaves your body impaired, and this will ultimately damage your metabolism. These toxins have not only made us fat; they've made us sick. Our hormones have turned against us.

I often get food as gifts from colleagues, friends, and patients, even though they all know I'm on this diet 24/7. It's very generous of them and I know they mean well, but I simply do not eat any processed food. Most of the time, it goes in the garbage. Let me give you an example.

One day a colleague sent me a "healthy" bag full of treats in gratitude for taking care of his wife in the hospital. I picked up the first item: dark chocolate. Don't I love that? I looked at the ingredients. Sugar, high-fructose corn syrup, artificial colors, and partially hydrogenated oil. Garbage. The next item was turkey bacon. Ingredients artificial colors and flavors, preservatives, nitrites, and salt. Garbage. What a waste of money! Then, I always get a call asking if I enjoyed it. I always say it was delicious just to be courteous, but I would not touch this toxic food with a 10-foot pole.

But it is impossible for me to ask you to eat organic food all the time. Even if you can afford it, there will be times when you will run to your local supermarket or deli to get something to eat fast. Or maybe you'll get a "healthy" gift like the one I just described. Either one of these scenarios can sabotage your diet in no time flat. Hopefully, I've convinced you not to eat any processed food. Trust no one. If it's in a box, carefully read the label for all ingredients.

Being a savvy consumer is about reading the ingredients listed on processed food. I won't ask you to do anything else. Isn't this a simple and less complicated way to live? You don't need to carry a calculator or do any complicated math on the Perfect 10 Diet. I just want you to exercise and eat real food and natural fat—that's it.

The reason behind this approach is that all the food we eat can be used for energy or to repair cells. It's the artificial ingredients that can be harmful to our health and make us gain weight. In an attempt to make cheap, addictive foods that last forever on a shelf, food manufacturers load their products with sugar, high-fructose corn syrup, and chemicals our grandparents never ate. Processed food has little to no nutritional value and can lead to vitamin deficiencies. It's often loaded with colors, dyes, and artificial flavors to give it a near-natural taste. It often contains partially hydrogenated oils—deadly trans fats—to make it last longer on supermarket shelves. These additives are foreign substances the body doesn't know how to handle. In turn, all that junk creates a poisonous atmosphere for our glands and messes up hormones. There is no doubt in my mind that many types of cancer are related to these additives. There hasn't been nearly enough research to determine the cumulative effect of these additives on health.

While medical authorities advise the public to count saturated fat grams and limit the milligrams of cholesterol, I disagree with this advice. Recent research has rebuffed this myth. Your body makes plenty of saturated fat quite efficiently to store energy. The amount of saturated fat or cholesterol milligrams present in food you eat on a daily basis is irrelevant to your health. What you *should* avoid are chemicals, artificial dyes, partially hydrogenated oils, nitrites, sugar, and other added ingredients. Just because the label says it's good for you doesn't mean it really is.

## 1. Do Not Buy Low-Fat or Fat-Free Products

Low-fat and fat-free products are everywhere, but these products are processed. They are full of sugar and high-fructose corn syrup. They will raise your insulin levels, make you hungry, and prompt weight gain. Fat-free products will also negatively affect your cholesterol by raising your triglycerides and lowering your good cholesterol (C-HDL) level. Both are bad for your cardiovascular health when headed in these wrong directions. These products are processed and should have no place in your diet.

## 2. Do Not Buy Fat-Free Dairy Products

Low-fat and fat-free dairy are missing the good fats that help you lose weight. They mess up your insulin and sex hormones. Fat-free yogurt is loaded with sugar and high-fructose corn syrup. The added sugar will make you hungry, and prompt weight gain. Excess sugar will also negatively affect your cholesterol by raising your triglycerides and lowering your good cholesterol (C-HDL) levels. Again, both are bad for your cardiovascular health when headed in these wrong directions.

## 3. Do Not Buy Foods Made with Refined Polyunsaturated Oils or Hydrogenated Fats

Products made with refined polyunsaturated oils or hydrogenated and partially hydrogenated fats are toxic. They will negatively affect your health and lead to disease. Partially hydrogenated oils translate into trans fats. Trans fats equal disturbed hormones, clogged arteries, and cancer. To add insult to injury, many low-fat and fat-free products contain trans fats. Sugar and trans fats are a deadly combination when you include them in your diet in any amounts.

## 4. Do Not Buy Products that Contain Ingredients You Can't Pronounce

Ever heard of butylated hydroxyanisole (BHA)? How about butylated hydroxytoluene (BHT)? The rule of thumb on the Perfect 10 Diet is that if you can't pronounce the ingredients, leave the item on the shelf. These are most likely man-made chemicals that have unknown long-term health effects. BHA and BHT are found in baked goods and increase the risk of cancer. The list also includes, but is not limited to, brominated vegetable oil, hydrolyzed vegetable protein, propyl gallate, and potassium bromate. You may be wondering how you're going to remember the names of these harmful ingredients. But that's exactly my point: you don't have to remember these names at all. Just avoid products containing ingredients you can't pronounce or don't recognize regardless of any health claim or medical endorsement on the packaging.

## 5. Do Not Buy Low-Carb Products with Soy Protein Isolate

Do you like sugar-free foods and low-carb goodies? These products are the latest food gimmick being pushed on the public. While many of these foods contain less sugar, many contain soy protein isolate. I previously discussed that soy protein contains MSG, a neurotoxin, as well as nitrites. Nitrites cause cancer. Low-carb products also contain chemicals, sugar alcohols, and partially hydrogenated oils. All of these mess up your hormones and are toxic to your body.

## 6. Do Not Buy Food Made with Natural and Artificial Flavors

When a food item contains this message on its label, it means it contains chemicals. Chemicals are added to give food a near-natural taste and a prolonged shelf life. No one knows what these chemicals are except the food manufacturers themselves. If you're going to eat it, you deserve to know what it is. Avoid any food that includes natural and artificial flavors.

## 7. Do Not Buy Food Items that Contain Unspecified Spices

When the average consumer sees the word "spices" in fine print, he or she may be intrigued, believing the food is tasty and flavorful. However, many chemicals found in processed food are allowed to be called spices under government regulations. These are not spices; instead, they're manmade chemicals. If the food contains garlic, pepper, or other real spices, it will say so on the package.

## 8. Do Not Buy Products Containing Sodium Nitrites

Processed meats such as deli cold cuts, bacon, Canadian bacon, sausage, hot dogs, and corned beef contain nitrites. Many frozen entrées do as well. The presence of nitrites, even in small amounts, has a strong correlation with an increased risk for developing cancer. I realize these protein choices are sometimes advertised as meeting the American Heart Association's criteria of a diet low in saturated fats, and that they are encouraged by low-carb diet gurus who sell millions of books. In reality, it is still baloney. Take action. Do you want to drop the pounds and have a perfect 10 body, or do you simply want to drop dead? No ham, bacon, or Canadian bacon is allowed on the Perfect 10 Diet.

## 9. Do Not Buy Products with Monosodium Glutamate (MSG)

Many people are aware that MSG can cause headaches and seizures, the so-called Chinese restaurant syndrome. But many do not realize MSG can also make you gain weight. If the label lists spices, natural flavorings, citric acid, or anything hydrolyzed or autolyzed, it probably contains MSG. Like I said, MSG is a neurotoxin. It is present in frozen entrées, commercial salad dressings, and bottled sauces, and you should completely avoid it.

## 10. Do Not Buy Products with Artificial Sweeteners

Artificial sweeteners found in diet sodas and low-carb products have no calories, but artificial sweeteners are more dangerous than sugar. Why? Because research done on animals indicates that artificial sweeteners may lead to more weight gain than eating sugar. NutraSweet and Equal also contain aspartame. When ingested, one of aspartame's ingredients, methyl alcohol, converts into formaldehyde, a deadly neurotoxin. Aspartame causes cancer in rats. Sweet'N Low is no better. It contains a coal tar compound. Splenda was invented to kill ants. Artificial sweeteners will make you crave sugar and will make your body highly acidic. It is commonly believed that cancer cells thrive in an acidic environment. No artificial sweeteners are allowed at all on the Perfect 10 Diet.

By now, I hope you get the picture. Don't trust anyone but yourself. The food manufacturers have one goal, and that is to make profits. They have to produce food with the cheapest ingredients, preserve it for the longest shelf life, and sell it at the highest profit. Have no faith in government agencies, either. Labels are designed to fool you into thinking you are making healthy choices. As a result, many of the products that you think are wholesome are anything but. Stay clear of all processed foods, and always choose whole, organic, and fresh foods.

CHAPTER 9

# The Perfect 10 Diet in Your Daily Life

A successful diet must be a balanced diet. However, achieving optimal balance or perfection isn't a static state. Who among us is really disciplined all the time? There will be days when you'll make healthy choices, and others when you won't. Being able to embrace the good days and keep focused on the goal of balanced, healthy choices will sustain good health.

In order to help you navigate the ebbs and flows of eating in the real world, I have divided foods up into 4 major groups so you make healthy and smart choices at all times. If you forget what's good and bad from this book, just ask yourself if the food was around 200 years ago. If it didn't exist then, you shouldn't eat it. The four major groups include:

1. Foods that are very healthy and that you should eat on a daily basis to prevent disease
2. Foods that are healthy and that you can include in your diet
3. Foods that are moderately healthy but that can be dangerous when eaten frequently or to excess
4. Foods that are unhealthy and dangerous and that should be avoided at all times

## 1. Foods That Are Very Healthy and That You Should Eat on a Daily Basis to Prevent Disease

Foods in this category keep you healthy and free from diseases. I realize that the food choices may be harder to find in your local supermarket, but this food contains all the nutrients that your body needs. It's full of the vitamins, minerals, enzymes, and amino acids you need for optimal health. Very healthy food is, of course, mostly from organic sources.

### VERY HEALTHY CARBOHYDRATES

- Fiber-rich vegetables (raw, organic, unsprayed, and non–genetically modified)
- Organic vegetable juices (all vegetables except carrots and beets, as they rapidly break down into sugar)
- Organic whole grains, such as rye and pumpernickel bread and noninstant oatmeal (in Stages Two and Three)
- Fruits (organic, unsprayed, non–genetically modified, and ripe)

### VERY HEALTHY PROTEIN

- All pasture-fed, organically raised fowls (chicken, duck, and turkey)
- Eggs (from pasture-fed chicken and high in omega-3 fatty acids)
- Fish (deep-water ocean fish, not farm-raised fish, and with no added colors)
- Organic legumes (except genetically modified soy)
- Organic organ meats
- Organic mushrooms
- Ocean-caught shellfish (not farm raised)

### VERY HEALTHY FATS

- Organic flaxseed oil
- Organic ghee
- Organic extra-virgin coconut oil and coconut milk
- Monounsaturated oils (cold-pressed, extra-virgin olive oil, avocado oil, macadamia oil)
- Nuts (raw and unsalted)
- Raw organic butter from grass-fed cows

#### VERY HEALTHY DAIRY

- Full-fat, raw organic goat and cow dairy from reputable sources (in small amounts)
- Kefir

### 2. Foods That Are Healthy and That You Can Include in Your Diet

These foods are not as nutrient dense, but are still healthful. You can still eat food from this category on a daily basis, and rest assured that you're providing your body with high-quality food.

#### HEALTHY CARBOHYDRATES

- Nonorganic and non–genetically modified vegetables (without sprayed insecticides)
- Fiber-rich vegetables (nonorganic or canned with no added sugar, salt, or preservatives)
- Nonorganic and non–genetically modified whole fruits (without sprayed insecticides)

#### HEALTHY PROTEIN

- Farm-raised fish (with no added artificial colors)
- Organic poultry
- Eggs from organically raised poultry
- Preservative-free deli turkey

#### HEALTHY FATS

- Nonorganic coconut oil
- Nonorganic ghee
- Unsalted butter from nonorganic sources
- Olive oil

#### HEALTHY DAIRY

- Full-fat, organic, pasteurized dairy (in small amounts)

## 3. Foods That Are Moderately Healthy but That Can Be Dangerous when Eaten Frequently or to Excess

Food in this category may be incorporated into your diet, but you should not eat it on a daily basis, as it has been linked to disease when eaten frequently or to excess.

### MODERATELY HEALTHY CARBOHYDRATES

- Starchy vegetables in small amounts (such as potatoes, which are high on the glycemic index and can lead to a spike in insulin levels if the sugar is not used)
- Genetically modified fruits
- Genetically modified vegetables

### MODERATELY HEALTHY PROTEIN

- Red meat, pork, and lamb (organically fed animals are better for your health than farm raised)
- Organic non–genetically modified soy
- Large fish (may contain mercury)

### MODERATELY HEALTHY FAT

- Peanuts, in small amounts
- Cold-pressed polyunsaturated oils in small amounts extracted with no chemicals (use only over salads, and do not use for cooking)

### MODERATELY HEALTHY DAIRY

- Nonorganic, full-fat, pasteurized dairy (may contain antibiotics or hormones)

## 4. Foods That Are Unhealthy and Dangerous and That Should Be Avoided at All Times

These are the foods that you should not eat at any time. Avoid food in this category, regardless of any health claims or medical endorsements.

### UNHEALTHY CARBOHYDRATES

- All products with sugar or high-fructose corn syrup, such as soda and condiments (jelly, ketchup, and barbecue sauce)
- All kinds of sugar with different names (dextrose, molasses, honey, maple syrup, or maltose)
- All carbonated beverages
- Bleached and unbleached white flour and its products (cakes, refined cereals, crackers, and all low-fat and fat-free baked products)
- Fruit juices with added sugar

### UNHEALTHY PROTEIN

- All nitrite-containing products (bacon, Canadian bacon, corned beef, ham, hot dogs, and sausage)
- Imitation shellfish
- Deep-fried chicken and fish
- Frozen entrées with preservatives, soybean oil, or partially hydrogenated oil
- Low-carb snacks and shakes made with soy protein isolate

### UNHEALTHY FAT

- All refined polyunsaturated oils (when used for cooking and consumed in excess)
- Polyunsaturated oils heated several times, such as in the fast-food industry
- All rancid, monounsaturated or polyunsaturated oils
- All hydrogenated or partially hydrogenated fat and oils
- All salad dressings containing soybean oil or partially hydrogenated oil
- Animal fat from nonorganic sources (contains toxins, pesticides, and hormones)
- Mayonnaise made with soybean oil
- Margarine (hydrogenated and non-hydrogenated)
- Vegetable shortening

### UNHEALTHY DAIRY

- All fat-free and reduced-fat dairy
- Ice cream and frozen yogurt with added sugar
- Powdered milk with partially hydrogenated oil
- Vegetarian cheese made with soy protein isolate or partially hydrogenated oil

## Rules to Follow on the Perfect 10 Diet

1. Eat food primarily from the first two groups.
2. Eat food sparingly from the third group.
3. Try to include more food from organic sources.
4. Eat plenty of fresh vegetables for lunch and dinner.
5. Eat whole fruits, with the skin intact.
6. Include more monounsaturated fats in your diet, especially from nuts and extra-virgin olive oil.
7. Do not fear saturated fats, such as butter. Use them frequently when cooking. They are good for your sex hormones and DHEA.
8. Do not cook in polyunsaturated oils (corn or vegetable oil) or any type of margarine.
9. Avoid processed food at all times.
10. Carefully read labels and avoid all processed foods, especially foods containing partially hydrogenated oil, trans fats, sugar, or high-fructose corn syrup.

CHAPTER 10

# Eating Out the Perfect 10 Diet Way

We work very long hours and spend very little downtime at home. As a result, we tend to eat out quite frequently. This leaves us dependent on others to prepare our meals. This could be both a blessing and a curse. The blessing is that you can experience and benefit from delicious and healthy cuisines from around the world; the curse is that it can be detrimental to your weight-loss efforts since you will have no control over the quality of ingredients or cooking methods.

But we all can make the best out of our lifestyles by being savvy consumers. Eating out the Perfect 10 Diet way can be an enjoyable and healthy experience. Eat any cuisine in the world on the Perfect 10 Diet, but keep in mind that you must:

- avoid sugar
- avoid refined carbohydrates
- avoid foods with any trans fats

Break some rules, if you have to, as long as you don't do it every day. Enjoy a healthy snack at home 30 minutes before you go out to eat. By doing this, you will decrease your hunger by the time you arrive at the restaurant. This way, you don't end up ordering an appetizer, an entrée, and dessert.

Also, choose a type of cuisine that suits whatever stage of the Perfect 10 Diet you are currently in (for example, no pasta-laden Italian restaurants in Stages One or Two). No Mexican restaurants either. Tortilla chips, burritos, and mixed drinks are all tough on hormones. Do not fear high-fat cuisines, such as French or Thai.

Once you get to the restaurant, immediately order a bottle of water and drink a full glass right away. Ask the waiter to remove any white bread from the table and to bring a dish of cheese and olives instead. If you have company, push the white bread to the side. Stay away from any breaded appetizers or entrées. Avoid all fried food choices, as they are probably loaded with killer trans fats.

If you have your heart set on a steak and haven't eaten red meat for a while, go ahead and enjoy it, but have it cooked rare or medium rare. Regardless of what you're ordering, always ask your waiter how your food is prepared. Do they use margarine, vegetable oils, or butter? If the waiter is uncertain, ask to speak to the chef. Don't be embarrassed, because it's your health we're talking about. Don't hesitate to request that a specific dish be cooked in butter rather than vegetable oil. Unless you speak up, no one will look after you. Also, if your selection comes with a side order, such as French fries or a potato, ask the waiter to replace it with a green salad or a side order of steamed vegetables.

An easy way to control portion size away from home is to order an appetizer for each person and share an entrée with a companion if he or she is also dieting. If you're still hungry, a delicious fruit cup can fill you up nicely. It is a good way to eat less and have a variety of healthy foods. If you aren't all that hungry, don't eat everything on your plate. Ask for a doggie bag and eat the rest the next day. Bon appétit!

## American Restaurants

American cuisine does not have to be unhealthy or fattening. Apart from fast food, we have an international diet. American restaurants offer a large selection of foods, so you're guaranteed to find something acceptable and satisfying.

| CHOOSE | INSTEAD OF |
|---|---|
| A vegetable omelet with decaffeinated coffee | Pancakes with bacon or sausage, home fries, and orange juice |
| Turkey burger, no bun (Stage One) or on whole-grain bread (Stages Two and Three) | Hamburger with bun and French fries |
| Broiled salmon with lemon and butter | Fried fish fillet and curly fries |
| Grilled jumbo shrimp salad | Pasta with shrimp and clams |
| Grilled chicken with a spinach salad | Chicken Parmesan on white bread |

## Chinese Restaurants

Chinese food is a favorite cuisine on the Perfect 10 Diet as long as the menu items are steamed or grilled. You can also choose an entrée that is stir-fried. This is acceptable since it's different from deep frying. This method sautés the food with a small amount of peanut oil and minimizes the risk of cholesterol oxidation. I am not a big fan of peanut oil, since it's refined and contains an excess of omega-6, but eating Chinese food cooked in peanut oil once in a while is fine as long as you don't overdo it. Always avoid food choices containing MSG, and skip all deep-fried foods on the menu.

| CHOOSE | INSTEAD OF |
|---|---|
| Chicken with steamed vegetables | Chicken fried rice |
| Garlic shrimp with mixed vegetables | Shrimp fried rice |
| Stir-fried chicken with garlic sauce and mixed vegetables | Fried chicken with fries |
| Chicken with mushrooms | Chicken lo mein (pasta) |

## Cuban Restaurants

Cuban food has been influenced by many traditions, owing to the complex history of the Caribbean area. Cuban cuisine is a fusion of Spanish, French, African, Arabic, Chinese, and Caribbean cuisines. Most of the food is sautéed or slow cooked over a low flame. Very little is deep-fried, and there are no heavy sauces. Many dishes use a sofrito as their base. The sofrito consists of an onion, green pepper, garlic, and oregano mixture quick-fried in olive oil. Meats and poultry are usually marinated in citrus juices. Vegetables in Cuban cuisine include yucca and malanga, which are very starchy and should be avoided on the Perfect 10 Diet.

| CHOOSE | INSTEAD OF |
|---|---|
| Coconut chicken | Egg-breaded steak |
| Spanish Oysters | Arroz moro (white rice and beans) |
| Cuban-style sea bass | Veal scallops with bacon |
| Shrimp casserole with sofrito | Cuban lamb shanks with crushed potatoes |

## Fast Food and Pizzerias

You don't have to skip fast-food chains or pizzerias on the Perfect 10 Diet, but avoid fried choices, please. Trans fats are notorious for messing up hormones. In fast-food chains, salads or chicken sandwiches without the bun or fries are acceptable. No diet can be perfect without pizza. Look for pizzerias offering vegetable-topped options made with whole-grain crusts in Stages Two and Three of the Perfect 10 Diet.

If they don't offer an option like that, stick with salads. The salad listed in the following table is perfectly acceptable on the Perfect 10 Diet, but skip the croutons and ask for olives instead. Avoid oil and vinegar as dressing, because vinegar is bad for your hormones and the oil might be hydrogenated. Instead, specifically request extra-virgin olive oil.

| CHOOSE | INSTEAD OF |
|---|---|
| Chicken salad with olives | Hamburger with fries |
| Grilled chicken sandwich on rye bread (Stages Two and Three ) | Chicken nuggets with fries |
| Vegetable pizza, without a crust, or whole-wheat pizza | Regular pizza |
| Chicken on a whole-wheat wrap (Stages Two and Three) | Chicken Parmesan on white bread |

## French Restaurants

Vegetable dishes are plentiful in French cooking. Many dishes, however, are made with heavy cream sauces. This is certainly acceptable, but I recommend that you ask for the sauce on the side so that you can keep calories in check. Several menu items also contain potatoes. Ask for an acceptable substitute, such as a green salad. French desserts? Sorry. Eat the fruit, but skip the starchy crusts and the jam.

| CHOOSE | INSTEAD OF |
|---|---|
| Escargots (snails) in butter | Charcuterie (cold cuts with nitrites) |
| Orange duck | Steak with French fries |
| Vegetable soup | Cream of potato soup |
| Chicken with mixed green salad | Chicken and a baked potato |
| Duck with mixed green vegetables | Duck with fries |
| Coquille St. Jacques | Crepe of any kind (refined flour) |

## Indian Restaurants

Who's afraid of rich Indian curry sauces made with ghee? On the Perfect 10 Diet, bring it on! Indian curry sauces are full of turmeric, a natural oxidant. Laboratory studies have found that turmeric inhibits the development of cataract, lymphoma, and both breast and colon cancer. Turmeric has also been found to lower cholesterol.

However, many Indian dishes come with white rice. If you want to make a big impression, don't be tempted. Ask for brown or basmati rice instead. Brown rice in Stage Two is perfectly acceptable in moderate amounts. Unlike other white rice varieties, basmati rice has a relatively low glycemic index, and you can eat small amounts in Stage Two on the Perfect 10 Diet. However, Indian breads, such as poori, paratha, and chappati, are made with refined flour and may be fried, so avoid them.

Many Indian restaurants now use refined vegetable oils instead of ghee (a clarified butter) for cooking, so be cautious. Ask your waiter or the chef how your food is prepared, and don't be shy about asking for it to be cooked in ghee. If they can't accommodate your wishes, stick to a grilled protein or vegetable choice with no cooking fat at all and a side salad.

| CHOOSE | INSTEAD OF |
|---|---|
| Roasted eggplant | Pakoras (fried vegetables) |
| Mulligatawny soup | Any refined white bread |
| Shrimp/mushroom tandoori | Shrimp biryani (a rice dish) |
| Chicken tandoori | Chicken biryani (a rice dish) |

## Italian Restaurants

Okay, if you really want to be thin and fit in the latest Milan fashion, reserve Italian restaurants for Stage Three only on the Perfect 10 Diet. White pasta is never an option on the Perfect 10 Diet, and temptations to cheat with what is forbidden can set you back in no time flat. If you must eat in Italian restaurants at any stage of the diet, make wise and healthy choices.

| CHOOSE | INSTEAD OF |
|---|---|
| Baked clams | Prosciutto (processed ham) |
| Grilled shrimp | Pasta with meatballs |
| Chicken Marsala | Veal Milanese (breaded and fried) |
| Stracciatella (Roman egg-drop soup) | Tortellini in broth |
| Zuppa fredda all menta (chilled mint soup) | Potato gnocchi |
| Baked salmon | Risotto |

## Japanese Restaurants

Seafood is the staple of the Japanese diet, and that makes their diet heart-healthy. Fish is also good for your thyroid and sex hormones. You will make a wise choice with most menu options, whether it's sashimi (fish without rice) or shellfish. However, some menu items, such as the popular California roll, contain imitation crab and white rice, both of which are fast-digesting carbohydrates. Avoid these as they are bad for your insulin. Limit tofu and other soy choices, since they may be genetically modified. Many Japanese people suffer from elevated blood pressure because of their high soy sauce consumption (soy sauce has too much sodium in it). Enjoy the fish, but skip the soy sauce.

| CHOOSE | INSTEAD OF |
|---|---|
| Fish with mixed vegetables | Fish teriyaki and white rice |
| Sashimi (raw fish without rice) | Sushi (raw fish and white rice) |
| Avocado or chicken salad | Beef noodle soup |
| Dragon roll (without the rice) | California roll |

## Middle Eastern Restaurants

Middle Eastern cuisine is vast, wide, and rich in its choices. In the United States, the term "Middle Eastern cuisine" is used arbitrarily to include Moroccan, Turkish, Persian, and Israeli cuisines. Many of these countries are not in the Middle East, but there are some similar dishes that the Perfect 10 Diet includes as part of the plan. Of course, white bread and pastries such as baklava and ladyfingers are never part of the Perfect 10 Diet.

| CHOOSE | INSTEAD OF |
|---|---|
| Chicken shawarma with a salad | Falafel on pita bread |
| Baked eggplant, tomatoes, and peppers | Kibbe (fried ground meat) on pita |
| Mixed grill with salad | Couscous |
| Fruit | Any heavy, sugar-loaded pastry |

## Mexican Restaurants

Many Mexican dishes are made with white flour. This means all tacos and tortillas should be avoided. Ask your waiter to substitute starchy tortillas with lettuce for your guacamole. Avoid frozen mixed drinks like margaritas and daiquiris, because they contain a lot of sugar.

| CHOOSE | INSTEAD OF |
|---|---|
| Grilled fish with vegetables | Any burrito |
| Jumbo shrimp with vegetables | Shrimp enchilada |
| Baked chicken wings with full-fat blue-cheese dressing | Chicken taco/nachos |

## Russian Restaurants

Russia is a country with long-lasting, frigid winters. The foods included are designed to give warmth. The essential components of Russian cuisine are those that provide more carbohydrates and fat rather than protein. Fresh fruits and vegetables are rarely used, so you have to be careful to ask your server for substitutions.

| CHOOSE | INSTEAD OF |
|---|---|
| Stuffed squash with mixed vegetables | Moscow chicken with rice |
| Duck liver with mango | Ham with potatoes |
| Chicken with prunes | Potato zrazy (potatoes, onion, and beef) |
| Chicken with vegetables | Ham in the dough |

## Starbucks, Dunkin' Donuts, and Similar Cafés

Starbucks, Dunkin' Donuts, and similar cafés offer many varieties of salads, eggs, and whole-grain bagels. However, I want you to steer clear of all pastries and doughnuts. Also, avoid specialty drinks such as chocolate mochas and frappuccinos. For example, a large Starbucks white chocolate mocha has 580 calories. These drinks not only contain massive amounts of sugar, but many also contain hydrogenated fats from the syrup. While these chains are making efforts to eliminate trans fats from their menu, this could take years. In addition to the trans fats, sugar is also toxic to your body. Choose decaffeinated teas or coffee, or once in a while, treat yourself to a small organic full-fat latte or a cappuccino.

| CHOOSE | INSTEAD OF |
|---|---|
| Decaffeinated coffee with or without small amounts of whole milk or half-and-half | Coffee with fat-free milk |
| Decaffeinated tea with lemon, or regular tea | Soy chai latte |
| Small organic latte | Chocolate mocha, frappuccino, or caramel macchiato with fat-free milk (sugar and hydrogenated fats) |
| Egg omelet | Croissant/doughnut or pastry (sugar and hydrogenated fats) |
| Whole-wheat bagel with butter or cream cheese (Stages Two and Three) | Plain bagel with jelly or honey |
| Fruit platter | Doughnut |

## Steak Houses

If you think you'll have to avoid steak houses on the Perfect 10 Diet, think again. With a variety of choices at these restaurants, you can still lose weight while enjoying a healthy meal. There are no deprivations on the Perfect 10 Diet: treat yourself to steak if you want, as long as it's only once in a while.

| CHOOSE | INSTEAD OF |
|---|---|
| Caesar salad | Fried onion rings |
| Shrimp cocktail | Fried calamari |
| Petite filet (8 ounces), cooked rare, with a side salad | Porterhouse steak (21 ounces), cooked well done, with French fries |
| Fresh seasonal berries | Apple crumb tart with vanilla ice cream |

## Thai Restaurants

Thai cuisine uses a range of exciting ingredients. Some common flavors include fresh ginger, garlic, mint, onions, and shallots. Some less common elements are lemon-grass, galangal, and chiles. Many of theses herbs and spices have medicinal properties. Many recipes are cooked in coconut oil, a healthy and rich saturated fat. However, you should always avoid any fried food and white rice. Thai desserts other than fruit are not usually served at a Thai meal; they're just for special occasions. If you must eat dessert in a Thai restaurant, choose mango with sticky rice and just eat the fruit.

| CHOOSE | INSTEAD OF |
|---|---|
| Shrimp in coconut curry | Shrimp pad Thai (noodles) |
| Chicken in coconut curry with bamboo shoots | Chicken fried rice |
| Fish with mixed veggies | Fried fish tempura |
| Thai salad | Pork/sausage fried rice |

## Vietnamese Restaurants

The emphasis in Vietnamese cuisine is on vegetables, fresh herbs, and dipping sauces. The Vietnamese have a number of vegetarian dishes influenced by Buddhist beliefs. The most common meats in Vietnamese cuisine are chicken, shrimp, and pork. Duck and beef are less common.

| CHOOSE | INSTEAD OF |
|---|---|
| Mussels with coconut sauce | Spring roll |
| Shrimp with ginger and scallions | Deep-fried shrimp in sweet-and-sour sauce |
| Chicken with mixed vegetables | Beef with rice noodles |
| Salad Vietnamese style | Shrimp on rice vermicelli |

## Tips for Dining Out

Follow these simple tips, and you will be rewarded with good health and weight loss.

1. Eat an acceptable snack 30 minutes before you go out. Yes, it's okay to break the Perfect 10 Diet rules here. A fat or protein food is preferred, such as nuts, an avocado, or 2 slices of cheese to avoid over-ordering at the restaurant.
2. Do not skip meals before dining out.
3. Avoid "all-you-can-eat" restaurants. It's no bargain when you pay the price in pounds. There are plenty of food choices on the Perfect 10 Diet, but please don't have them all in the same meal.
4. Drink 1 or 2 glasses of water before dining out.
5. Select grilled, broiled, or baked entrées, and never anything deep-fried.
6. Ask about chef's specials, since they are usually the freshest market finds.
7. Have your waiter or chef explain how your meal is prepared. Don't hesitate to ask for changes or substitutions, or to send your food back if it doesn't meet your specific requirements.
8. Don't be afraid of a rich buttery sauce, but ask for it on the side to avoid excess calories. Use a fork to drizzle it on your meal.
9. Eat half your entrée and then drink a glass of water before you decide whether you want the second half.
10. Don't order a dessert until you've finished your meal, and then opt for fresh fruit. If you can't resist a rich, sugary dessert, share it with your companions.

CHAPTER 11

# The Right Strategy to Becoming a Perfect 10

The right journey to good health is about determination. Your health is the most important thing in the world. It has to be a "10." You need to lose weight to achieve optimal health and prevent disease. So what's standing between you and the perfect 10 body you dream of? Boredom? Lack of motivation? Stress? Self-esteem? You need to take action. Once your hormones become balanced, weight loss follows. To have perfect 10 hormones and a perfect 10 body:

- Eat right
- Value your health
- Relax
- Follow a healthy lifestyle

## Eat Right

If you want to have a perfect 10 body, your goal is to imagine it and go after it. You can't go back to your old eating habits. Salt, sugar, chemicals, and junk food will damage your satiety and make you addicted. I am constantly amazed when I go to supermarkets and see what others have in their shopping carts. Okay, maybe they don't know that orange juice has a lot of sugar, or that margarine is really bad, but come on! What about those large bottles of soda and those big bags of French fries? Learn to buy fresh vegetables and fruits each and every time you go to the supermarket.

Europeans have an advantage to eating fresh food daily because they tend to own smaller refrigerators. They shop for vegetables and fruits almost every day. In the United States, we have bigger refrigerators, and we love stainless-steel appliances better suited to a restaurant than a house. We shop for a whole week, or for a whole month. If your food buying revolves around saving trips, you're buying food that has little to no nutritional value. Instead, visit markets that sell organic food frequently.

Buy a small amount of food every few days. I'm always in the express lane in the supermarkets with few items, while most people are in the slower lanes with full carts that carry more food than their weight. I see these disturbing shopping habits everywhere I go.

It is important to eat natural food in order to support a healthy metabolism. The Perfect 10 Diet is rich in its food choices and will never make you bored. The following are the top 10 foods that will help you become a perfect 10.

## *The Top 10 Perfect Foods*

1. **Eggs.** A daily omelet has been found to lower your chance of developing diabetes. Eggs are low in the glycemic index and easy on insulin.

2. **Shellfish.** Oysters in particular are rich in zinc and can help balance your sex hormones. Include oysters in your diet two to three times a week.

3. **Dark meat.** Dark meat from poultry has higher zinc and is more favorable than white meat. Zinc helps support your sex hormones.

4. **Wild salmon.** A protein source with one of the highest sources of omega-3 fatty acids is a no brainer on the Perfect 10 Diet. Wild salmon

can regulate leptin, your hunger hormone, and help you support your sex hormones. Of course, as with other seafood, wild salmon is great for thyroid health.

5. **Cruciferous vegetables.** Those wonderful vegetables (Brussels sprouts, cabbage, cauliflower, rutabagas, turnips, collard greens, kale, bok choy) are great to support a healthy estrogen metabolism, and this can prevent cancer. Just make sure to have them cooked a little if you suffer from a sluggish thyroid.

6. **Oranges.** Oranges and other citrus fruits can help balance cortisol levels with their high vitamin C content.

7. **Oatmeal.** Oatmeal has one of the highest satiety levels of any food. It is great to support a healthy insulin metabolism and keep you hunger free for hours.

8. **Butter.** Butter can balance your sex hormones and DHEA. It can also prevent heart disease and cancer. What are you waiting for? Include butter in your diet right now.

9. **Olive oil.** Use olive oil frequently to dress all your salads. It is a great way to include more monounsaturated fats in your diet. Olive oil is great for your sex hormones, and it also lowers cholesterol.

10. **Whole milk.** I know I told you milk is not needed past childhood, but in moderation, having a little milk is okay as long as it is organic whole milk. Milk can help you balance your sex hormones and insulin. If insulin is balanced, weight loss follows.

# Value Your Health

I'll admit I'm no Dr. Phil, but if you have always struggled with your weight, I'm willing to bet you medicate with food most of the time. Why? It's simple. Food can act as a quick stress reliever. It can easily provide comfort and consolation when you are worried, annoyed, lonely, bored, or depressed.

So let me ask you this: How do you feel about yourself? Do you value your appearance? Do you have low self-esteem? Do you want to live a long and healthy life and be around for your children, grandchildren, and other loved ones? Remember, good nutrition goes hand in hand with good health.

## Are You an Emotional Eater?

- Do you like to snack all the time?
- Do you feel that eating makes you less angry?
- Do you feel guilty after most meals?
- Do you have low self-esteem?
- Do you procrastinate when it comes to your health and tell yourself you'll start dieting next week, or next month?

If you answered yes to any of these questions, you may be an emotional eater. Unfortunately, many people do get high on food all day long. For breakfast, they'll have a doughnut, muffin, or a roll with jelly with a large cup of coffee with sugar. Then, they'll have a burger, French fries, and soda for lunch—more bad carbohydrates from white bread and starches, as well as caffeine flooding to their bloodstream to create more insulin. Next, a venti fat-free latte to chase away the afternoon blues. Finally, they'll finish it off with a big pasta meal or white rice for dinner, followed by a pint of ice cream while watching TV. For many, that's not the end of it. Some of us even add alcohol, nicotine, or both.

People who tend to eat like that and don't think about their health are using food to control their insulin level. They eat sugar to get a quick fix for their fluctuating levels. They also eat sugar to feel happy, since sugar also raises serotonin levels in the brain. This neurotransmitter increases when you ingest sugar, so you feel better. But then serotonin comes crashing down along with your falling insulin, and you have to fix this declining level. Didn't I tell you sugar is like crack?

So let me ask you another question: What is this sugar and food addiction doing to your body and overall health? Do you love yourself? Do you want to be healthy? If you hate yourself, ask yourself why. Confront your inner critic. Go to therapy if necessary, because it's definitely worth the money.

Analyze why you have such low self-esteem. Silence your inner critic, who puts you down all the time. Would you let anyone else hurt you like that? So why would you do it to yourself? Love yourself and your body even if you are overweight. Treat your body well. Give yourself permission to live and make changes in your life beyond dieting so you can enjoy life now and every single day. You have to live a happy life, and you have to eat just to live, and not live to eat. Treat poor dietary habits just like any other addiction, such as drugs or gambling. You deserve the best in life, and nothing less.

Don't give yourself excuses, or tell yourself that cheating "just once" won't hurt. Breaking the rules will lead you to nowhere but poor health. Did you know that just thinking about food can actually trigger the hormones that stimulate your appetite? Your goal is to change the way you think about food. Eat on a predictable schedule—3 meals a day, and that's it. I eat at 7 a.m., 2 p.m., and 7 p.m., and then I forget about food the rest of the time unless I'm really hungry or find myself at a gathering with food. In those cases, I have a snack.

Think twice before you put anything in your body that you think is bad for your hormones and health. If you are used to putting something fattening in your mouth out of boredom or to get relief instead of engaging in a nonfood activity to calm yourself, make a switch to do something that's good for you! Take the dog for a walk, or start knitting. I don't care what it is, as long as it isn't dangerous or bad for you, and it takes your mind off food.

You should stick to the Perfect 10 Diet all the time, and *especially* on weekends. Why? Because we tend to consume more calories and alcohol Friday through Sunday than during the rest of the week, and this can easily add on pounds. The Perfect 10 Diet is a 7 days a week diet. In summary, stop putting off your health goals or saying I will start next week, next month, or next year. Life is too short to put any resolution off, especially when it comes to your health. It's time for you to be a perfect 10 in health right now.

Of course, I don't expect you to change overnight. Start slow. First, change your shopping habits. Try making sure you've got 10 items or less in your cart at the supermarket. Anytime you start going crazy in the supermarket, ask yourself why you need such a big shopping cart.

### Tips for Weight Loss

1. Never go to the supermarket hungry. You'll end up shopping like there's no tomorrow.
2. Stick to 3 meals every day.
3. Do not snack unless you are really hungry or know you'll be hitting the gym to burn the excess calories.
4. Make wise food choices all the time, and value your body and appearance.
5. Your mom was right: always eat slowly and take time to chew your food.
6. If you are so busy that you have no time for lunch at work, take a 5-minute break. Eat a small meal or a have a piece of fruit rather than eating a big meal while working and not concentrating on amounts.
7. Praise yourself for your daily accomplishments.

## Relax

Are you juggling work, raising children, and managing a home? This can leave you stressed or even burned out in no time at all, and stress can kill any diet. During moments of tension, the brain stimulates the production of ghrelin, a hormone that acts as an antidepressant. It calms your nerves, but it also makes you hungry. Of course, there will always be stress in life, so you must find a different way to deal with it. Whenever you feel stress kicking in, take a deep breath and say to yourself, "I can handle this." This strategy pulls your body away from the response of rapid breathing and tension, which can lead you to run to food for comfort.

Also stress—particularly when it is unresolved or prolonged—forces your body to produce cortisol, the stress hormone. Remember, cortisol gives you a boost to run from danger, but it's dangerous in large amounts since it can lead to central obesity, the most dangerous type. Cortisol is secreted every time you watch a horror movie, encounter problems in a relationship, have a bad day at work, or find yourself stuck in traffic. Chronic high levels of cortisol can also lead to disease development and premature aging.

Relax. I've had the opportunity to treat several centenarians in my practice. When asked about the secret to their longevity, they all responded, "We don't get stressed out." Try to identify the sources of stress in your life and learn to manage them better. Moving to a tropical island would be nice, but it may not solve all your problems. While fear may stop you from making some radical changes, a healthy life will not start until you take action.

That may include finding a new job, getting out of an unhealthy relationship (or getting into a healthy one), and having a spiritual attitude in your life. You should live your life all the way, and enjoy every single day. Also, make sure you get plenty of rest and relaxation, and find time to meditate. Only you control your emotions, and you can choose to see the glass as half full or half empty. Your perception and the way you see any situation can affect your stress level. You have the power. The freshness of a positive attitude can keep you from falling apart and drifting away from the Perfect 10 Diet.

Is there a relationship between stress and hormonal disturbance? You bet. Progesterone is the building block for many other major hormones. Cortisol, testosterone, and estrogen are all made from progesterone in a process that begins with cholesterol. Take a look at the following chart of the metabolic pathway (Fig. 11.1). These hormones are present in our bodies to varying degrees at all times, but only progesterone is readily converted into its sister hormones if needed. If we are under a lot of stress and our adrenals are pumping out cortisol, our bodies will take any available progesterone and divert it to meet that demand. If too much progesterone gets diverted for cortisol, this can make you develop belly fat. With too much progesterone shunted to make cortisol, there will be a disturbance in all sex hormones. No wonder we feel sick, lethargic, and uninterested in sex when we're under stress! Stress also causes insulin and leptin resistance. Relax to be a perfect 10.

**Figure 11.1:** How Hormones Are Made in the Body

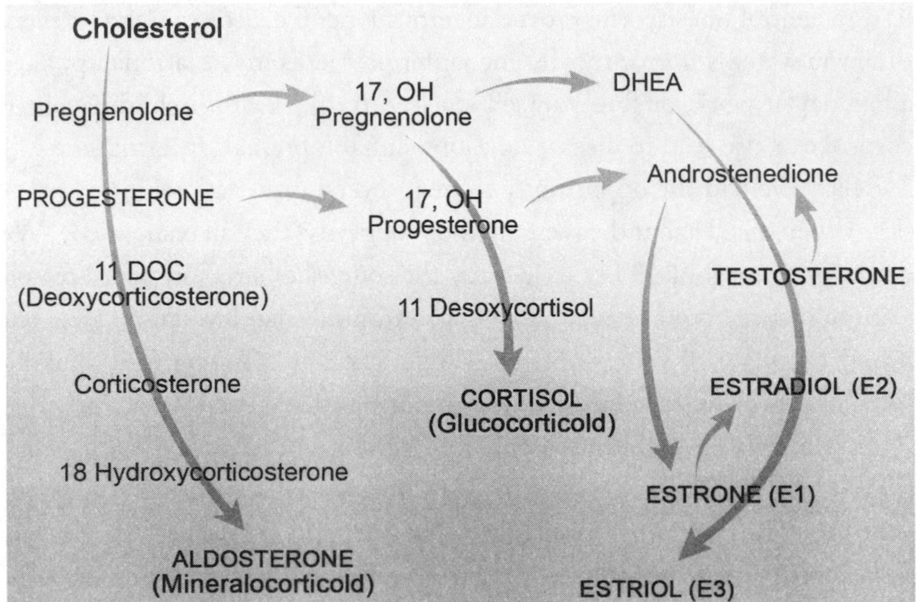


If you find yourself stressed and worried, especially if you resort to food for comfort, I suggest the following:

1. Take a bath rather than a shower. It's a great way to relax and energize yourself after a stressful day.
2. Sit in a quiet place and imagine yourself on a beach or a tropical island. Hear the waves, smell the ocean breeze, and feel the sunlight. Research indicates that the brain can be tricked into thinking what you imagine is the real thing. This can reduce your stress level and reduce your cortisol level.
3. Hug your family members, and stroke your pet. The sensation of touch can even boost your immune system.
4. Take a 1- to 2-minute time-out. If you're having a bad day, stop for 1 to 2 minutes. Take time out to think about something pleasant—real or imaginary. This will help calm you down in no time.
5. Listen to soothing or classical music. Research indicates that listening to soothing or classical music after performing a stressful task can lower blood pressure.

6. Take slow, deep breaths. Stress causes you to breathe heavily, which makes stress worse. Get control of your breathing. Take the time to inhale slowly and deeply and repeat for a few minutes.
7. Laugh a lot. Watch a comedy show or go to a yoga laughter club. Laughter clubs are gatherings where people meet and fake laughter. The brain cannot recognize real laughter from fake laughter. Laughing reduces cortisol and boosts endorphins to make you happy. I do few laughter yoga sessions from time to time and I always find myself laughing for real just by watching people. I feel energized by the time I leave.
8. Get a massage. Have you ever wondered why you are able to sleep much better after a great massage? It is the reduction in cortisol that leaves you relaxed.
9. Write down what you need to do each day, and prioritize what must be done first. Do the things that are most important first, and let the less important things go. Concentrate on doing 1 task at a time. Once you have finished, take a moment to let yourself feel good about getting it done. Take a rest, if you need to, and then move on. Time management is a key step in reducing stress levels.
10. Relax and do nothing for a few minutes each day.

All these measures will help lower your cortisol level and, in turn, lead to weight loss.

## Follow a Healthy Lifestyle

You need to follow a healthy lifestyle in order to balance your hormones and become a perfect 10.

1. Exercise regularly. If you're overweight, don't just sit there—do something about it. Excess weight is bad for many of your hormones, and it's a sign that you have too much insulin.
2. Quit smoking. You can't continue to smoke and expect to be a perfect 10. Cigarettes are especially bad for your sex hormones and DHEA. They also contain a chemical called thiocyanate which can disturb the

thyroid gland. Nicotine leads to premature aging. Cigarettes will also damage your skin, stain your teeth, and make you look unattractive long before you develop emphysema or lung cancer.

3. Limit your alcohol intake. Habitual drinking raises your insulin level and shuts down your sex hormones. Alcohol also makes you age faster. If you need help quitting, contact Alcoholics Anonymous or ask your doctor for medications. Many prescription pills to help you quit are now available.
4. Do not use recreational drugs. They mess up your sex hormones long before they make you an addict. Get help.
5. Get some sun. A little bit of sun helps your body make vitamin D to support your sex hormones. But be careful—if you're a sun worshipper or if you get too much midday sun, you won't be young looking for long. To protect yourself from the sun, use coconut- or cocoa butter–based sunscreens and not synthetic oils. After prolonged sun exposure, apply aloe vera gel to your skin.
6. Don't stay up too late. You need to sleep at least eight hours a night to get a perfect 10 body. A lack of sleep may disrupt the hormones that control your weight. If you don't get enough sleep, your production of growth hormone, the hormone that keeps you young and fit, shuts down. You can also impair the production of leptin, the hormone that controls your hunger. Getting enough sleep is the cheapest and simplest advice I can give for losing weight.
7. Have sex regularly. Research indicates that people who have sex regularly have increased sex hormones, have improved immunity, stay younger, feel happier, and live longer. In fact, having one hundred orgasms per year can add eight years to a person's lifespan. It also increases endorphins by over 200 percent for several hours postsex. For those of you who are not in a committed relationship and want to act on my final hormone makeover suggestion: practice safe sex, please.

## *Fiona's Story*

Fiona is a 42-year-old nanny who had emigrated from Ireland more than 20 years earlier. She was a pretty girl, but looked unhealthy. At 5 feet, 4 inches tall, Fiona weighed 170 pounds. Her face was round, her skin was thin, and her waist was much bigger than her hips. Fiona came to see me for chronic insomnia and wanted some sleeping pills. Even without the benefit of lab results, I could tell that Fiona was suffering from typical symptoms of excess cortisol production, which leads to central obesity. Her diet was poor—fast food, baked potatoes, soda, and a few drinks on the weekend. It's no wonder she had insomnia with all that excess sugar stimulating excessive cortisol production. The excessive cortisol was shutting down her production of melatonin, the sleep hormone.

I convinced Fiona that sleeping pills were not the answer; they would only mask a serious underlying problem. What needed to be addressed was her excess cortisol. I advised Fiona to follow the Perfect 10 Diet, with no alcohol whatsoever, and to implement some changes in her lifestyle.

Fiona began going to bed no later than 10 p.m., instead of staying up late watching TV. She shut her curtains tightly and slept in total darkness to shut down the cortisol production that is stimulated by any type of light. She was advised to take melatonin to help her sleep until her body began to produce less cortisol.

Ten months later, Fiona came to see me again. She was much thinner, looked much healthier, and said, "I'm sleeping better, and now I'm just here for my yearly physical." I love to see patients with no complaints. It makes my day much easier.

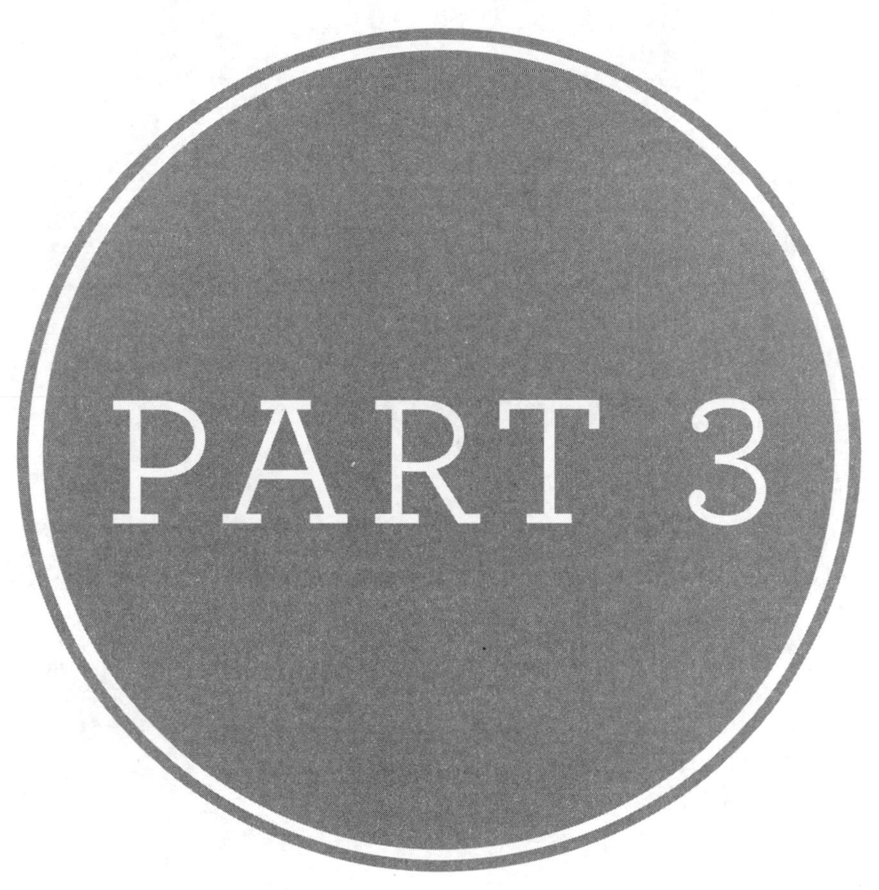
PART 3

CHAPTER 12

# Exercise and the Perfect 10 Diet

Having big dreams of being the next perfect 10 top runway model, like Tyra Banks or Heidi Klum? Or do you simply want to be thin and show off your new figure in tiny Prada pants? Let me tell you a little secret: I couldn't care less if you have a figure to die for. I just want you to be healthy and reasonably fit. But true perfection has its price, boys and girls, and you have to sweat if you want to be flawless. Give up the notion that you can have a perfect 10 body while being sedentary. Diets that promise you miraculous weight loss without exercise will ultimately deceive you. Join a gym. Short on dough? Join the YMCA. And if you're the kind of person who is not into gym routines, how about dancing for an hour every day? Turn on your CD players, iPods, and iPhones, and let's burn some calories, Perfect 10 Diet followers.

Exercise will do more than help you lose excess weight. It will positively affect your energy, endurance, and stamina. It raises the brain's level of serotonin, the neurotransmitter that makes you happy.

But the true power of exercise lies in its hormonal power (Fig. 12.1). When you exercise, you lower your insulin level and increase your glucagon level. Remember, glucagon is the fat-burning hormone that opposes insulin action. Glucagon goes up when you exercise, creating the perfect scenario for losing weight. When these two hormones are in balance, you shed the pounds.

With exercise, you also increase the production of growth hormone (HGH) (Fig. 12.2). Growth hormone helps repair tissues and build muscle mass. The combined effect of having these 3 hormones in perfect harmony dramatically improves your ability to lose weight, but you have to go to pain level to get some HGH in your bloodstream. The lactic acid created by intense workouts and related muscle fatigue boosts HGH secretion, and this can improve body composition and well-being.

As you continue to work out, you increase your muscle mass, which can lead to further improvement in insulin sensitivity. The amount of exercise you get on a regular basis will strongly affect your weight, because muscles burn more calories. Having muscles is like having a machine burning calories 24/7.

However, many people start exercising, and then they give up. Don't expect immediate gratification. Exercising inconsistently may make dropping the

**Figure 12.1:** How Exercise Affects Hormones

| HORMONE | RESPONSE TO EXERCISE | EFFECT |
|---|---|---|
| *Catabolic Hormones* | | |
| Cortisol | Increases | Increases fat breakdown |
| Glucagon | Increases | Increases fat breakdown |
| *Anabolic Hormones* | | |
| Insulin | Decreases | Allows fat to melt |
| HGH | Increases | Mobilizes fat for energy |

**Figure 12.2:** Type of Exercise and HGH Effects

| TYPE OF EXERCISE | INTENSITY | EFFECT ON HGH |
|---|---|---|
| Walking | Slow | None |
| Jogging | Moderate | None to moderate |
| Running | High | Moderate |
| Stationary bike | Moderate | Moderate |
| Weight training | High | Maximal |

pounds more difficult. Continuous exercise on a regular basis is essential to continued weight loss success on the Perfect 10 Diet.

## What Is Your Activity Level?

### CHECK THE BOX THAT APPLIES TO YOU

- ❑ I make no effort to get regular exercise.
- ❑ I live an active life and get my workouts walking and running errands.
- ❑ I work out 2 times a week for at least 45 minutes.
- ❑ I work out 3 to 4 times a week for at least 45 minutes.
- ❑ I work out 5 times or more a week for at least 45 minutes.

In reality, the fastest way to results is a minimum of 4 days of training per week. If you checked one of the first 2 boxes, you're not providing your body with the stimulation it needs to burn fat. If you checked the middle box, make an effort to increase your workout schedule to 3 to 4 times a week. If you checked one of the last 2 boxes, you're doing just fine.

Exercise will not just help you lose weight. Each hour of exercise can add 2 hours to your life. Amazing, isn't it? It will increase your flexibility level, improve your cardiovascular health, prevent osteoporosis, and improve your overall energy level. Figure out what kind of physical activity you enjoy, and go for it. This may be walking at a rapid pace, dancing, playing tennis, or swimming. It can also mean a workout at the gym 3 times a week. The goal should be to engage in a half hour of rigorous, sweat-inducing activity each day.

On the days that you don't go to the gym, incorporate 30 minutes of daily exercise into your daily routine. Don't think you can spare a half hour? Then divide the 30 minutes into three 10-minute blocks. Do 10 minutes of sit-ups or push-ups in the morning before going to work. Walk briskly for 10 minutes on your lunch break, or get off the train or bus 1 or 2 stops short of your destination and walk the rest of the way home. Take the steps, and not the elevator, at work or in the train station. After work, lift dumbbells for 10 minutes while watching TV. Light exercise, like a last stroll around the block before you go to bed, is also okay.

Heavy exercise should not be done before you go to bed, as it's bad for cortisol production and can keep you up at night. Cortisol is the enemy of melatonin, the hormone that puts you to sleep.

When traveling, always check to see if there is a gym or pool at the hotel where you're staying. Combining different types of fitness can make all the difference in your ability to lose weight and keep it off, not to mention in how strong your overall health will be. But don't start any exercise program before obtaining a comprehensive physical from a knowledgeable physician.

## 1. Slow Rhythmic Movements

Do you want to have the slim body of a Victoria's Secret underwear model? How about walking? It may not get any HGH going in your bloodstream, but it's great if you're really overweight or are a little intimidated by starting a heavy exercise routine. Take baby steps and start to walk every day before engaging in a heavy exercise routine. When you walk, you get the benefits of slow, rhythmic movements and improve your circulation while expanding lung capacity. If you walk regularly, you will lose weight.

Walking should be a pleasant experience rather than a chore. If possible, you should try to walk at least a mile a day. If you live in a warm climate, walk outdoors. Fresh air can take the edge off a stressful day and can make you feel more relaxed. This can help reduce cortisol, the stress hormone.

## 2. Stretching

Stretching will improve the flexibility of your muscles, tendons, and ligaments. Do some stretching exercises for about 5 minutes before and after you engage in any type of strenuous activity. It's a great way to ease into exercising and relieve muscle tension after a good workout.

## 3. Posture

Strike a pose. This type of exercise requires you to maintain a certain posture for a prolonged period of time. The most common forms of such exercise are yoga and Pilates. The benefits of posture exercises are relaxation, meditation, and improved flexibility. This type of exercise also reduces cortisol.

## 4. Aerobic Exercise

Want to have the perfect 10 body of Maria Sharapova or David Beckham? How about doing what they are doing? Aerobic exercise increases heart and respiration rates and causes your body to use oxygen. This includes brisk walking, jogging, dancing, brisk bicycling, using stationary machines (such as treadmills), skiing, and engaging in sports (such as tennis, basketball, hockey, and soccer). This is an ideal type of exercise for burning fat.

## 5. Anaerobic Exercise

When we think of anaerobic exercise, we think of heavy, bulky weights, clunky barbells, and Mr. Olympia or Mr. Universe. It doesn't have to go that extreme, but if you like beef, go for it. I mean muscles, folks, not red meat. This is the Perfect 10 Diet here. Anaerobic means "without air" or the type of exercise that makes you breathe so hard you can hardly talk—like heavy weight lifting. This type of exercise places your body in survival mode due to a lack of oxygen. Anaerobic activity helps rid the body of cellular toxins and builds a beefy look while greatly boosting HGH.

## 6. Resistance Exercise

Do you ever fantasize about having the 6-pack abs of a Calvin Klein or Abercrombie & Fitch underwear model? Don't dream it, go for it! Resistance exercise is ideal for building muscle and sculpting that perfect 10 body.

This type of exercise puts resistance on muscles. It involves using either your own body (performing sit-ups or squats), or using dumbbells and/or exercise machines. Contrary to common belief, weight training does not mean you have to do 3 sets of weight-resistance exercise back to back. You can train different groups of muscles one set at a time, such as focusing on abs and then moving on to legs, and then back to abs. Changing it up can give you the power to do more. This type of exercise is also great for boosting HGH production, especially when muscles get fatigued. Resistance training is beneficial for preventing osteoporosis and increasing muscular strength. Multiple repetitive movements with moderately heavy weights are preferred over less frequent repetitions with very heavy weights. This will help prevent injuries while building strong muscles.

## What If I Choose Only Running to Lose Weight?

I recommend a combination of exercises in order to maximize HGH secretion. This includes aerobic, anaerobic, and stretching exercises. Start with a warm-up, like doing 10 minutes on the elliptical machine. Then, follow it by some resistance training for a good 20 to 30 minutes. Next, return to some aerobic exercise for 20 minutes. As you lose weight and build muscles, you'll burn more calories.

Don't limit your exercise routine to running alone. I do not believe excessive running—such as marathon running—is very healthy. Humans were not built to run for long periods of time; we were designed to run to escape predators, and to walk for long distances. Long-distance runners create more free radicals and are more predisposed to colds and infections. They can also end up losing muscle mass and tend to suffer from many knee and ankle injuries. Running and jogging should be intermittent and should be part of a comprehensive exercise program.

## I Have a Physical Job. Do I Still Have to Exercise?

The answer to this question will depend upon the type of work you do. If your job includes anaerobic activity, such as lifting boxes or furniture, add some aerobic activity to your routine. If your job includes walking, such as mail delivery, include some anaerobic activity to achieve a chiseled, defined body. If your job is very physical and you add more exercise to it, make sure you take in enough calories to meet your increased nutritional needs.

## How Much Do I Need to Exercise?

Fitness experts agree that most people should burn between 1,000 to 1,400 calories a week through exercise. Guess how many calories you have to burn a week on the Perfect 10 Diet? That's right, a minimum of 1,400 calories to aim for true perfection in health. This requires that you walk at least 1 hour a day or go to the gym for about 45 minutes at least 3 to 4 times a week. I encourage you to keep a log of how much time you spend exercising. In fact, counting exercise time is the only math you'll need to do on the Perfect 10 Diet.

## Carbohydrate or Fat Loading Before Exercise

There are great misconceptions in sports nutrition about which fuel source is best to enhance muscle performance. Many experts believe eating carbohydrates before exercise will provide instant energy. I disagree. Research indicates that eating fat before exercising improves performance as well as endurance. Fat provides twice the energy needed for heavy exercise and triggers less of an insulin response before a workout, so you're better able to sustain the workout. If you eat too many carbohydrates before exercising, your blood sugar level will spike, and this will stimulate the release of insulin. This forces your body to burn your last meal rather than your fat.

You're less likely to lose weight in this scenario. Fat gives you the endurance to exercise longer, and it improves performance. Eating carbohydrates *after* a workout is a better option, as it will replenish the depleted glycogen stores in your muscles and liver. For example, have a full-fat yogurt or some olives with cheese for a snack before a workout, and then have a meal with slowly digesting carbs after. Also, I recommend you eat some protein after heavy workouts to boost HGH production.

## I Suffer from Elevated Blood Pressure. Should I Exercise?

Yes, if you suffer from hypertension, I still encourage you to exercise, but don't limit your workouts to anaerobic activity alone. Include more aerobic activity in your routine. Research indicates that hypertensive people do better with aerobic exercise alone or a combined aerobic/anaerobic exercise routine.

## Body Mass Index (BMI)

You've begun the Perfect 10 Diet, but your weight hasn't budged. Even worse, maybe it's gone up. Don't be alarmed. Muscle weighs about 20 percent more than fat, so even a dramatic fat loss may not translate into a dramatic dip in body weight. Gauge your weight by how well your clothes fit. The body mass index (BMI) is the percentage of fat in the body, and it's more important than weight alone. It's a more accurate way to determine measurements of body weight. For example, a 200-pound weight lifter with a BMI of 6 percent can be confident that most of his body weight is muscle. He certainly does not need to lose any weight, since he is in perfect shape. A sedentary person who weighs 170 pounds and has a BMI of 28 percent is carrying an unhealthy amount of fat, and he or she needs to lose weight.

The BMI can be measured with calipers that determine the thickness of skin folds, or by a process where an electric current is passed through the body. Fat has a poor conductivity compared to muscle, so the process measures the proportion of fat to muscle.

BMI measurement can be performed at a gym or in a physician's office. People with a BMI of 30 percent and above are considered to be obese, people with a BMI between 25 and 30 percent are considered to be overweight, and people with a BMI under 20 percent are considered to be in shape or average.

But who wants to be average in health? This is the Perfect 10 Diet here. I hope Perfect 10 Diet followers will go for fitness levels that are a few points lower. Now, *that's* hot.

## *Ronald's Story*

Ronald, 49 years old, 6 feet, 2 inches tall, at 240 pounds, was out of shape when I first saw him. With a BMI of 31 percent, he was truly obese.

Ronald had been on a low-fat diet all his life. His weight had begun to affect his blood pressure, despite the fact that Ronald exercised rain or shine and ran at least 5 days a week. It was Ronald's habit to eat two bananas on his cereal before he exercised and to drink orange juice after his workout. Ronald was disappointed that he was not losing any weight despite his heavy exercise routine. I advised him to eat an avocado or a slice of rye bread with cheese, or a full-fat yogurt before his workout, and to reserve the banana for after his workout.

Ronald was shocked when he realized that what he ate before working out was actually keeping him from losing weight. Instead of burning fat during the workout, his body burned the sugar from the bananas.

The presence of high insulin levels in Ronald's bloodstream before the workout interfered with his weight-loss efforts. In 14 months on the Perfect 10 Diet, Ronald was down to 170 pounds, and his BMI was down to 15 percent.

## Tips for Staying Active

1. Make it your practice to park your car a distance away from your destination. The walk will do you good.
2. Get off the bus or train 1 to 2 stops before your final stop and walk the rest of the way.
3. Join a gym with a friend; this will motivate you *and* your friend.
4. Have a plan for stormy days, such as indoor exercise, going to the gym, or walking around the mall.
5. Skip the elevator. Take the stairs at work throughout the day and on your breaks.
6. Buy some dumbbells and do an exercise routine at home.
7. When you travel, check to see if your hotel has a gym before making a reservation.
8. If you can afford it, hire a personal trainer to keep you motivated and on schedule.

CHAPTER 13

# Becoming a Perfect 10 with a Little Help

I had doubts about including a chapter dedicated to hormone replacement when *The Perfect 10 Diet* is simply a diet book. There have been countless books written for people with specific hormone problems, such as diabetes, thyroid disease, and cortisol imbalances, but that would mean reading multiple books (with conflicting information) since they are all geared toward a specific topic. This would only lead to confusion.

At the end, I realized that the Perfect 10 Diet is the crown jewel of all diets, and it must address all hormonal imbalances that plague our society today and all the health issues related to nutrition. For this reason, we must all aim to balance these ten hormones because their impact on each other and overall health is huge.

If you're a perfect 10 by now because you followed everything I told you to do, great. But what if you're only an 8 or a 7? That's not good. Chances are that when you get older, this number will go down to 6 or even 5. Don't despair. The Perfect 10 Diet can give you a makeover at any age. Becoming a perfect 10 is easy and achievable with a little help. No, I'm not talking about a new wardrobe, a stylish haircut, or plastic surgery. (That's not my field.) I am talking about balancing your ten hormones with supplements or hormones when the Perfect 10 Diet is not enough.

You see, when you're young and healthy, your hormones are in balance. Sure, they can get messed up prematurely because of a poor diet or disease, such as diabetes or a thyroid problem. But what about when you get a little older and hit menopause, or its male equivalent, andropause? Your sex hormones will simply disappear, and DHEA and HGH will go, too. The Perfect 10 Diet will help, but it may not be enough. You still need all your hormones, regardless of your chronological age.

Throughout history, medical science has maintained that aging, along with its chronic problems, is an unavoidable process of nature we must learn to live with and accept without question. But as a member of the American Academy of Anti-Aging Medicine, I became convinced that becoming old and weak, suffering from numerous aches and pains, and becoming depressed does not have to happen.

We must not accept that the diseases that occur with aging are a normal process. You can stay younger longer by balancing your hormones. You see, when hormones decline or become unbalanced, disease develops. But you can delay the aging process with hormone supplementation in case the Perfect 10 Diet is not enough. It's okay to get an extra help to be a perfect 10. I always talk and listen to top doctors from all over the world and get the latest information on breakthrough medicine. Didn't I tell you the Perfect 10 Diet is truly an anti-aging diet?

## Decoding Your Deficiencies or Hormonal Problems

### Body and Weight

- If you are struggling with your weight, you may have problems with insulin, glucagon, leptin, thyroid hormone, cortisol, HGH, DHEA, estrogen and progesterone (women), and testosterone (men).
- Does your face look round or swollen? You may have a cortisol or thyroid problem.
- Do you have a double chin even though you're in shape? This usually indicates a combination of hormone deficiencies—mainly HGH.
- If your breasts are too large: For women, you may have a progesterone

problem. For men, you may have a testosterone problem that is causing it to break down into the female sex hormone, estrogen.

- Are you underweight because of a lack of muscle mass? You may have a problem with HGH, thyroid, DHEA, insulin, and estrogen (in women) or testosterone (in men).

## Bones and Joints

- If you have been diagnosed with bone loss or osteoporosis, you may have a problem with estrogen (in women) or testosterone (in men), HGH, thyroid hormone, or cortisol.
- If you have been diagnosed with osteoarthritis, you may have a problem with estrogen (in women) or testosterone (in men), thyroid, or HGH.
- Do you have rheumatoid arthritis? You may have a problem with estrogen or progesterone (in women), thyroid, or HGH.

## Hair

- Is your hair dry or unmanageable? You may have a thyroid problem.
- Do you have brittle, slow-growing hair? You may have a thyroid problem.
- Is your hair dull and without natural highlights? You may have an HGH deficiency.
- If you're a man losing hair from the top of your head, suspect a declining testosterone level, together with an excess of dihydrotestosterone.
- If you're a woman losing hair from the top of your head, this may be an indication of low female sex hormones, estrogen and progesterone, high testosterone, low thyroid, or all of the above.
- Is your hair disappearing in circular patches? You might have a deficiency in cortisol.

## Energy

- Does even the least amount of stress leave you weak, anxious, and shaky? You may have a cortisol problem.
- Are you always tired, regardless of the amount of hours you sleep? You may have a thyroid, estrogen or progesterone (in women), testosterone (in men), or HGH problem.

- If you feel shaky after a big pasta meal, you may have low blood sugar levels due to a disturbance in your insulin.

## Eyes

- Is your vision decreasing? You may have a low HGH level.
- Do you have bags underneath your eyes? You may be deficient in HGH.

## Mood

- Do small things set you off, and do you find you can't deal with stress? You may have a cortisol problem.
- Do you feel sad all the time, or have you been diagnosed with depression? You may have a sluggish thyroid, low progesterone (in women) or low testosterone (in men), or an HGH problem.

## Sex

- If you have a hard time getting aroused, you may have a cortisol problem.
- Do you lack sexual desire? You may have a problem with estrogen (in women) or testosterone (in men and women), DHEA, or HGH.
- Do your genitals (penis or clitoris) seem less sensitive? You may have a testosterone problem (men and women).
- For men, are your erections not firm enough? You may have a problem in testosterone, cortisol, or both.

## Skin

- If you have age spots, you may be deficient in HGH, DHEA, or both.
- If you have wrinkles around your eyes (crow's feet), your sex hormones may be low.
- If you have deep wrinkles on your face (especially falling cheeks), you may be HGH deficient.

## Sleep

- If you have trouble falling asleep, you may have too much cortisol shutting down your production of melatonin, the sleep hormone.
- If you don't dream a lot, you may have HGH deficiency.

If you suspect a deficiency or an excess in one or many of your hormones, see your physician and ask him to check the levels.

## Insulin

Insulin should improve on the Perfect 10 Diet as you start to eat more natural fats and eliminate bad carbs. But if you can't skip a snack, or you feel dizzy if you don't eat every 2 or 3 hours, suspect an insulin problem. Ask your doctor to check your fasting insulin level, which means no eating for at least 9 hours. Note the result.

Check your level in the morning, right after an overnight fast. A fasting insulin level should be 5 units or lower. A higher level, which is very common in the United States, may indicate that you are suffering some degree of hyperinsulinemia. Two-thirds of Americans have it, and that's why many of us have a hard time losing weight. Are you one of them?

Ignore the normal lab reference range (up to 20) since it refers to the average American who has high levels to begin with, considering the massive amount of sugar and refined carbohydrates we eat in this country. If your insulin levels are high, you will have a hard time losing weight. Following the Perfect 10 Diet is a good way to start, but you may need additional help to get your insulin level down—especially if you have strained your pancreas for a long time.

Chromium's importance in the regulation of blood sugar has been recognized since the 1950s. Chromium has also been shown to facilitate weight loss. I recommend 4,000 to 5,000 micrograms of chromium picolinate per day as part of the Perfect 10 Diet program initially. You should take that much until your sugar cravings go away, and at that point, you can reduce your intake to 1,000 micrograms. If the problem still exists, your physician may prescribe a diabetic drug to increase insulin sensitivity, and this may help you shed the pounds.

However, if you're a diabetic, a word of caution: your diabetic medications may need to be adjusted lower, now that you're on the Perfect 10 Diet. The same holds true if you are taking insulin shots, as your sugar levels will be reduced.

If you are a diabetic on insulin, you may not be able to lose a lot of weight on the Perfect 10 Diet. Why? Your insulin level in this situation is not regulated by your diet; instead, it's regulated by the amounts of insulin you inject. It's important to get off insulin injections, if your body is still able to make it, to achieve weight-loss results. But how can you do that? Check your insulin level in your doctor's office after a meal that includes sugar, such as a doughnut or a glass of orange juice. (It's a one-time deal on the Perfect 10 Diet before you kiss sugar good-bye.) If your insulin level is over 10 after this sugary meal, your pancreas is still making insulin. That means that you can control your diabetes simply by following the Perfect 10 Diet alone, and you won't need insulin injections. Oral diabetic medications may be sufficient, and that can help you lose the stubborn pounds.

## Glucagon

Glucagon, the fat-burning hormone, is not routinely checked unless a pancreatic tumor is suspected. You don't need to worry about fixing your glucagon level via supplements; it should regulate on the Perfect 10 Diet after you fix the insulin disturbance.

## Leptin

I check leptin levels for many of my patients, especially when they have an insulin problem, since both hormones go hand in hand. Many, but not all, laboratories perform leptin analysis. Within 2 to 3 weeks after beginning the Perfect 10 Diet, nearly everyone will experience a dramatic decline in leptin levels. Younger people have quicker results than older people, who have more damage to undo.

The most reliable test for monitoring leptin levels is the radioimmunoassay (RIA). This test will tell whether or not you have leptin resistance. The optimal fasting leptin level is between 4 and 6 ng/dL. If your fasting leptin is over 10ng/dL, you have a leptin problem, and that's not good. Most overweight and obese people have extremely elevated leptin levels: 20, 30, or even 40 ng/dL!

If your levels do not fall as quickly as they should on the Perfect 10 Diet, you have to lower them by taking supplements. First, add a dose of fish oil at 3 grams per day. Next, add Gymnema Sylvestere, an herb that has been a standard of ayurveda, a traditional Indian medicine, since 600 BC. It decreases the absorption of blood sugar into the blood, and it possibly regenerates the beta cells of the pancreas. It's great for people with both insulin and leptin problems. Make sure you use a brand that is guaranteed to be standardized for 25 percent gymnemic acid, the herb's most active constituent.

## Thyroid

You eat seafood, seaweed, vegetables, and fruits, but you still feel tired. Could it be a thyroid problem? If you suspect a sluggish or overactive thyroid, ask your doctor to check your thyroid hormone levels. To check for thyroid, you will need a blood test for a hormone called thyroid stimulating hormone (TSH). Do not go by the lab reference, which states up to 5 mIU/L is normal. This is an old reference. Your TSH level should be below 2, or even below 1. If the TSH is higher than 2, you have a sluggish thyroid. However, TSH, the standard test, is inaccurate and can miss a sluggish thyroid. I like to check the free T3. Free T3 is a more accurate test. It can tell you how much of the active part of the hormone is available to do its job. Check the reference range; it should be in the higher limit. If you have an underactive thyroid, a prescription for thyroid hormone can easily fix the problem and help you become a perfect 10.

## Human Growth Hormone (HGH)

Following the Perfect 10 Diet is a great way to boost your HGH levels since exercise is an integral part of the diet, together with the right protein amounts. If you still suspect a growth hormone problem, get to know your levels, especially if you are over 60 or if you have symptoms (Fig. 13.1). People fear that if they supplement HGH they will turn into the wrestler Andre the Giant, who stood at 7 feet, 4 inches and weighed 500 pounds. This is not the case. Many of us are really deficient and we need HGH as we get older. Hollywood stars and celebrities, who never seem to age like we do, have a special secret; they stay vital with HGH.

The gold standard test to diagnose growth hormone deficiency is a challenge test, but it's flawed. The challenge test assumes the higher control center, the hypothalamus, to be normal. Many studies refute the challenge test as inaccurate, and they believe it produces very inconsistent results.

A good way to start is to ask your doctor to measure another hormone called insulin-like growth factor, or IGF-1, since it's a more reliable test. However, you must consult a doctor experienced in anti-aging medicine, since additional testing may be needed.

If your IGF-1 level is a little less than 150 mcg/l, there is good chance that you may be deficient in HGH. Take 2 grams of glutamine after every workout or right before sleep. This can boost your growth hormone level naturally. L-arginine is also an important supplement; the proper dose is about 1 gram, twice a day, on an empty stomach. In addition, Perfect 10 Diet followers should eat at least 25 grams of protein after each intense workout. The protein will help build ripped muscles and boost HGH production naturally.

I've seen levels of HGH go up 60 to 100 points in my patients as they dropped the pounds and incorporated exercise into their lives. Awesome.

But let's say your IGF-1 level is 125. If so, there's a higher chance that you really are HGH deficient, and you will need further testing. You may need the real deal—HGH injections. In general, doctors are reluctant to prescribe growth hormone because of its abuse by athletes. This is unjustified, because many of us, as we get old, are really deficient. But before you

**Figure 13.1:** Growth Homone Decline with Age

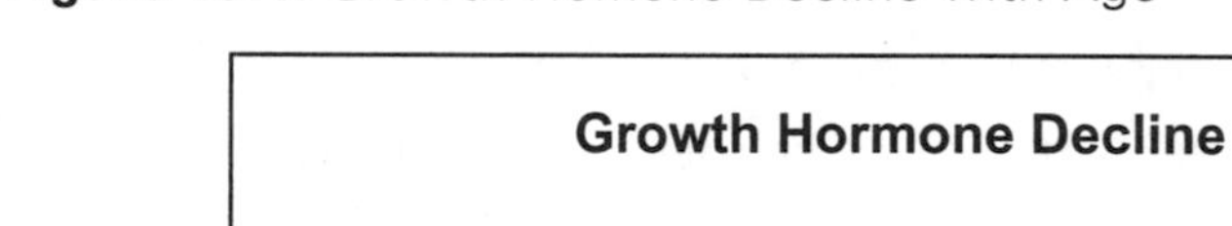


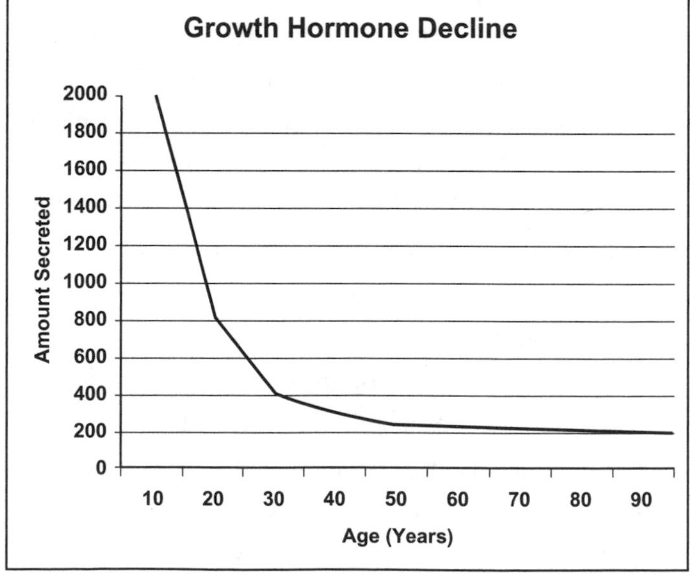

get HGH injections for a presumed deficiency, make sure that all your other hormonal abnormalities have been corrected. Fixing other hormone problems alone can boost growth hormone levels by 20 to 50 percent.

If, however, you truly are deficient and start to take HGH, you can really say hello to a perfect 10 body. Taking growth hormone is not just about being fit or wrinkle-free without botox. The benefits of growth hormone supplementation include increased energy, increased sex drive, improved vision, reduced body fat, increased muscle mass, strengthened immune system, lowered cholesterol, restored deep-sleep patterns, and much, much more. For more information on growth hormone, read *Grow Young with HGH* by Dr. Ronald Klatz. Dr. Klatz was the first to shed light on the importance of HGH to the world, and he brings it into the spotlight in this sensational book.

## Cortisol

You eliminated sugar and refined carbs once you adopted the Perfect 10 Diet, but you might still feel stressed or emotional, or might even sometimes feel your heart pounding in your chest. These are symptoms of a high cortisol level. Cortisol is the only hormone that goes up as we age. Total blood cortisol levels are around 180 ng/mL between 8 and 9 a.m., and around 45 ng/mL between 4 and 8 p.m. A random blood test, administered whenever your appointment at the doctor's office happens to be, may not be accurate. The best way to measure cortisol is to do a saliva test at various times during the day. If you have high levels, you may be stressed out. If you have low levels, your adrenals have burned out. Remember, cortisol is a stress hormone that gives you energy, so to check for cortisol, the test must be done in sedentary conditions. This means no intense activity, driving in heavy traffic, or vigorous exercise for 24 hours before the test.

Lowering your cortisol level can be tough if you're always stressed. Implement the suggestions that I discussed earlier, because a de-stressed mind can lead to a perfect 10 killer body. Some research suggests that phospahtidyl serine (PS) can be helpful. PS, which is a phospholipid consisting of a lipid attached to an amino acid and an L-serine molecule, is present in every cell of your body. Taking 300 milligrams of PS as a supplement can suppress your cortisol level considerably. A dose of 50 milligrams or 100 milligrams a day of 5-hydroxy tryptophan may also help. If you feel anxious or can't deal with stress, you may not have enough cortisol. It is possible your adrenals have burned out and you need cortisol. You need to relax and take vitamins and adrenal extract.

## Dehydroepiandrosterone (DHEA)

The role of DHEA in weight loss is controversial, but as I previously discussed, correction of DHEA can lead to an improvement in many of your other hormones. How do you know if you have low levels? How's your sex drive? Are you fatigued all the time, but your doctor hasn't figured it out yet? The problem could be DHEA. If you suspect a DHEA problem, a simple blood test for DHEA sulfate level will reveal the answer. For men, normal levels are 400 to 500 mcg/dL. For women, normal levels are 370 to 430 mcg/dL. When we get old, DHEA levels drop (Fig. 13.2). Supplementation is necessary. You can purchase DHEA in pill form (25 to 50 milligrams per day) over the counter, but don't take DHEA if you have a history of genital cancer with metastasis. Also, keep an eye on your levels. If you take too much, you may experience oily hair and skin, and maybe even acne. Women who are deficient are less likely to tolerate high doses of DHEA supplementation ion, so smaller doses may be necessary.

**Figure 13.2:** DHEA Levels with Age

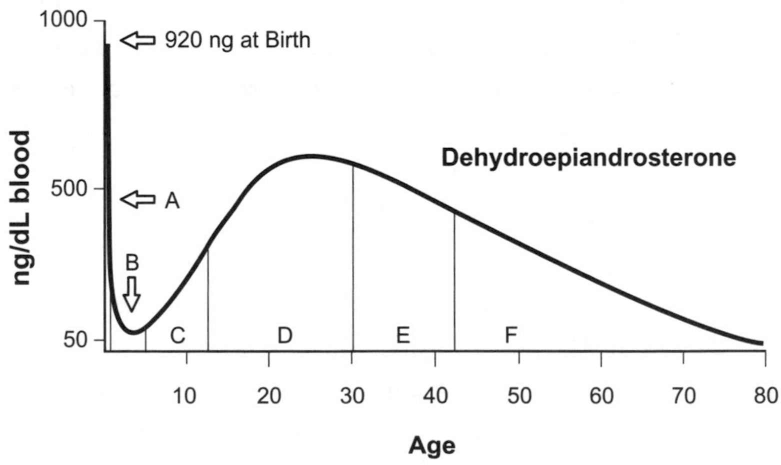

## Estrogen and Progesterone

The Perfect 10 Diet will help you improve your female sex hormones, since it encourages natural fats that have been avoided in this country for decades and discourages sugar. But what about after you hit menopause? The Perfect 10 Diet will definitely help, but it will not get you to the levels you had when you were a 20-year-old.

Lots of women would kill to stay young forever. They spend countless dollars on expensive wrinkle creams, filler injections, Botox, and even drastic plastic surgeries. What if I told you there was a way for you to stay younger looking longer? It's true.

In her landmark books, *Ageless* and *The Sexy Years,* actress Suzanne Somers brought bioidentical, or natural, hormone replacement to the spotlight. If you're a woman living with menopausal symptoms, or a young woman with disturbed sex hormones, bioidentical hormones can help relieve your symptoms by balancing your hormones while helping you to stay younger looking longer.

As a woman, do you need estrogen and progesterone supplementation on top of the Perfect 10 Diet? It's possible. If you're premenopausal and your periods are irregular, you may have a disturbance in estrogen or progesterone, or both. Also, if you're living with menopausal symptoms, you need supplementation. You need to balance these important hormones with professional medical help.

You see, during and after menopause, estrogen and progesterone levels decline precipitously (Fig. 13.3). That's not good for either health or weight. Hot flashes and night sweats are some of the other annoying symptoms. Centuries ago, most people didn't live past the age of 40 or 50, but now, many women live well into their 80s or 90s. You don't have to suffer or live a dull life without your sex hormones. Even if you're older, you should have the hormones of a 20- or a 30-year-old woman in order to stay healthy. Believe me; you can delay aging, and you don't have to suffer as you get older thanks to natural hormone replacement.

My menopausal patients complain all the time: "But I don't care about libido. I don't want to have sex anymore." It's not about sex. If you have unbalanced sex hormones at any age, you are more likely to develop diseases.

A woman's estrogen levels are close to 200, and her progesterone level is around 20 when she is in her reproductive years.

Believe me; it's perfectly okay to have your sex drive back in your sixties or seventies. Why? Because balanced sex hormones tell your heart and cells, "Hey, I'm young and reproductive, so no heart disease or cancer for me." What kind of hormones? Natural, of course, and not synthetic. Unfortunately, many doctors treat young women with hormonal problems with contraceptive pills. Contraceptive pills are synthetic. The same goes for menopausal women who are treated with drugs like Premarin or Prempro, which are also synthetic. Both are not only poor choices, they are plain dangerous.

"Premarin" stands for pregnant ("pre") mares ("mar") urine ("in"), and that's exactly where it comes from: horses. Prempro is estrogen's "premarin," with progesterone. Drug manufacturers tell us that these hormones are natural. They are not. Premarin and prempro are not natural hormones unless your food is hay. In 2002 a large study conducted by the National Institute of Health showed that postmenopausal women taking estrogen plus progestin have an increased risk of heart attack, stroke, breast cancer, and blood clots. Of course, these dangerous drugs also make you gain weight. Premarin is 50 percent estrone sulfate, 25 percent equilin, and others. That's not the kind of estrogen you want. Equilin metabolites damage DNA and can increase the risk of cancer.

If your periods are irregular, or if you're a woman living with menopause symptoms, I urge you to learn more about bioidentical hormones

**Figure 13.3:** Declines of Estrogen and Progesterone with Age

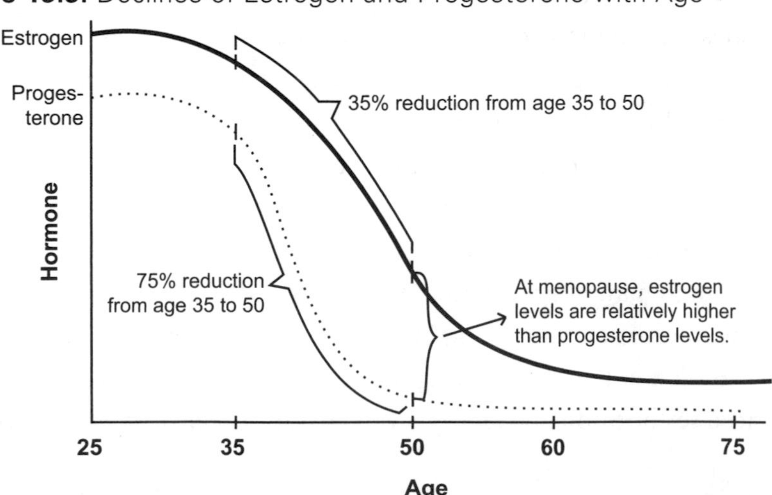

and how they can help get you back on track. Bioidentical hormones are extracted from yams, but they have a similar structure to human hormones. A good source to learn more about bioidentical hormones is *The Wisdom of Menopause* by Christiane Northrup, MD (Bantam, 2000).

Unfortunately, many doctors are in the dark about these types of natural hormones. I hope that over the next few years, more and more doctors will start to learn about bioidentical hormones, but it may take a long time. Why don't more doctors know about them? Medical schools and training programs don't teach about natural remedies because they get grants for research from pharmaceutical companies—which, of course, sell only patented drugs like the horse hormones. No wonder we are sick as a society.

A discussion on bioidentical hormone treatment and balancing your own sex hormones through supplementation is well beyond the scope of this diet book. To learn more, log on to the American Academy of Anti-Aging Medicine at www.worldhealth.net. The American Academy of Anti-Aging Medicine is the leader in bioidentical hormone replacement, and they can help you find a doctor familiar with the therapy and specific labs where you can get your levels checked. When your sex hormones are in perfect balance, you'll feel great and you'll be preventing old-age diseases.

## Testosterone

Testosterone is one of the most misunderstood hormones. Body builders have tarnished its reputation by putting large amounts of synthetic testosterone into their bodies. Don't get testosterone online or from pharmacies overseas.

For men, a normal testosterone level ranges from 300 to 826 ng/mL. Most testosterone is bound to a protein called serum hormone binding globulin (SHGB) and can't be readily used. A small percentage of testosterone is free and does all the actions. Each person's body chemistry is different, so a person whose testosterone level is at the low end of the range may still have enough free testosterone to function and feel good. On the other hand, someone whose testosterone is at the high end of the range may still have a slight deficiency with respect to his normal level because most of his testosterone is attached to the protein.

The Perfect 10 Diet will help you support this important hormone. But what do you do when your testosterone level starts to decline? What do you do if you have a chronic illness, such as diabetes, or you're overweight? This negatively affects this hormone. And what about when you get older and your testosterone level naturally starts to decline? The Perfect 10 Diet may not be enough to fix this problem.

Male andropause—and, for that matter, the whole topic of male aging—rarely gets mentioned in doctors' offices because it's assumed that many of the symptoms of andropause are just part of getting older. But men, just like women, experience sharp hormonal drop-offs, and they have to take andropause seriously.

As we get older, the testicular cells that make testosterone die and produce less. There is also an increase in the protein (SHBG) that holds testosterone, so less of the hormone becomes available. Men usually begin to notice these hormonal changes around age 40. Between the ages of 25 and 50, a man's testosterone level decreases by approximately 50 percent. As the level falls, the result is a decreased libido and erection problems. Hello, Viagra!

After that point, low levels can cause high blood pressure and heart disease. As the process continues, men begin to experience benign enlargement of the prostate, and they start to wake up several times during the night to urinate. Lower testosterone levels can even mean a higher risk of mortality, so you have to supplement this important hormone as you age. It is the difference between life and death.

Equal rights for men now. Suzanne Somers shed the light on the benefits of natural bioidentical hormone replacement for women in menopause; I'd like to do the same for my fellow men. I hope this book sheds light on this important topic for doctors and the public. Testosterone replacement therapy, which is also known as TRT, has a potent anti-aging effect, and it has shown tremendous benefits. A good age to start testosterone replacement therapy is in your 40s. That's if your levels are low of course.

Low testosterone levels are prevalent among older men, yet this condition is often ignored or goes undiagnosed for years. Men with low testosterone are often misdiagnosed with fatigue of an unknown cause, depression, or anxiety. In reality, the problem is a low level of testosterone.

The benefits of testosterone supplementation therapy outweigh the potential drawbacks, especially with the appropriate delivery, dose, and monitoring. To get started, get to know your levels. Testosterone level should be measured in the morning, since it tends to be lower (by about 15 percent) in the afternoon. If your total testosterone level is 270, which is low, your doctor may tell you, "It's in the normal range." Normal for whom? An 80-year-old man? You need to have much higher levels to feel good, have harder erections, and have the energy of a 20-year-old man. You always need to compare your level to the reference range of a young man in his 20s, not the lab reference for your age group. Do you want to have the normal testosterone level of an 80-year-old man? I don't think so.

The most common imbalance in aging men is a decrease in testosterone while the levels of estrogen, the female sex hormone, remain the same or sometimes increase. Your wife may appreciate this feminine side of you she's never seen, but it's not a good sign if your estrogen level is higher than hers. A testosterone-estrogen imbalance is the direct cause of many of the problems associated with aging, including benign enlargement of the prostate. You can also develop enlarged male breasts and that can affect your social life.

I know this is the Perfect 10 Diet, but my concern here is not how society perceives you. I'm more concerned about your declining testosterone levels and this estrogen excess. Low testosterone can translate to early Alzheimer's disease, hip fractures, and incontinence caused by an enlarged prostate. That certainly doesn't fall into perfect 10 health.

So what do you do if you're a guy with a testosterone-estrogen imbalance?

You need to follow the Perfect 10 Diet so that you can lose weight; this prevents the conversion of testosterone to estrogen. You should stop drinking coffee altogether, because coffee can accelerate the conversion from testosterone to estrogen by 60 percent. Alcohol should go too.

You also need supplementation to keep testosterone from further breaking into estrogen. How do you do that? Take zinc, 100 milligrams a day. The mineral zinc inhibits the aromatase enzyme that converts testosterone to excess estrogen. Seafood is rich in zinc, so now you know why seafood is a favorite protein source on the Perfect 10 Diet. I also recommend taking chrysin, a bioflavonoid that has shown potential as a natural aromatase inhibitor at a dose of 750 milligrams, along with piperine at a dose of 7.5 milligrams. A supplement called SuperMiraForte from Life Extension can provide them.

Male pattern baldness is a completely different scenario, and it's related to genetics. This means that testosterone is breaking down to dihydrotestosterone (DHT), a potent type of testosterone. This usually happens to men in their twenties or thirties. Does this mean you need testosterone supplementation? Yes and no.

If you have low testosterone levels, and symptoms such as erection problems, you may benefit from testosterone supplements. If you don't—oh, well, it's just your appearance. I'm reluctant to recommend hair loss pills, since they shut production of pregnenolone, a hormone that affects mood. While no one has the answer to prevent hair loss, zinc at a dose of 100 milligrams a day can block the conversion of testosterone to DHT without shutting pregnenolone altogether, but just make sure your total zinc intake does not exceed 100 milligrams a day. Now you're a perfect 10 hunk.

If you think testosterone hormone is just a guy thing, think again. For women, a normal testosterone level is around 75 ng/dL. If a woman's testosterone level is much higher, she can develop male pattern baldness and other traits of masculinity. A prescription for a diuretic from your doctor can easily fix this problem and get your levels in the right range. If you have a low sex drive as you get older, your levels may be too low. Believe it or not, as women age, they can also become deficient, and they need a little testosterone too to feel young and sexy. A prescription for a very low dose of testosterone cream can easily fix the problem.

## *Sandra's Story*

Sandra, age 47, is a senior mortgage broker well known for her stable character and charming, gracious personality. However, in recent months, her periods had become irregular. Over the course of 7 months, Sandra gained more than 20 pounds with no change in her diet. She experienced mood swings, and she frequently lost her temper with her clients and her family. Hot flashes and night sweats had become the norm, preventing her from getting any restful sleep. Sandra's usual boundless energy was simply gone.

She saw me for anxiety medication to help her calm down and function in her job. During the examination, I found that her breasts were tender and causing her pain. She also had some hair loss on the top of her head. I explained to Sandra that her symptoms were related to menopause and a loss of her female sex hormones. She needed to start bioidentical hormone therapy to replace her lost sex hormones, and she needed to follow the Perfect 10 Diet.

After 1 week on bioidentical hormone therapy, her hot flashes disappeared, as well as her mood swings. In less than 6 months, Sandra was her usual self again and back to her original weight.

## *Jeffrey's Story*

Jeffrey, a 45-year-old mail carrier, always considered himself to be a strong macho man. However, he'd recently put on 30 pounds over a few months. His muscles were not as firm, and his belly was not as flat. Jeffrey felt depressed, and he lost a lot of self-confidence. At times, he would lose his erections, and at times he could not even attain an orgasm. He lost his interest in his wife and all other women, even though he was not gay.

Jeffrey was interested in addressing his erection problem. His lack of sexual desire was putting a strain on his marriage, since his wife suspected he was having an affair. Jeffrey also wanted to try a new antidepressant that he'd seen advertised on TV. He was too tired to exercise, and his diet was horrible.

All of his symptoms were suggestive of testosterone deficiency rather than depression. I put Jeffrey on the Perfect 10 Diet to lose weight and boost his testosterone level, but that wasn't enough. He also needed supplementation of this quite misunderstood hormone. I prescribed a testosterone cream and closely followed his progress.

Jeffrey began going to the gym on a regular basis again. After a few weeks, he regained sexual interest and felt much happier. Looking at him now, I can see that Jeffrey is fit and back in the game.

CHAPTER 14

# Staying the Course

Every single meal should be perfect to help you balance your hormones, but it's not just hunger or temptation that can get you derailed from a dietary plan. Very often, it's the ordinary ups and downs of daily life. Stress, anxiety, and boredom are just a few examples of what might send us back to our old dietary habits. If you stumble, refocus and get on track again.

So what should you do if you have a strong craving for pasta or pizza instead of the acceptable food choices on the Perfect 10 Diet? The first thing I suggest is to drink a full glass of water and then wait a few minutes to see if you still have the craving. If you still do, drink another glass of water. This should curb the craving for good.

Still tempted? Have a cup of tea. In the event that you're still hungry—which isn't likely—it's okay to have a snack on the Perfect 10 Diet. Eat some nuts, some olives with feta cheese, or a boiled egg. Making a poor food choice should never be caused by weakness or a lack of preparation. You should never be in a situation where you just say, "Oh, well, screw it." Once your body gets rid of sugar, eating it will make you feel bad, as it will mess up your hormones in no time at all.

If you do slip up and eat a meal with too many starchy carbs, you can resort to what I would call Plan B. You can compensate by doing an immediate 30-minute workout before the sugar raises your insulin to dangerous levels.

It's also important to have support from family members, friends, or coworkers in order to stay motivated. The Perfect 10 Diet is not about excluding foods (except sugar, refined carbs, and trans fats). If you want to treat yourself to sweets in Stage Three, doing so should be a calculated, scheduled, and premeditated choice, and the portion size should be less than you would have planned to eat. You should be able to enjoy and follow the Perfect 10 Diet for life.

## At Home

If you cook your meals yourself, you'll have a lot of control over how closely you can monitor your diet. But if someone else in your family cooks or prepares your meals, you'll have to educate them about what's acceptable and what's not. Make sure your kitchen is stocked with fruits and nuts. You should select snack foods that are full of fat or protein since it stabilizes your sugar level. If someone other than you prepares your meals, make sure they cook with butter or extra-virgin olive oil, and not polyunsaturated vegetable oils or margarine. Watch your portion sizes, and stick to just 3 meals a day.

## At Work

Cake and cookies will always be part of office life. So will bagels and doughnuts. The fact that these foods are often in the office pantry doesn't mean that you have to eat them. Plan ahead and bring your own snack or lunch. Nuts are easy to carry, and you can always keep them handy in your briefcase, purse, or desk drawer.

## With Friends

Friends are often the unwitting saboteurs of diets. We gather with friends to celebrate, blow off steam, get away from stress, or have a good time. These encounters frequently involve food. If you're joining friends for lunch or dinner, make wise menu choices. Tell them you're on a diet. Ask if you can bring your own food. Resist the first or second drink when meeting for cocktails, and have a glass of mineral water with a twist instead. Stay away from cake, cookies, and ice cream. Friendships are sweet, but you should do your best to keep sugar out of the relationship.

## During Travel

Many people let travel become an excuse for falling off a diet, especially when it's a vacation. The Perfect 10 Diet does not restrict your choices with its wide, varied, and rich selection of foods. Remember, the goal of the Perfect 10 Diet is to reprogram your body to burn fat as your primary source of energy. Master your willpower and don't sabotage your hard work when you travel, because it can set you back in no time.

Whenever you're away from home, continue to follow the principles of the Perfect 10 Diet. For example, always go for rich breakfast choices. Many hotels offer a cheap or free continental breakfast that consists mainly of refined carbs, such as croissants, cereal, jam, bagels, and sweet pastries. You should always pass on this food, even if it's the Ritz Carlton or the Four Seasons. Please don't eat this sugar-filled breakfast just because it came with the price of your room. Instead, request boiled eggs or an omelet. Substitute cereals with berries and add full-fat milk. Don't sabotage your hormones and dietary efforts with other people's selections.

## On the Road

When you're on the road and can't eat in a restaurant, reach for healthful snacks. Fresh fruit is a perfectly acceptable snack on the Perfect 10 Diet, as are all nuts. Pack something along, so you don't find yourself stranded without any alternatives but a candy bar from a vending machine in a gas station.

## Parties

Parties, holidays, and work events lure people away from their healthy eating plans. At parties, scan the offerings and find something healthy to eat. Boiled shrimp or chicken skewers are perfectly acceptable choices. Vegetables dipped in guacamole or cream cheese are also acceptable. The fat and protein in finger foods will help delay the absorption of sugar you may take in from any alcoholic beverages. The Perfect 10 Diet is about luxury and indulgence all the way. How about some caviar, if it's served? It's rich in omega-3 fatty acids, which are good for your sex hormones and overall health. When it's time to cut the cake, reach for some berries with whipped cream, if available, or go back to the appetizer or main course. You want to miss the sugar, and not the fun.

CHAPTER 15

# Overcoming Sluggish Weight Loss

Some of my patients have lost 200 pounds on the Perfect 10 Diet, and others have lost only a few pounds. Those already close to their ideal weight have greatly improved their health. Even after balancing their diets, some people still have trouble triggering their metabolism to switch from burning sugar to burning fat to lose any weight. This is related to a variety of reasons I will discuss in this chapter.

## I Am Following the Perfect 10 Diet but I'm Unable to Lose Weight—What Am I Doing Wrong?

If you do not lose weight, or if you even start to gain a few pounds, on the Perfect 10 Diet, don't be alarmed. One common reason is that you are building muscle, which weighs more than fat. Judge your weight loss by how well your clothes fit rather than by the weight on the scale.

Another possibility for diet failure may be that you're not following the Perfect 10 Diet correctly, or that you're eating more than you need and not watching your portion sizes. Let's examine these two diet killers in more detail.

## Incorrectly Following the Perfect 10 Diet

It's extremely unlikely that you will not lose weight if you follow the Perfect 10 Diet correctly. The Perfect 10 Diet includes fiber-rich vegetables, the right fats, and healthy protein sources. If you adhere to these choices and exercise regularly, you will definitely lose weight. If you are not losing weight, and you have no existing underlying problem, such as a sluggish thyroid or insulin resistance, you may be doing something wrong.

One of my patients, Catherine, lost weight during her first 3 weeks on the Perfect 10 Diet, and then plateaued. Catherine was very disappointed that the diet seemed to have stopped working for her after she began adding 1 serving a day of a whole-grain cereal. All her hormone levels were normal. She reassured me that she had entirely cut out soda, fruit juices, pasta, and white bread. I told her to keep a food diary and return in 3 weeks.

Sure enough, something popped up in her food diary that explained why she wasn't losing weight: Catherine was consuming 3 servings of fat-free dairy a day (milk in cereal and coffee, and fat-free yogurt). She also ate snacks every day, instead of occasionally. When I say snacks are optional, that doesn't mean you can have them all the time. When I say milk is okay, I don't mean 3 servings of dairy. A fat-free yogurt has 50 grams of sugar. The sugar Catherine was eating from fat-free dairy alone was sabotaging her insulin and her efforts to lose weight.

If you find that you're not losing weight on the Perfect 10 Diet, pay closer attention to what you're actually eating. Read the fine print to see that there is no added sugar in your whole-grain cereal, or exchange it for a slice of rye bread that has less than 8 to 9 grams of sugar per slice. Unless you're very close to your ideal body weight, you're probably eating something you shouldn't.

## Eating More Than You Need

Eating rich, delicious food does not mean indulging or eating to excess. I have not asked you to count anything on the Perfect 10 Diet. You don't have to count calories, fat grams, or net carbs, but portion control is definitely important. If you eat too much, you still can make too much insulin. Make it a habit to fill your plate just to the rim with fiber-rich vegetables. When I say that you should eat natural fats to lose weight, I'm talking about moderation.

For instance, when I say you may have nuts once in a while for a snack or to sprinkle on top of your salads, I'm talking about a small handful, not a whole jar. When I say eating chocolate made with cocoa butter with reduced sugar is okay, I mean having a bite or two, not eating the whole bar.

## Metabolic Resistance

If you're doing everything correctly but still not losing weight, it may not be your fault. Your body may be resisting your weight-loss efforts, which is known as metabolic resistance. Have your doctor check the levels of many of the hormones I've discussed—insulin, TSH for thyroid, leptin, IGF-1 for growth hormone, estrogen and progesterone for women, testosterone for men, and DHEA-sulfate. (Estrogen and progesterone are best measured 3 weeks after your period.) Next, check with your doctor to see if any of the medications you are on are interfering with your weight loss.

## Medications

Many medications can cause weight gain—the list is quite extensive. Always ask your physician for a natural alternative before he or she prescribes a drug you may have to take on a long-term basis. I make it a habit to exhaust all natural alternatives before prescribing a drug for any prolonged period of time. You will be surprised that many diseases can improve with a good diet and natural alternatives alone. However, don't stop any medications before consulting your physician.

### SYNTHETIC HORMONES

Synthetic female sex hormones, such as Premarin and Prempro, make you gain weight. The list also includes many oral contraceptives. Read more about bioidentical hormones and how they can help you. If you're a woman who takes contraceptive pills, consider using condoms or a diaphragm instead.

### ANTIDEPRESSANTS

These drugs often have serious side effects, one of which is weight gain. Tricyclic antidepressants and selective serotonin reuptake inhibitors are the most likely offenders, especially paroxetine (Paxil). Check if you have a hormonal problem causing the depression, such as low sex hormones or cortisol. If all are normal, take SAMe. A study examining the natural substitute SAMe showed that it was just as effective as other antidepressants with no weight gain or sexual side effects.

## DIABETIC DRUGS

The list of diabetic drugs is quite extensive and includes insulin. As discussed, it's important to get off insulin injections if your body is still able to make insulin. Oral medications may be sufficient.

If you're on an oral diabetic drug, it's important to ask your doctor how the drug works. Many diabetic drugs promote insulin secretion, which can lead to weight gain. Drugs that increase insulin sensitivity, such as Metformin, should always be prescribed first, rather than drugs that promote insulin secretion. Discuss this with your physician since insulin resistance is the real underlying issue in the early stages of diabetes. If you need insulin, watch your diet more carefully to decrease insulin demand.

## ARTHRITIS DRUGS

Many arthritis patients are prescribed steroids, which may cause weight gain. Ask your physician to put you on the lowest dosage possible if you need to be on steroids for any prolonged period of time. Take DHEA to prevent some of the unpleasant side effects associated with steroid use. Also, take daily supplements, such as borage or evening primrose oil. This may help with your symptoms.

## HYPERTENSION DRUGS

Some hypertension drugs, such as beta-blockers, promote weight gain. Limit foods that are high in sodium, such as olives, cheese, and pickles. Supplementation with fish oil (2 to 3 grams daily), C-12 peptide (50 milligrams daily), potassium, calcium, and magnesium can also help lower your blood pressure. And don't neglect to add aerobic exercise to your daily routine.

## Tips to Overcome Sluggish Weight Loss

While you may lose more weight on the Perfect 10 Diet compared to other diets that have failed you in the past, it's not prudent to lose more than 1 to 2 pounds weekly after the initial big weight loss in Stage One. But if you're not losing weight or facing resistance, don't give up. Take a closer look at your efforts, and take the necessary steps to correct them.

### LOOK FOR HIDDEN CALORIES

Gum and most condiments, such as ketchup, barbecue sauce, and salad dressings, all contain sugar or high-fructose corn syrup. These calories are bad for your hormones. Are you eating food that's not allowed on the Perfect 10 Diet?

### LOOK FOR FORGOTTEN CALORIES

Avoid eating while watching TV, reading, or writing, as this usually leads to overeating. Stick with your regimen: eat 3 meals and concentrate on *what* you eat.

### CUT BACK ON PORTION SIZE

Skip a slice of whole-grain bread or an extra serving of brown rice, and you will be rewarded with further weight loss. If these measures still fail, your calorie needs may simply be less than you assumed. The Perfect 10 Diet permits 3 meals daily, so if you're used to snacking every day, limit it to just once in a while.

### LIMIT CAFFEINE AND ALCOHOL

Caffeine increases insulin secretion and leads to weight gain, so stick to decaffeinated beverages. Alcohol is used up for energy when it's consumed, so cut down to 1 to 2 drinks per week or stop completely until you reach your desired weight.

### INCREASE YOUR EXERCISE

Go to the gym for an additional session or increase your daily exercise routine by another 10 minutes.

### KEEP A FOOD LOG

Write down every single thing you eat, and how much of it you eat. You may be surprised at what you find written down at the end of the day.

### DRINK PLENTY OF WATER

This will do more than just keep your body hydrated—it will curb your appetite, too.

CHAPTER 16

# The Tests That Can Change Your Life

No diet is truly successful unless it helps you fight disease and makes you live a long and healthy life. The Perfect 10 Diet will deliver on all its promises. It will improve your overall health while you lose weight. The proof will be not only in how you feel and your energy level, but also in the improvement you'll see in risk factors for many diseases. Ask your doctor to perform these tests during your next visit or yearly physical.

## 1. Cholesterol

The quest for lower cholesterol has become an obsession in this country and around the world. Public health officials are urging millions of people to get on cholesterol-lowering drugs at increasingly younger ages. Why is it that everyone who is around the age of 45 or 50 needs a statin drug, such as Lipitor, Zocor, or Crestor? Why now when our grandparents never had this problem?

The higher your cholesterol level, the more likely you are to die from heart disease or stroke. That's the information promoted by medical research and drug manufacturers. They demonstrate their data with graphs and TV commercials. In truth, it's only half the story. Except for a few people with certain genetic diseases, or about 1 percent of the population, cholesterol level has little to do with the degree of atherosclerosis. Also as we get older, loss of HGH and sex hormones lead to higher cholesterol levels.

It's estimated that 50 percent of heart attacks occur in people with normal cholesterol levels! Surprised? I bet. The relationship between cholesterol levels and heart disease is minuscule, but the data is greatly exaggerated in order to get more people on cholesterol drugs. While we are told to lower cholesterol levels aggressively with drugs, taking these will not help you live longer. Patent-statins or cholesterol drugs are awful. Your brain and cells need cholesterol to function. Cholesterol drugs deplete the body of coenzyme Q10, a natural substance needed by your body. Coenzyme Q10 is a fat-soluble antioxidant that acts independently, protecting against DNA damage and other forms of oxidative damage. None of the patent cholesterol drugs on the market come with coenzyme Q10.

When you shut down your cholesterol, you affect how your brain functions, because it needs cholesterol. Memory lapses are now anecdotally linked with the regular use of statins drugs. Statins also kill your sex drive by shutting down your sex hormone production, and the pharmaceutical companies know it. Cholesterol is the parent from which these hormones are made. These drugs don't even come with a warning that they will shut down these hormones for life.

Oh, one more thing—statins drugs or a lowered cholesterol level can possibly increase your risk of cancer. In the summer of 2007, researchers from Tufts University reported in the *Journal of the American College of Cardiology* that lowering cholesterol as much as possible may reduce the risk of heart disease, but with a price—it could raise the risk of cancer. The issue is still unsettled.

I rarely bother with my patients' cholesterol levels unless they are greatly elevated. Believe it or not, most cholesterol abnormalities can be corrected with a proper diet and natural hormone supplementation (if you're deficient), not statins drugs.

## What Is Cholesterol, and Why Do We Need It?

Cholesterol is essential for survival. It's made in your body when glucose is converted into a two-carbon molecule to make acetyl-Co; later, it's fully converted into cholesterol. Therefore, it's naturally produced in our bodies. It is used to make sex hormones and stabilize cell walls.

**Figure 16.1:** Functions of Cholesterol

- Formation and maintenance of cell membranes (helps cells resist changes in temperature and protects and insulates nerve fibers)
- Formation of sex hormones (estrogen, progesterone, testosterone) and cortisol
- Production of bile salts, which help digest food
- Conversion into vitamin D when the skin is exposed to sunlight

We've already discussed the terms bad cholesterol and good cholesterol, but let me explain further. Cholesterol is not soluble, so it gets around in the bloodstream by being carried by a protein called LDL. This LDL is portrayed as bad cholesterol, even though it's essential since it carries cholesterol to the cells and tissues. Cholesterol is recycled back to the liver by another protein called HDL, which is also known as good cholesterol.

The ratio of bad cholesterol to good cholesterol is more important than your total cholesterol levels alone. In other words, if you have enough good cholesterol to remove the bad cholesterol to be recycled, you're fine. At times, a glitch can happen and cholesterol stays at the surface to clog the arteries. This may be related to a diet that's heavy in refined carbohydrates, sugar, and trans fats. It's also possible that it's related to an infectious etiology that can trigger inflammation in the arteries. But this inflammation is not caused by eating too much saturated fat, animal products, or cholesterol-rich foods.

High cholesterol in the bloodstream is a manifestation of the body's needs at the time, an inflammation in the arteries, or a hormone deficiency as we grow older. Cholesterol can be compared to firefighters who come to a burning building to extinguish a fire. The firefighters didn't cause the fire, they came to extinguish it. The cholesterol comes to heal the tissues, and clogs may form. Cholesterol by itself is not the real culprit, but when oxidized, it may clog the arteries.

As I've mentioned, cholesterol becomes damaged when it's oxidized from your consumption of heated polyunsaturated oils, eating too much sugar, or smoking. These things make cholesterol sticky and cause it to adhere to the arterial walls. In the presence of a poor diet, a lethal cascade goes through the body and turns "on" the inflammation button. You need to radically change your diet if you want to lower your cholesterol.

## Follow a High-Fat/Low-Carb Diet to Lower Cholesterol

I know I've been telling you to eat more fat all along in this book, and you may be wondering about your cholesterol level on the Perfect 10 Diet. It will be much lower on the Perfect 10 Diet than on a low-fat diet. When you follow a low-fat/high-carb diet, the metabolized sugar is converted into triglycerides. Triglycerides are really bad components of the cholesterol profile, and a high level is a risk factor for heart disease. Paradoxically, triglyceride levels go down on high-fat/low-carb diets.

On the other hand, low-density lipoprotein (LDL), which gets all the attention, is not that important. It's hard for most people to believe that a higher-fat diet is superior to a lower-fat diet when it comes to improving cholesterol levels, but it's true.

You see, insulin and glucagon play a role in the synthesis of cholesterol. Insulin stimulates a key enzyme called HMG-CoA reductase to manufacture cholesterol, while glucagon inhibits it. People who have a chronically elevated insulin level almost always have a high cholesterol level. Glucagon, on the other hand, does the exact opposite and acts like a cholesterol-lowering drug. These two hormones will be in perfect balance on the Perfect 10 Diet as you eat more natural fats.

Let's say you follow the Perfect 10 Diet with a preference toward French cuisine; that's perfectly okay with me. As a matter of fact, it's better for your sex hormones, and you don't have to worry about your cholesterol. The French have higher cholesterol than Americans, but have fewer heart attacks. Here's why: your bad cholesterol, C-LDL, may go up because you're eating more cheese and butter, but so will your good cholesterol, C-HDL; therefore, the effect is neutral. The ratio is what's important, not the total cholesterol level alone. If you have enough HDL, you can remove

**Figure 16.2:** Comparing Different Diets

| | LOW-FAT/HIGH-CARB | HIGH-SATURATED-FAT/LOW-CARB |
|---|---|---|
| LDL cholesterol | 150 | 160 |
| HDL cholesterol | 35 | 48 |
| Ratio LDL/HDL | 4.29 | 3.3 |
| Triglycerides | 200 | 120 |

the excess cholesterol left by LDL. Any elevation of LDL is on the fluffy or large LDL, which does not clog the arteries. An optimal ratio of LDL to HDL should be below 3. In the same time, your triglycerides level will fall down precipitously when you cut sugar from your diet. That's what I like to see as a doctor.

On the other hand, if you follow a low-fat/high-carbohydrate diet, both your LDL and HDL will go down (Fig. 16.2). At the same time, your triglycerides level will rise because of the excess sugar. Your LDL will be mostly small type because of the excess sugar, and this type of small LDL clogs your arteries. Thus, a low-fat diet increases your chance of developing heart disease.

## Which Cholesterol Profile Would You Rather Have?

The cholesterol profile is more favorable on a high-fat/low-carb diet than on a low-fat/high-carbohydrate diet. From Figure 16.2, you can see that you're less likely to be on a cholesterol drug when you follow a high-fat/low-carb diet, even if it's skewed toward saturated fat.

Don't just take my word for it. Probably the most famous dietary guru of all time was Dr. Robert Atkins. Dr. Atkins promoted a high-protein/very-high-fat/very-low-carb diet for decades. He was ridiculed for it, with critics claiming that a diet high in saturated fat would dangerously raise cholesterol levels. They were wrong.

His diet had other problems, but Dr. Atkins was smarter than his critics. Dr. Atkins clearly and smartly understood that his diet would not only promote weight loss, but would also dramatically lower cholesterol. The amount of total fat on the Atkins Diet is approximately 60 percent of total calories, and the saturated fat level is a whopping 20 percent, or twice the amount of saturated fat recommended by the American Heart Association. The amount of carbohydrates allowed on the Atkins Diet is minuscule—no more than a few grams in the initial stage. (On Atkins, you limit carbs even from vegetables and fruits.) Countless recent research studies have indicated that the Atkins Diet is indeed superior to the American Heart Association's low-fat diet in lowering cholesterol and even to the Mediterranean diet.

Surprised? I'll bet you are, since you've always been told that saturated fats raise cholesterol. However, repeat the same studies without sugar and refined carbs, and you'll get the exact opposite results. I found that out 10 years ago based on my observations of cholesterol levels in patients who were following the Atkins Diet—long before all these studies exonerated this doctor.

Dr. Atkins was definitely on the right track to go against the low-fat advice, but not necessarily right about how his diet can mess up hormones. In other words, it's not the eggs; it's the potatoes and orange juice, my friends, that you should worry about. It's not the burger and cheese; it's the soda and white bread. Sugar and refined carbs cause more negative cholesterol abnormalities than any amount of saturated fat or cholesterol-rich products you can possibly eat. Yet we are still told that a low-fat diet is the best way to lower cholesterol!

Don't get me wrong. By no means am I advising you to follow a high-protein/very-low-carb diet filled with bacon and sausages that mess up your hormones or increase your risk for cancer. The point I'm making is that a cholesterol profile is more favorable on a high-fat diet (even when high in saturated fat) than a low-fat diet. The Perfect 10 Diet will help you achieve even better cholesterol levels with its balance in all food groups and with its diversity in good fat choices.

## 2. Highly Sensitive C-Reactive Protein (hs-CRP)

Inflammation is part of your body's response to injury and disease. However, inflammatory chemicals are often elevated in the blood of people who are not overtly sick or injured. Low-grade chronic inflammation is associated with an increased risk for heart disease, diabetes, cancer, and other health problems.

One of the best markers for systemic inflammation is highly sensitive C-reactive protein (hs-CRP), a protein that is produced during inflammation. This newly discovered marker is much more important than the bad cholesterol, C-LDL. Evidence has shown that inflammation is closely tied to insulin and leptin resistance. Your level of hs-CRP should be below 1 mg/L. Ask your doctor to run the highly sensitive C-reactive protein test, rather than the standard, less sensitive C-reactive protein test. You should see an improvement in your hs-CRP level as you follow the Perfect 10 Diet, which is rich in seafood and includes more omega-3 fatty acids in your diet. If your levels are higher than 1, add extra omega-3 fatty acids in pill form. Just like your cholesterol, if you correct underlying hormonal problems, your hs-CRP should fall.

## 3. Fasting Sugar

A diagnosis for diabetes is made when a fasting sugar level is over 126 mg/dL. But if your fasting sugar level is over 70, you may be prediabetic and at risk for developing diabetes. It's important to not go by the lab reference range, which indicates that 70 to 126 mg/dL is normal. Eliminate sugar from your diet and implement the Perfect 10 Diet plan to see an improvement.

CHAPTER 17

# Does This Sound Like You?

Since I founded the Midtown Integrative Center in 1998, thousands of people have adopted the Perfect 10 Diet. Many tell their success stories, and the impact that the Perfect 10 Diet has had on their health, lives, and families. Many were able to reduce the amount of medications they were taking, or were cured from many chronic illnesses. Weight loss, reversal of diabetes, and improved blood pressure, just to name a few, are some of the benefits of the Perfect 10 Diet. Hormones control your health.

Are you overweight? Are you a diabetic? Do you have an underactive thyroid? Are you a young woman with irregular periods? Are you a woman in menopause? Are you a man in andropause? Are you a body builder interested in getting bigger? Are you a senior citizen interested in fighting the progression of aging? It doesn't matter who you are—the Perfect 10 Diet is for you. The Perfect 10 Diet addresses all hormones.

For this reason, I've seen the diet successfully work for all kinds of people, from competitive athletes to sedentary older people. The secret to the success on the Perfect 10 Diet is that it offers the right kind of nutritional balance for everyone. It's designed to improve your hormones, unlike low-fat and low-carb diets, which greatly disturb them. This makes me confident that the Perfect 10 Diet can work for you, too. It will give you the perfect 10 health you deserve after you've been lied to for decades.

Following are the stories of several of my patients who found great success on the Perfect 10 Diet. You may see yourself in one (or several) of them.

## Kevin's Story

Kevin is a 42-year-old pharmaceutical representative who weighed 240 pounds when he came to see me for excessive fatigue. Kevin related that he found himself rushing out of his apartment every morning and relying on coffee and a bagel from the street vendor or local deli. Since he never had time for lunch, he'd end up grabbing a slice of pizza or a couple of hot dogs on the road. He assured me that on weekends, he tried to eat healthy—by having low-fat bran muffins and pasta! While his weight was creeping up, his energy level was plummeting.

I met with Kevin and explained to him that both his fatigue and weight gain were related to his poor diet. On weekdays, he should eat boiled eggs instead of low-fat muffins—and they don't even require much time to prepare. For lunch, he should be eating a salad or turkey breast on a whole-grain wrap instead of pizza.

Kevin started on the Perfect 10 Diet. As his weight decreased, his energy level increased. Kevin's weight was down to 180 pounds in 12 months, and his fatigue vanished. His insulin and leptin levels, once very high, normalized.

## Larry's Story

Larry is a 55-year-old banker who has worked hard his whole life. When he came to see me, he complained of feeling worn out most of the time. He found that he could barely make it through the hours of a normal workday, and his employer had begun to notice the change in his work performance.

Although he was sleeping 7 to 8 hours a night, Larry never could regain his energy. He was eating lots of carbs—from bagels in the morning to pasta for lunch—and not enough protein. Larry's cheeks sagged, and his young looks were just about gone. At 5 feet, 7 inches tall, he was overweight at 196 pounds, and he lived a sedentary life.

Larry was suffering from typical symptoms of growth hormone deficiency. Of course, his insulin level was also sky high from all the bad carbs he ate. He was placed on the Perfect 10 Diet and advised to exercise regularly.

After 8 weeks on the diet, Larry's energy level was back. He lost 15 pounds, and his complexion was glowing. His insulin level dropped precipitously, and his growth hormone level was as high as that of a 30-year-old man.

## Joan's Story

Joan is a 32-year-old FedEx employee with a hectic schedule and little time to work out. When I first met Joan, her weight was 385 pounds. Joan was so desperate to lose weight that she was contemplating bariatric surgery. She had followed a low-fat diet all her life, and she would lose weight often, only to gain it back—and then some.

Joan followed the principles of the Perfect 10 Diet and lost 175 pounds in 16 months. In June 2006, I invited Joan to join me in talking about the dangers of high-fructose corn syrup on the *CBS Evening News*. Joan was gracious enough to share her story and let a camera crew follow her around a local supermarket.

## Jonathan's Story

Jonathan is a 36-year-old teacher who stands 5 feet, 8 inches and was severely overweight—230 pounds. He came to see me for problems with frequent urination and erectile dysfunction. His blood work revealed a fasting blood sugar of 315, which meant that Jonathan was suffering from type II diabetes. His testosterone level was also way too low, which is typical in many diabetics.

Jonathan's previous physician had advised him to limit all fat without really giving him any specific details or plans. He ate cereal and baked potatoes, believing he was making healthy, low-fat food choices. He believed that drinking freshly squeezed orange juice was good for him because of its high vitamin C content. He snacked on unsalted pretzels, believing that they would lead to greater weight loss than nuts.

Jonathan was definitely misled by the low-fat recommendations. I counseled Jonathan extensively and put him on the Perfect 10 Diet. I advised him to increase his natural fat intake and eliminate refined carbs from his diet.

Jonathan lost 60 pounds in 18 months. Since losing the weight, his blood sugar and insulin levels have normalized. I also prescribed a natural testosterone cream to boost his level, and his erections returned, along with a soaring libido. Jonathan's diabetes is controlled without the use of any drugs, and he sees me only for his routine annual physical.

## Elizabeth's Story

Elizabeth is a 52-year-old businesswoman who came to see me for weight loss. She had recently divorced a successful attorney who had offered her no emotional support for years. Her weight had gone up from 130 pounds to 180 pounds since her last visit 2 years before.

"Elizabeth, why do you want to lose weight?" I asked.

"My knees and back hurt, and I think if I lose weight, I'll feel better."

"How have you been doing since your divorce?"

With a surprised look, she replied, "Doctor, why do you ask?" and burst into tears.

We are all designed to seek safety, and if we do not feel safe, we crave other things, like food. I held her hand as she cried.

"I feel alone and insecure. I eat to compensate for the void I feel inside. I can't stop eating French fries. I'll eat an entire quart of vanilla fudge ice cream, and a whole bag of chocolate chip cookies. I think these foods compensate for the lack of intimacy in my life."

Elizabeth was very depressed, and her food addiction to these carbs and sugars stemmed from the effects of sugar on mood. Her insulin and cortisol levels were sky high. I placed Elizabeth on the Perfect 10 Diet, and within 10 months, her insulin and cortisol levels had normalized. Her depression was gone and she was down to 130 pounds, and involved in a new relationship.

## Susan's Story

Susan is a 50-year-old financial planner who came to visit me after seeing me as a guest speaker on a TV program. Susan complained of a little fatigue, but she was in good shape and did not need to lose weight. However, Susan told me that she was interested in improving her diet since her thyroid was sluggish. She also had a history of breast cancer that was in remission.

When I asked Susan about her diet, she told me that she ate soy products 3 to 4 times a week. She added that she cooked only with corn or mixed vegetable oils. I educated Susan about the dangers of eating soy in view of her history of breast cancer as well as the dangers of refined vegetable oils. She immediately gave up both. Five years later, she remains cancer-free, and her thyroid hormone level is perfect with a small, stable dose of thyroid hormone.

## Richard's Story

Richard is a 42-year-old magazine editor who has been HIV positive for more than 17 years. Although his HIV viral load was undetectable when he came to see me, he was showing signs of HIV lipodystrophy, a condition associated with HIV infection that is characterized by elevated cholesterol and sugar, insulin resistance, abnormal fat deposits in the neck and trunk, and facial wasting. The condition may be related to the HIV virus, and HIV drugs.

Although Richard exercised vigorously, he ate as he pleased—large fruit smoothies for breakfast, fast food, and pizzas on a daily basis. His insulin level was too high, and his testosterone level was too low. Again, low testosterone is common with serious illnesses such as HIV, and it's aggravated by the absence of saturated fat from the diet.

I put Richard on the Perfect 10 Diet and advised him to follow a high-fat/low-carb diet to improve his insulin resistance. I also prescribed a natural testosterone cream for him. I emphasized to Richard that he should avoid the hydrogenated and trans fats since they interfere with the proper body synthesis of his disease-fighting T cells. After following the Perfect 10 Diet for 5 months, Richard's sugar and cholesterol levels normalized without drugs. His insulin and testosterone levels became perfect. Richard's immune system also improved significantly.

## Gina's Story

Gina is a 33-year-old hairdresser who came to see me for irregular menstrual periods. She told me that she had seen several doctors for an infertility problem during the preceding 5 years.

After taking an extensive history, I asked Gina about her diet. She told me that she stuck to a low-fat diet at all times, joking that she even suffered through constant stomach cramps because of her attempts to get 3 servings of fat-free dairy daily.

Gina's diet was poor, even though she believed otherwise. I ordered an insulin level for Gina, and I wasn't surprised when it came back extremely high. Her estrogen and progesterone level were also unbalanced.

A pelvic ultrasound revealed multiple cysts on her ovaries. Gina had polycystic ovary syndrome, which caused her irregular periods and infertility. The condition is related to insulin resistance. It was clear that Gina's disease was aggravated by her diet. When I told Gina about the dangers of fat-free dairy on ovulation and its bad effect on female sex hormones, she broke down into tears and confided that her infertility problem had put a strain on her marriage.

Gina started on the Perfect 10 Diet. After just a couple of months, Gina's periods became regular. She was able to conceive within a year.

## Pam's Story

Pam is a 43-year-old single real estate broker who had suffered from severe asthma for 12 years. She had been placed on cortisone to control her shortness of breath. After years of this treatment, she had lost muscle mass and felt tired, depressed, and anxious. Although Pam had learned to live with her disease, she had become concerned that her libido was almost nonexistent, and she felt no attraction to men of any type.

Pam's symptoms were consistent with DHEA and testosterone deficiencies. She needed supplementation, but that wasn't enough. Pam needed to change her diet. She told me she had avoided saturated fats for as long as she could remember, and she only used margarine instead of butter. Pam was advised to follow the Perfect 10 Diet and avoid all fake fats. After 4 months, her mood had greatly improved, and she was happily dating.

CHAPTER 18

# Frequently Asked Questions

I have counseled thousands of patients throughout the years, and many asked very insightful questions about the Perfect 10 Diet. I have included some of the most frequently asked questions here to share with you.

**Q** *I suffer from diabetes. Is the Perfect 10 Diet safe for me?*

**A** Absolutely. The Perfect 10 Diet is beneficial for diabetics, as it will help stabilize your blood sugar levels and lower your insulin demands. It's balanced in all food groups. Diabetics in particular should eat more natural fats and should not follow a low-fat diet.

**Q** *Can I eat any nitrite-free bacon, Canadian bacon, ham, or sausage on the Perfect 10 Diet?*

**A** No, these protein sources have been linked to gastrointestinal cancer even without nitrites. They contain a lot of salt, which raises blood pressure. Bacon and sausage are often fried, which produces harmful oxidized cholesterol. The link to colon cancer appears to be related to the protein itself, not just the nitrites. If you must eat nitrite-free bacon, Canadian bacon, ham, or sausage, do so infrequently and in very small amounts. If you do, bake them rather than fry them.

Q *Which fruit juices are best to drink?*

A None except for tomato, which is rich in lycopene. Fruit juices can contain more sugar than soda. Vegetable juices are better alternatives, except carrot and beet juices, as they contain a lot of sugar.

Q *What can I eat instead of baked potatoes since they are so high in sugar?*

A Any fiber-rich vegetable is a better substitute for white potatoes—even sweet potatoes. Sautéed cauliflower has a similar taste to potatoes and is a perfectly acceptable substitute. I've provided a delicious cauliflower recipe in this book.

Q *How is the Perfect 10 Diet different than the Mediterranean diet?*

A The Perfect 10 Diet embraces the principles of the Mediterranean diet in its amounts of and types of fat, but the Perfect 10 Diet greatly expands on it. The Perfect 10 Diet, of course, has less whole grains than the Mediterranean diet, and it includes a wider range of healthy fats, such as butter and coconut, that are eaten frequently in other cuisines. The Perfect 10 Diet is truly an international delight.

Q *I stopped smoking and gained a lot of weight. What do you suggest?*

A One cigarette burns 5 calories, so smoking a pack (20 cigarettes) a day means your body burns an extra 200 calories. You need to substitute the smoking habit with a healthy calorie-burning activity. That's why exercise is a core part of the Perfect 10 Diet.

*I would like to occasionally replace one of my meals with a protein shake when I am busy. Any recommendations?*

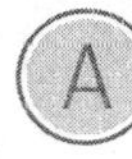
Whey protein is a high-quality protein powder made from cows' milk. Milk has two proteins: casein (approximately 80 percent) and whey protein (approximately 20 percent). Whey protein is more soluble than casein, and it also has a higher quality rating. Look for shakes made with whey that have no added artificial ingredients or artificial sweeteners. Avoid shakes made with soy protein isolate, as they are chemically treated.

*I work night shifts. How can I follow the Perfect 10 Diet?*

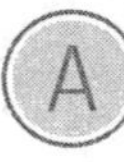
Just switch your meals to match your schedule. When you wake up at night, eat breakfast, and then in the morning, have your dinner. Follow the Perfect 10 Diet by eating 3 meals a day.

*Do I really have to exercise on the Perfect 10 Diet to lose weight?*

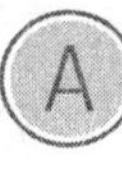
Of course. Did you think I was going to lie to you? The good news is that you will need to work out much less on the Perfect 10 Diet than you would on other diets because your hormones will be working with you, not against you.

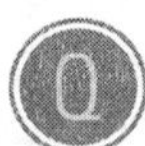
*What can I eat at the movies?*

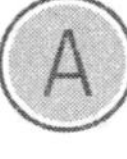
Bring your own nuts or snacks, and stay away from the stands. Movie snacks are loaded with sugar. Also, stay away from movie popcorn as it's probably made with hydrogenated oils.

*I follow the Perfect 10 Diet, but I still feel hungry after meals. What can I do?*

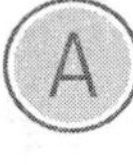
If you eat 3 meals but still feel hungry, your daily calorie requirements may be higher than you think or you may have an insulin problem. Go ahead and increase your portion sizes at meals. Eat until you feel full. You have the option to eat snacks if necessary.

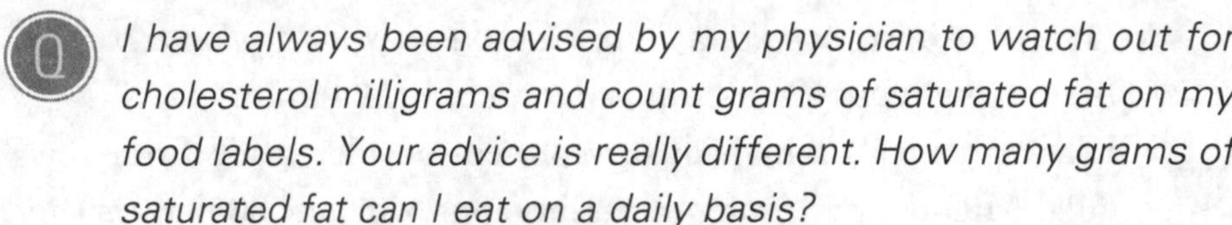

Q *I have always been advised by my physician to watch out for cholesterol milligrams and count grams of saturated fat on my food labels. Your advice is really different. How many grams of saturated fat can I eat on a daily basis?*

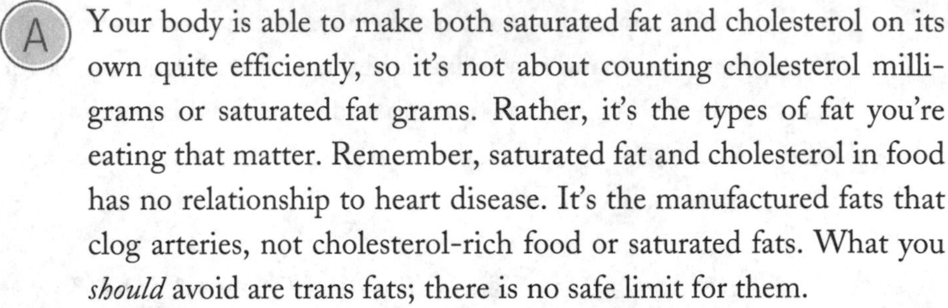

A Your body is able to make both saturated fat and cholesterol on its own quite efficiently, so it's not about counting cholesterol milligrams or saturated fat grams. Rather, it's the types of fat you're eating that matter. Remember, saturated fat and cholesterol in food has no relationship to heart disease. It's the manufactured fats that clog arteries, not cholesterol-rich food or saturated fats. What you *should* avoid are trans fats; there is no safe limit for them.

Q *I like to eat French fries once in a while. How should I cook them?*

A I discourage eating deep-fried food at all times. If you must fry any food, use ghee, coconut oil, palm oil, or butter. I also recommend macadamia oil, which has a neutral taste and a high burning point.

Q *How much red meat (including beef, lamb, and pork) or processed meat can I eat?*

A Researchers define high consumption of red meat and its relationship to colon cancer as 3 or more ounces of red meat per day for a man. This is the size of a fast-food hamburger. For a woman, the amount is 2 or more ounces. For processed meat (bacon, sausage, hot dogs, ham, and cold cuts), the amount is only 1 ounce. A slice of bologna weighs 1 ounce, as do 3 slices of cooked bacon. If you're eating red meat on a daily basis, try to cut this back to once every 2 weeks. If you're eating red meat weekly, try to scale it back to once every 3 to 4 weeks. When you do eat red meat, have it rare or medium, and never well done. Avoid processed meat at all times.

Q *I usually eat breakfast after leaving home. Any tips on how to eat on the run?*

A Boil a few eggs the night before and keep them in the refrigerator. Have them with a piece of cheese for breakfast, and you won't have to eat something fast when you're in a rush. Another idea is to always keep fresh fruit in the house and take some with you when you leave home.

Q *I've begun the Perfect 10 Diet and have increased my fat intake; however, I've gained weight and feel bloated. I'm scared to continue. What are your suggestions?*

A Your body and digestive enzymes need adequate time to adjust to this new way of healthy eating. Don't be scared; continue to follow the principles of the Perfect 10 Diet. Keep portion size under control and exercise regularly, and you will achieve success.

Q *Are egg whites better than whole eggs for my health?*

A No. Egg whites are devoid of the heart-healthy omega-3 fatty acids found in the yolks. Eat eggs with their yolks regularly, especially from pasture-fed and free-range chickens in order to avoid hormones and antibiotics.

Q *Where can I find macadamia butter, almond butter, and coconut milk?*

A Supermarkets are beginning to stock these products. If you cannot find them, health-food stores are your best bet for these healthy fats.

Q *Which fruits are preferred on the Perfect 10 Diet?*

A All fruits are permitted on the Perfect 10 Diet. However, berries, cherries, and cantaloupes are favored, as these fruits have less sugar. High-fat fruits, such as coconut, are encouraged for those who have trouble losing weight, since they can stabilize insulin levels.

Q *Do you recommend low-fat or low-carb condiments on the Perfect 10 Diet?*

A Neither. I am not a fan of any processed food. Low-carb condiments contain sugar and alcohol, which can cause bloating, as well as artificial sweeteners. I am also disturbed by the use of partially hydrogenated oil in many of these low-carb products. If you must buy a low-carb condiment or product, look for one that doesn't contain partially hydrogenated oil or soy protein isolate.

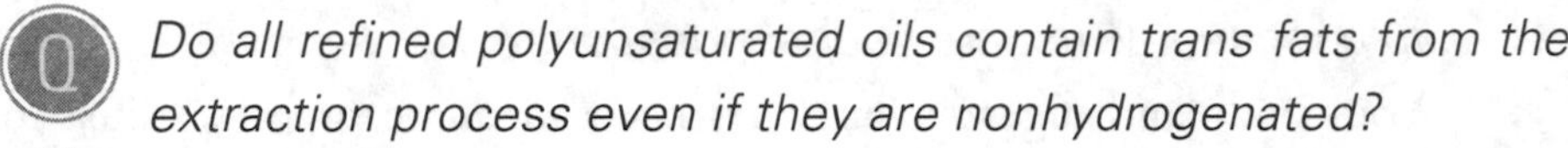

Q *Do all refined polyunsaturated oils contain trans fats from the extraction process even if they are nonhydrogenated?*

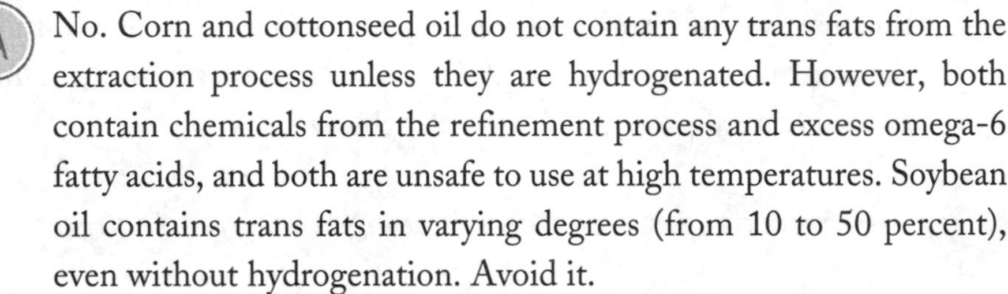

A No. Corn and cottonseed oil do not contain any trans fats from the extraction process unless they are hydrogenated. However, both contain chemicals from the refinement process and excess omega-6 fatty acids, and both are unsafe to use at high temperatures. Soybean oil contains trans fats in varying degrees (from 10 to 50 percent), even without hydrogenation. Avoid it.

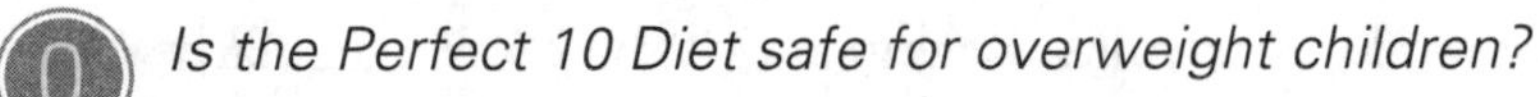

Q *Is the Perfect 10 Diet safe for overweight children?*

A Absolutely. The Perfect 10 Diet is optimal for overweight children, except when it comes to seafood (because of mercury). All children need to include more fat in their diets, especially saturated fats for their developing brains.

Q *Is the Perfect 10 Diet safe for pregnant women?*

A Yes. Pregnant women can follow Stage Three on the Perfect 10 Diet, with proper calcium supplementation and also with appropriate cautions about seafood. Although the Perfect 10 Diet is nutritionally sound for most adults, a pregnant woman has additional nutritional needs, such as iron and calcium, that must be accommodated.

Q *Can I eat pasta on the Perfect 10 Diet?*

A Of course. Whole-wheat pasta cooked al dente is perfectly acceptable in Stages Two and Three of the Perfect 10 Diet.

*What is your opinion about over-the-counter diet pills?*

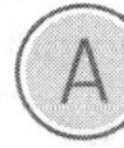

I am reluctant to suggest any over-the-counter diet pills, since many contain caffeine, which can lead to heart palpitations. I am also not a fan of the fat-blocking pills, as they can lead to vitamin deficiencies. Hoodia, which has been shown to curb appetite, has to be taken from the plant rather than in a pill form to achieve results. I have listed natural supplements at the end of the book that may help with weight loss. If you have little willpower when it comes to food, ask your doctor for a prescription drug that is suitable for you.

*Which breads are recommended on the Perfect 10 Diet?*

All whole-grain breads are good, but rye and pumpernickel breads are the best since they contain the least amount of sugar and the highest fiber content. Read the label carefully to make sure there is no enriched flour, molasses, or hydrogenated oil used in the manufacturing process.

*The Perfect 10 Diet appears to be restrictive when it comes to certain foods. How can I stay on track every day?*

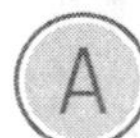

In truth, the Perfect 10 Diet is only restrictive when it comes to refined carbohydrates, sugar, and partially hydrogenated oils. Most foods are permitted, including red meat, pork, and lamb on occasion. Very little is off limits. Once you learn to replace refined carbs and sugar with healthy food choices, the Perfect 10 Diet will become second nature.

*I am allergic to fish and do not like chicken. What can I eat instead?*

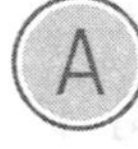

Protein can come from any animal source, including turkey, goose, or duck. Eggs, mushrooms, and beans are also excellent sources of protein. You can also eat red meat, and non–genetically modified soy on the Perfect 10 Diet, but in moderation.

*I heard that butter and animal fat contains some trans fats. Is this true?*

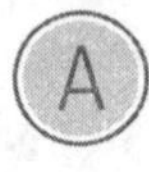
Yes, butter and fat from ruminate animals contain negligible amounts of trans fats. However, these natural trans fats have been reported to prevent cancer and do not interfere with hormones or cellular communications. They are completely different from the artificial trans fats found in margarine and hydrogenated vegetable oils. Those manufactured trans fats are carcinogenic.

*I get very bored on diets. How can the Perfect 10 Diet keep me motivated?*

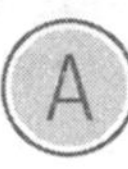
Experiment with different kinds of cuisine, such as French, Thai, Vietnamese, Middle Eastern, Japanese, Spanish, or Greek. Mix up your protein and vegetable sources, and be creative with herbs, spices, and other non-restricted condiments.

*I'm allergic to fish. How can I get omega-3 fatty acids into my diet?*

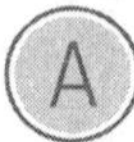
Add a teaspoon of flaxseed oil to your diet every day. Eat nuts and eggs from pasture-fed or free-range birds regularly.

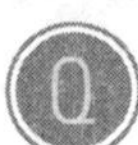
*Will the Perfect 10 Diet have any effect on my complexion?*

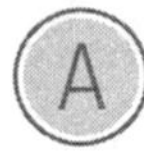
Absolutely. The Perfect 10 Diet will help you have a glowing complexion. Sugar and polyunsaturated vegetable oils have a huge negative impact on complexion. Both damage collagen underneath the skin, just like they clog the arteries. As you eliminate polyunsaturated oils and sugar from your diet, you stop the damage. A balanced diet with the right amounts of natural fats will actually improve your complexion. Your body will be able to absorb the fat-soluble vitamins, including vitamin A. Vitamin A has a great influence on the complexion. By following the Perfect 10 Diet, your complexion will gradually improve. And let's not forget the positive effect of optimized sex hormones and HGH on skin.

*Is it true that a high-fat diet can lead to an aggravation of acne?*

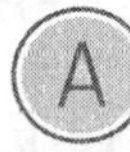

No. Fat in food does not promote acne; it's a myth. However, if you break out in acne pimples after eating dairy products, there could be a link to the hormones present in cows' milk. Stop dairy altogether for 3 weeks. If your acne clears up, it's related to dairy. If your acne doesn't clear up, it's probably not related to dairy, and you should consult a dermatologist.

*Can I drink an occasional diet soda on the Perfect 10 Diet?*

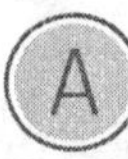

No, absolutely not. I do not encourage diet sodas on the Perfect 10 Diet because of their artificial sweeteners. If you really crave soda, have a regular organic soda made with real sugar, rather than high-fructose corn syrup, and hit the gym before the sugar screws up your hormones.

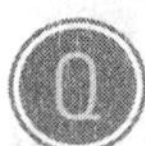

*Can I chew sugar-free gum on the Perfect 10 Diet?*

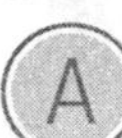

No. It contains artificial sweeteners. If you must chew gum, choose a reduced-sugar variety.

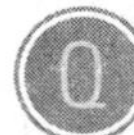

*I travel frequently. What can I eat on planes?*

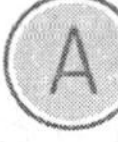

Airlines are notorious for their bad food. And I'm always given sweets or margarine with my meals. Pack a snack, or buy some nuts or an apple at the airport to take on board. On planes, choose an entrée that has protein as the main food rather refined carbs (chicken instead of pasta, for example).

*Which supplements should I take?*

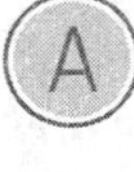

For most people, a whole-food pill with all the vitamins and minerals should be sufficient. Everybody is different. But if you have any other medical conditions or hormonal imbalances, you may require additional supplements or hormones. Consult with your doctor.

*Will the Perfect 10 Diet help me keep the weight off?*

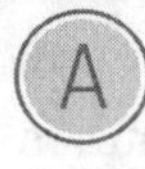

Of course. If you follow the principles of the Perfect 10 Diet correctly, your hormones will be balanced. You can eat more, work out less, and delay aging. By following the Perfect 10 Diet, you'll create healthy habits that will last a lifetime.

What a journey this has been! As I come to the end of this chapter, I want to sincerely thank you for reading *The Perfect 10 Diet*. It has been my great privilege to share this lifesaving information with you. Although I finished writing this book, I'm just getting started with this effort. I will keep you updated with the latest nutrition information and health research by newsletters on the Perfect 10 Diet's website: www.ThePerfect10Diet.com.

But I have few final thoughts to share with you. Where are we when it comes to knowledge and breakthrough information? What a sad state we've reached when the right information is not coming from our medical establishment, but from a doctor who took the initiative to write a book with the most up-to-date and nonbiased information. After all, I am neither a writer nor the surgeon general. I can't dwell on the past, though, because I believe that a revolution has begun as the Perfect 10 Diet takes off nationally and internationally. Is it a smooth takeoff, with so many imperfect diets blocking its runway? Of course not—it is going to be a long wait that may take years. You can't change 40 years of biased information overnight, or with one diet, but it's a start.

I certainly can't do it alone, so tell your family and friends. Make a difference in the lives of the people you care about. They need your help. I leave the message of the Perfect 10 Diet with you, and I know you will be safe. We are at a crossroads. We can either follow the same old road that took us nowhere, or head down a brand-new road that will take us to perfect 10 health. I've taken this new road along with my patients, and I'm so glad you have joined us. But everyone deserves better, so let's get loud enough for everyone to hear us. We have a lot of work to do. It's important to know that together, we can all make a difference. Social networking sites like Facebook, Twitter, and MySpace allow you to blog instantaneously and quickly spread information to the masses across the globe so that special interests, lobbyists, and the food industry can no longer suppress the truth.

I wrote *The Perfect 10 Diet* to share my knowledge and the latest nutritional research with you. I want to make a difference, and it was a most difficult journey. When I first started writing, some literary agents told me they weren't interested in my book because I'm not a published or established writer. Some pointed out that I'm neither a famous celebrity nor endorsed by Oprah. I didn't get it. You need a license to practice almost any profession, yet when it comes to our health, we are getting our information from nonprofessionals. I didn't despair, and I didn't give up after those rejections. In fact, they motivated me even more. I knew that the public, just like my patients, were in desperate need for clear guidance. Unlike the countless popular diets that made people face serious diseases from disturbed hormones, I knew the concepts of the Perfect 10 Diet would bring harmony and balance.

The Perfect 10 Diet's rhythms and rhymes are distinct from all the noise around. A new era is beginning as people start to listen. The Perfect 10 Diet is spreading beyond the United States. It's a greater achievement than I set out to accomplish. Destiny took me far, and I'm grateful.

Whether the Perfect 10 Diet makes a positive impact or falls on deaf ears for those who cling to dietary misinformation, I know that the Perfect 10 Diet will have a lasting impression on your health, appearance, and life.

# PART 4

## THE PERFECT 10 DIET RECIPES

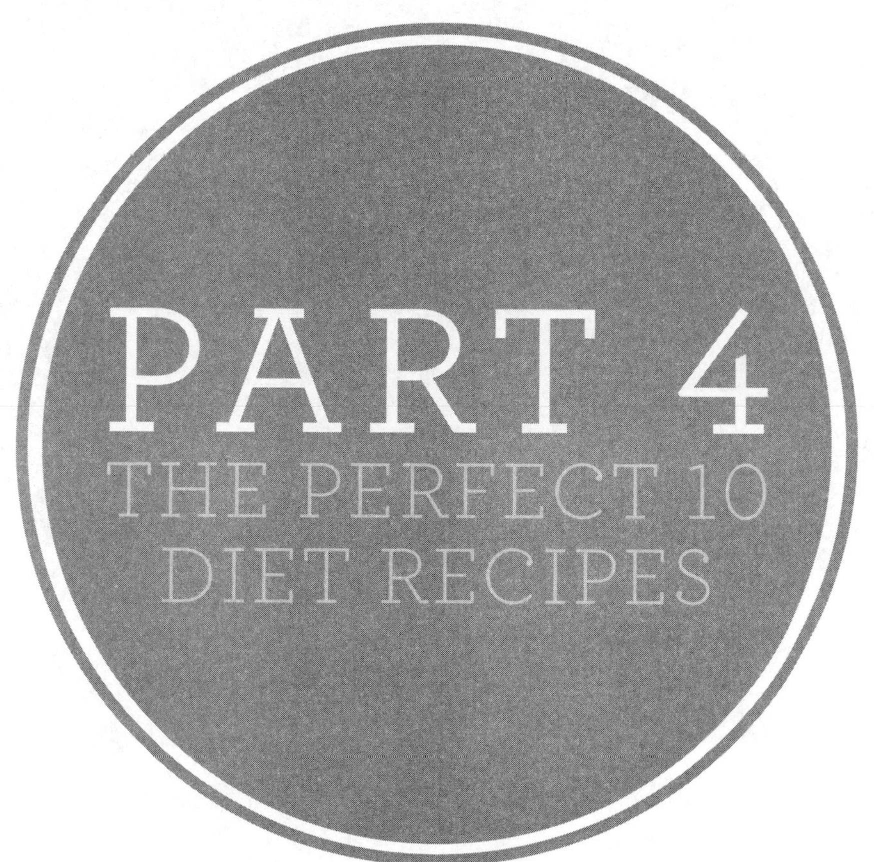

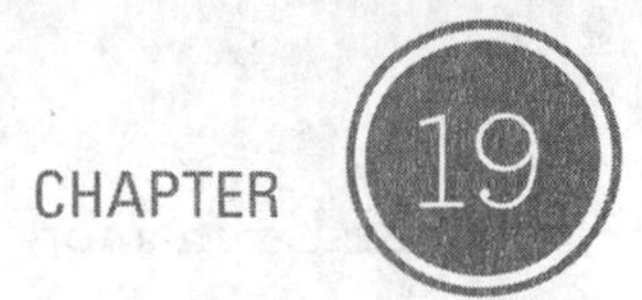
CHAPTER 19

# Recipes for Stage One

Stage One recipes do not contain any grains or alcohol.

## Breakfast

### French Cheese Omelet

SERVINGS: 1 to 2
PREPARATION TIME: 10 min.

INGREDIENTS

3 medium eggs
Pinch salt and freshly ground black pepper
½ tablespoon butter
¼ cup shredded Swiss, cheddar, or Monterey Jack cheese

DIRECTIONS

1. In a small bowl, combine the eggs, 2 tablespoons water, salt, and pepper.

2. Beat with a fork until ingredients are well mixed.
3. Heat a nonstick skillet over medium heat, and add the butter.
4. When the butter melts, add the egg mixture.
5. Stir eggs gently with a heat-proof, nonmetallic spatula.
6. Add the cheese, and cook until eggs are firm. Fold in half. Serve.

## Mushroom Omelet

SERVINGS: 1 to 2
PREPARATION TIME: 10 min.

INGREDIENTS

3 medium eggs
Pinch salt and freshly ground black pepper
1 tablespoon butter, divided
⅓ cup sliced fresh mushrooms

DIRECTIONS

1. In a small bowl, combine the eggs, 2 tablespoons water, salt, and pepper.
2. Beat with a fork until ingredients are well mixed.
3. Heat a nonstick skillet over medium heat, and add ½ tablespoon butter.
4. Add the mushrooms, and cook until tender. Remove from the pan, and set aside.
5. Add the remaining butter, and heat until melted.
6. Stir eggs gently with a heat-proof, nonmetallic spatula. Add the mushrooms, and cook until eggs are firm. Fold in half. Serve.

## Mediterranean Frittata

SERVINGS: 4 to 6
PREPARATION TIME: 30 min.

INGREDIENTS

8 medium eggs
Pinch salt
¼ cup whole milk or half-and-half
2 tablespoons extra-virgin olive oil, divided
½ cup chopped onion
½ cup chopped red peppers
1 teaspoon minced garlic
2 ounces crumbled feta cheese
¼ cup pitted olives
5 leaves fresh basil
Pinch freshly ground black pepper
2 tablespoons grated Parmesan cheese

DIRECTIONS

1. Combine the eggs, salt, and milk, and beat until ingredients are mixed.
2. In a large skillet, warm 1 tablespoon olive oil over low to medium heat.
3. Add the onion, red peppers, and garlic; cook until the onion is tender, but not brown.
4. Add the feta cheese, olives, basil, and black pepper.
5. Pour the egg mixture in the skillet.
6. Cook over medium heat. As the egg mixture sets at the bottom of the pan, lift the edge of the mixture with a spatula to allow the liquid mixture to run under and cook. Continue until the egg mixture is set.
7. Sprinkle the top of the frittata with the Parmesan cheese and remaining olive oil.
8. Place skillet under broiler, 4 inches from the flame. Heat frittata for 1 to 2 minutes, until firm. Cut into wedges and serve.

## Whitefish or Tuna Salad

SERVINGS: 2
PREPARATION TIME: 5 min.

INGREDIENTS

4 scoops tuna or whitefish (1 large can of tuna in water can also be used)
¼ cup chopped red onion
¼ cup chopped celery
1 teaspoon mayonnaise made with olive oil
Mixed greens
2 slices Swiss cheese, shredded

DIRECTIONS

1. Combine tuna/whitefish with the onion, celery, and mayonnaise.
2. Divide the mixed greens between two plates.
3. Divide the tuna/whitefish salad on top of the mixed greens.
4. Sprinkle the shredded cheese on the salads. Serve.

## Vegetable Quiche

SERVINGS: 4 to 5
PREPARATION TIME: 25 min.

INGREDIENTS

3 tablespoons extra-virgin olive oil, divided
1 small onion, diced
1 green pepper, chopped
1 red pepper, chopped
2 cups fresh, chopped spinach
8 medium eggs
½ cup whole milk
¾ cup shredded cheddar cheese

DIRECTIONS

1. Heat a large skillet; add 2 tablespoons olive oil.
2. Sauté the onion, peppers, and spinach for 6 to 7 minutes.
3. Remove the mixture from heat. Set aside, and let cool for 10 minutes.
4. Preheat the oven to 350°F, and coat a separated muffin pan with the remaining olive oil.
5. Mix the eggs with the milk, cheese, and sautéed onion mixture, and cook for 5 minutes.
6. Divide the mixture into the muffin pan, and bake at 350°F for 17 to 20 minutes. Remove from the oven and serve.

## Ricotta Muffins

SERVINGS: 6
PREPARATION TIME: 30 min.

INGREDIENTS

1 cup ricotta cheese
2 medium or large eggs
2 teaspoons agave
½ teaspoon vanilla extract
½ cup grated Parmesan cheese
1 ounce pignoli nuts
½ teaspoon butter

DIRECTIONS

1. Preheat the oven to 350°F.
2. Combine the ricotta and eggs in a bowl, and mix.
3. Add the agave, vanilla, cheese, and nuts.
4. Pour in a nonstick muffin pan brushed with butter.
5. Bake at 350°F for 15 to 20 minutes. Remove from the oven, and serve.

## Breakfast Smoothie

SERVINGS: 1
PREPARATION TIME: 5 min.

INGREDIENTS

½ cup whole-fat organic yogurt
5 strawberries, cut into small pieces
5 blueberries
2 packets stevia or 1 teaspoon agave
8 to 10 ice cubes

DIRECTIONS

1. Combine all ingredients in a blender, and mix on high speed.
2. Add water, if necessary, to make a drinkable consistency.
3. Serve with additional ice cubes.

# Salads and Entrées

## Salmon Salad with Artichokes

SERVINGS: 2
PREPARATION TIME: 15 min.

INGREDIENTS

2 tablespoons extra-virgin olive oil
1 tablespoon lemon juice
2 cloves garlic, minced
2 celery stalks, diced
1 small red onion, chopped
2 tablespoons chopped fresh parsley
1 ounce fennel, sliced

2 small artichokes
1 cup haricots verts or string beans
12 ounces salmon, cut into pieces
6 black olives, for garnish (optional)
1 lemon wedge, for garnish (optional)

DIRECTIONS

1. Mix the olive oil, lemon juice, garlic, celery, onion, parsley, and fennel.
2. Blanch the artichokes and haricots verts in hot water for 10 minutes; let cool, and chop.
3. Mix together all ingredients, except the salmon and garnishes, and toss.
4. Place the mixture on 2 plates with the salmon.
5. Garnish with the lemon wedge and olives. Serve.

## Spinach Niçoise Salad

SERVINGS: 2
PREPARATION TIME: 10 to 15 min.

INGREDIENTS

½ pound broad beans, shelled
1 cup baby spinach leaves, washed and patted dry
½ head lettuce
¼ cup olives, drained
1 cucumber, cut into strips
1 large onion, chopped
4 ounces cherry tomatoes
1 can solid light tuna in water, drained
2 hard-boiled eggs, peeled and halved, for garnish
Pinch freshly ground black pepper

DIRECTIONS

1. Blanch the beans in a pot of boiling water for 3 to 4 minutes, until tender. Chill.
2. Toss together the beans, spinach, lettuce, olives, cucumber, and onion. Dice the tomatoes, and add to the mixture. Divide the mixture onto 2 plates.
3. Divide the tuna atop the greens. Garnish with the eggs. Add pepper, to taste. Serve.

## Shrimp Salad

SERVINGS: 2
PREPARATION TIME: 10 to 15 min.

INGREDIENTS

2 tablespoons lime juice
1 tablespoon extra-virgin olive oil
2 tablespoons snipped fresh marjoram
Pinch salt and freshly ground black pepper
3 large tomatoes (red, orange, or yellow)
1 cup shredded yellow summer squash or zucchini
6 large shrimp, peeled, deveined, and cooked

DIRECTIONS

1. Preheat the oven to 350°F.
2. For dressing: Combine the lime juice, olive oil, marjoram, salt, and pepper. Refrigerate.
3. For salad: Cut the tomatoes into 6 slices, and place in a 2-quart baking dish.
4. Pour ½ the dressing over the tomatoes. Cover and bake for 4 minutes at 345°F.
5. Remove the tomatoes from the dish.
6. Set out 2 plates, and put 1 tomato slice on each plate. Top with 1 tablespoon shredded squash and 1 shrimp. Repeat, making layers, until the mixture has been completely used. Top with the tomato and reserved dressing. Serve.

## Vietnamese Salad

SERVINGS: 2 to 3
PREPARATION TIME: 20 min.

INGREDIENTS

1 head romaine lettuce, chopped
1 head butter lettuce, chopped
2 scallions
1 ruby-red grapefruit
1 packet stevia or 1 teaspoon agave
3 tablespoons fish sauce
3 tablespoons lime juice
½ teaspoon chili garlic paste
1 tablespoon chopped peanuts
½ cup chopped fresh cilantro
¼ cup chopped fresh mint

DIRECTIONS

1. Wash all ingredients. Divide the lettuce among 2 to 3 plates.
2. Slice the scallions, and place over the lettuce.
3. Divide the grapefruit into 3 pieces.
4. Mix together the stevia or agave, fish sauce, lime juice, and chili paste, and place over the lettuce, onion, and grapefruit.
5. Top the salads with the peanuts, cilantro, and mint. Serve.

## Scallop Ceviche

SERVINGS: 2
PREPARATION TIME: 1 to 2 hours

INGREDIENTS

½ pound bay scallops
1 (8-ounce) can tomato paste

1 plum tomato (medium-sized)
½ red onion
5 cilantro leaves
1 ounce lemon juice
Dash Tabasco sauce
Pinch salt and freshly ground black pepper

DIRECTIONS

1. Cook scallops for 20 to 30 minutes in boiling water and tomato paste. Drain.
2. Dice the tomatoes and onions, and chop the cilantro.
3. In a medium bowl, combine the tomatoes, onions, and cilantro with the lemon juice, Tabasco, salt, and pepper. Add the scallops and mix well.
4. Refrigerate for 1 to 2 hours before serving. Serve.

## Stir-Fried Oysters

SERVINGS: 1
PREPARATION TIME: 10 min.

INGREDIENTS

5 oysters (in shell)
1 leek
1 teaspoon butter
Pinch salt and freshly ground black pepper
Lemon wedge, for garnish (optional)

DIRECTIONS

1. Open the oysters (or have it done at the store), and refrigerate.
2. Wash the leek thoroughly, and slice thinly.
3. Heat the butter in a pan over medium heat. Add the leek, and cook for 2 to 3 minutes. Remove from heat, and set aside.

4. Add the oysters. Return to heat, and cook for 1 minute on each side.
5. Return the leek to the oyster pan. Stir once, and place on plate. Garnish with lemon. Serve.

## Tuna with Goat Cheese

SERVINGS: 2
PREPARATION TIME: 2 hours

INGREDIENTS

1 tablespoon extra-virgin olive oil
12 ounces cooked tuna (small type), diced into ½-inch pieces
Pinch freshly ground black pepper
3 ounces fresh goat cheese
1 tablespoon minced fresh chives
½ small clove garlic, chopped
½ teaspoon peeled, grated ginger root
Pinch cayenne pepper
1 cup arugula leaves, for garnish

DIRECTIONS

1. Drizzle the olive oil over the tuna in a glass baking dish. Add the black pepper.
2. Cover and refrigerate for 2 hours.
3. In a separate bowl, mash together the goat cheese with the chives, garlic, ginger, and cayenne pepper.
4. Toss the marinated tuna over the goat cheese mixture.
5. Garnish with the arugula. Serve.

## Sashimi of Salmon and Avocado Salad

SERVINGS: 2 to 3
PREPARATION TIME: 20 min.

INGREDIENTS

½ bunch cilantro, cleaned and stemmed
6 tablespoons extra-virgin olive oil
1 jalapeño pepper, halved
1 avocado
2 teaspoons lemon juice
Pinch salt and freshly ground black pepper
½ head lettuce
6 pieces salmon (sushi-grade), sliced into rectangles

DIRECTIONS

1. Blanch the cilantro in boiling water for 10 seconds. Remove and immediately place in ice water.
2. Remove the cilantro from the water, and place in a blender with the olive oil and jalapeño. Blend until fully incorporated.
3. Cut the avocado into 1-inch cubes, and place in a mixing bowl. Add the cilantro mixture, lemon juice, salt, and pepper, and set aside.
4. Arrange the lettuce in circles on 2 to 3 small plates, and place the avocado pieces in the center of each.
5. Place the salmon on top of the avocados. Pour the cilantro mixture over the top of the salmon. Serve.

## Chicken Wraps

SERVINGS: 4 to 5
PREPARATION TIME: 20 min.

INGREDIENTS

4 cups cooked, chopped skinless chicken breast, cooled to room temperature
½ cup sour cream
½ cup green onion, finely chopped
½ finely chopped teaspoon fresh parsley
Cayenne pepper, to taste (optional)
¼ teaspoon freshly grated nutmeg (optional)
½ cup toasted sunflower seeds
1 head butter lettuce leaves, separated, washed, and dried (to use as wraps)

DIRECTIONS

1. Combine the chicken, sour cream, green onion, parsley, pepper, nutmeg, and sunflower seeds in a large bowl.
2. Spoon the chicken mixture into butter lettuce leaves, and roll up. Serve.

## Chinese Sticky Wings

SERVINGS: 4 to 6
PREPARATION TIME: 6 to 7 hours

INGREDIENTS

1 teaspoon agave
1 tablespoon grated ginger root
1 clove garlic, chopped
½ teaspoon chili garlic paste
3 pounds chicken wings

DIRECTIONS

1. Preheat the oven to 375°F.
2. Mix together all ingredients, except the chicken wings.
3. Place the marinade in a sealed container, and refrigerate 3 to 4 hours.
4. Place the chicken wings in the marinade, and return to the refrigerator for 2 hours.

5. Remove the chicken wings from the marinade, and set marinade aside.
6. Arrange the chicken wings in a pan, and bake at 375°F for 15 minutes.
7. Remove the pan from the oven. Pour the marinade over the chicken wings, and bake for an additional 30 to 40 minutes. Serve.

## Grilled Chicken Paillard with Tangerine Butter

SERVINGS: 2
PREPARATION TIME: 90 min.

INGREDIENTS

2 chicken breasts
2 tablespoons extra-virgin olive oil
1 tangerine, peeled and cut into small pieces
1 cup fresh mixed herbs (tarragon, parsley, and thyme)
2 tablespoons lime juice
1 small head lettuce
3 medium cucumbers, sliced
1 teaspoon butter

DIRECTIONS

1. Clean the chicken breasts. Mix together the olive oil, tangerine, herbs, and lime juice. Marinate 1 hour.
2. Toss together the lettuce and sliced cucumbers. Set aside.
3. In a medium skillet, heat the butter over medium heat.
4. Sauté the chicken in a skillet for several minutes on each side, until thoroughly cooked.
5. Serve the chicken with the cucumber and lettuce salad.

## Sautéed Chicken with Shallots

SERVINGS: 2
PREPARATION TIME: 20 min.

INGREDIENTS

2 chicken breasts
3 teaspoons extra-virgin olive oil
1 teaspoon unsalted butter
½ cup shallots
2 cloves garlic, minced
4 roasted tomatoes, seeded and chopped
Pinch freshly ground black pepper

DIRECTIONS

1. Clean the chicken breasts.
2. Heat the olive oil and butter in a medium skillet over medium heat.
3. Add the shallots and garlic, and cook for 1 minute.
4. Add the chicken, and sauté for 7 to 10 minutes on each side, until thoroughly cooked.
5. Add the tomatoes, and cook for an additional 3 minutes.
6. Add pepper, to taste. Serve.

## Chicken Florentine

SERVINGS: 2
PREPARATION TIME: 20 min.

INGREDIENTS

2 chicken breasts
2 cups sautéed spinach
½ cup cream or water
1 tablespoon butter

1 cup mushrooms
½ medium red onion, chopped
Pinch salt and freshly ground black pepper

DIRECTIONS

1. Clean the chicken breasts. Cut a pocket into each chicken breast, and fill with the spinach.
2. Poach the breasts in cream or water for 15 minutes.
3. Heat the butter in a medium skillet. Add the mushrooms, and sauté for 3 minutes.
4. Add the onion, and cook for 3 additional minutes.
5. Add the chicken, and sauté for several minutes on each side, until thoroughly cooked. Add salt and pepper.
6. Spread the mushroom mixture over the chicken. Serve.

## Chicken with Tomato and Artichokes

SERVINGS: 2
PREPARATION TIME: 40 min.

INGREDIENTS

½ whole chicken
2 teaspoons macadamia oil
½ cup roasted tomatoes
2 cloves garlic, minced
½ cup artichoke hearts, chopped
¼ teaspoon chopped fresh tarragon
¼ teaspoon chopped fresh parsley
¼ teaspoon chopped fresh chervil
¼ teaspoon fresh chives
Pinch salt and freshly ground black pepper

DIRECTIONS

1. Preheat the oven to 350°F.
2. Place the chicken in a hot pan, and bake for 35 minutes at 350°F. Set aside.
3. In a skillet, heat the macadamia oil.
4. Add the tomatoes, garlic, and artichokes.
5. Sauté for 5 minutes, and add the tarragon, parsley, chervil, and chives.
6. Place the mixture on top of the chicken. Add salt and pepper and serve.

## Grilled Turkey Steak

SERVINGS: 2 to 3
PREPARATION TIME: 40 min.

INGREDIENTS

1½ pounds boneless, skinless turkey breasts
¼ cup Dijon mustard
Pinch freshly ground black pepper
Juice of 1 orange
1 teaspoon Worcestershire sauce
1 clove garlic, minced
1 tablespoon macadamia oil

DIRECTIONS

1. Place the turkey in a glass baking dish. Brush both sides of the turkey with the mustard, and sprinkle with pepper.
2. Mix together the orange juice, Worcestershire sauce, and garlic.
3. Pour half the orange juice mixture over the turkey, and reserve the remaining half. Turn to coat evenly. Cover, and refrigerate for 20 minutes.
4. Coat the grill rack with the macadamia oil. Preheat the grill to medium, and line it with aluminum foil.

5. Grill the turkey until thoroughly cooked, turning occasionally and brushing with the reserved orange juice mixture for 30 minutes.
6. Let stand 5 minutes.
7. Slice diagonally, and serve.

## Grilled Duck Breast

SERVINGS: 2
PREPARATION TIME: 10 min.

INGREDIENTS

2 teaspoons butter
2 duck breasts
Pinch salt and freshly ground black pepper
2 bunches watercress
1 cup frisée lettuce
1 red pepper, sliced

DIRECTIONS

1. Heat the butter in a pan over medium heat.
2. Season the duck breasts with salt and pepper.
3. Sauté the duck breasts for a few minutes on each side.
4. In a bowl, toss together the watercress, frisée, and red pepper.
5. Place the duck breasts on separate plates, and serve with the watercress salad.

# Snacks and Desserts

These recipes are acceptable for Stage One of the Perfect 10 Diet as optional midmorning or midafternoon snacks or desserts.

## Hummus

SERVINGS: 3
PREPARATION TIME: 3 to 5 hours

INGREDIENTS

1 cup dried chick peas (garbanzo beans)
⅓ cup tahini
3 tablespoons extra-virgin olive oil
Pinch salt and freshly ground black pepper
5 cloves garlic, finely chopped
¼ teaspoon ground cumin
½ cup fresh lemon juice
2 tablespoons chopped fresh parsley

DIRECTIONS

1. Rinse and drain chick peas. Soak in water for 4 hours or, preferably, overnight.
2. Drain and discard the water.
3. Place the chick peas in a saucepan. Cover the chick peas with 2 inches of water, and bring to a boil.
4. Cook on low heat for 1 hour, or until the skin cracks or the chick peas are tender.
5. In a blender, combine the chick peas, tahini, olive oil, salt, pepper, garlic, cumin, and lemon juice. Blend until smooth; if too thick, add water.
6. Sprinkle with parsley, and serve.

## Cocoa and Coconut Bananas

SERVINGS: 4
PREPARATION TIME: 10 min.

INGREDIENTS

4 teaspoons cocoa powder
4 teaspoons toasted unsweetened coconut
2 bananas, sliced

DIRECTIONS

1. Place the cocoa and coconut on separate plates.
2. Roll each banana slice in the cocoa powder, shake off the excess, then dip in coconut.

## Almond Ricotta Crème

SERVINGS: 1
PREPARATION TIME: 10 min.

INGREDIENTS

1 cup ricotta cheese
½ teaspoon almond extract
2 packets stevia or 1 teaspoon agave
2 teaspoons roasted almonds, chopped

DIRECTIONS

1. Mix together all ingredients, except almonds, in bowl. Sprinkle with the almonds.
2. Place in the freezer for 10 minutes.
3. Serve chilled.

## Pears with Blue Cheese

SERVINGS: 1
PREPARATION TIME: 3 min.

INGREDIENTS

1 pear, sliced
1 tablespoon crumbled blue cheese

DIRECTIONS

1. Top pear slices with blue cheese.

## Stage One on the Perfect 10 Diet Meal Plan

DAY ONE

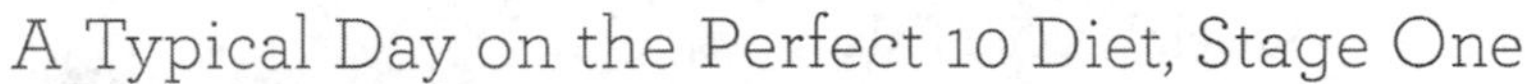

### A Typical Day on the Perfect 10 Diet, Stage One

**BREAKFAST:** Fresh Vegetable Juice and Eggs Copenhagen (Poached Eggs with Salmon)
**OPTIONAL MIDMORNING SNACK:** Lettuce Dipped in Hummus
**LUNCH:** Vietnamese Salad
**OPTIONAL MIDAFTERNOON SNACK:** Berries with 2 Teaspoons Unsweetened Whipped Cream
**DINNER:** Grilled Duck Breast with Side Salad

DAY TWO

### A Typical Day on the Perfect 10 Diet, Stage One

**BREAKFAST:** Breakfast Smoothie
**OPTIONAL MIDMORNING SNACK:** 2 Slices Turkey
**LUNCH:** Chicken Florentine
**OPTIONAL MIDAFTERNOON SNACK:** Stir-Fried Oysters
**DINNER:** Shrimp in Garlic Butter and a Side Salad

## A Typical Day on the Perfect 10 Diet, Stage One

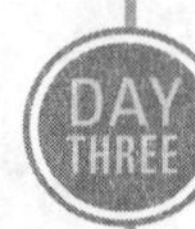


**BREAKFAST:** Vegetable Quiche and 2 Slices Watermelon
**OPTIONAL MIDMORNING SNACK:** ½ Cantaloupe
**LUNCH:** Sautéed Chicken with Shallots
**OPTIONAL MIDAFTERNOON SNACK:** ½ Cup Nuts of Your Choice
**DINNER:** Pan-Fried Crab Cakes

## A Typical Day on the Perfect 10 Diet, Stage One

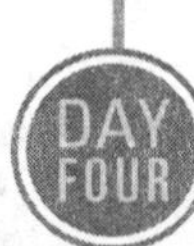


**BREAKFAST:** French Cheese Omelet with a Few Berries
**OPTIONAL MIDMORNING SNACK:** 2 Sticks Celery with 1 Tablespoon Cream Cheese
**LUNCH:** Grilled Turkey Steak with Mixed Greens
**OPTIONAL MIDAFTERNOON SNACK:** Avocado with Lime Juice
**DINNER:** Spinach Niçoise Salad

## A Typical Day on the Perfect 10 Diet, Stage One

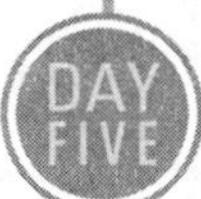


**BREAKFAST:** Strawberries Mixed with 1 Cup Almond Milk
**OPTIONAL MIDMORNING SNACK:** 3 Slices Turkey on Lettuce
**LUNCH:** Chinese Sticky Chicken Wings with a Side Salad
**OPTIONAL MIDAFTERNOON SNACK:** Some Cherry Tomatoes and 1 Tablespoon Almond Butter
**DINNER:** Shrimp with Mushrooms

## A Typical Day on the Perfect 10 Diet, Stage One

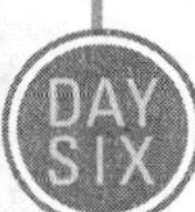


**BREAKFAST:** Mixed Fruit Salad

**OPTIONAL MIDMORNING SNACK:** 1 Scoop Tuna

**LUNCH:** Scallop Ceviche

**OPTIONAL MIDAFTERNOON SNACK:** Almond Ricotta Crème

**DINNER:** Grilled Chicken Paillard with Tangerine Butter

## A Typical Day on the Perfect 10 Diet, Stage One

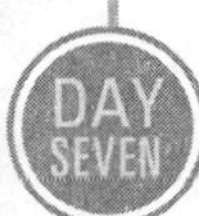


**BREAKFAST:** Mediterranean Frittata

**OPTIONAL MIDMORNING SNACK:** Few Olives

**LUNCH:** Grilled Chicken with Mixed Vegetables

**OPTIONAL MIDAFTERNOON SNACK:** 2 to 3 Dates in Shredded Coconut

**DINNER:** Salmon with Sautéed Mushrooms

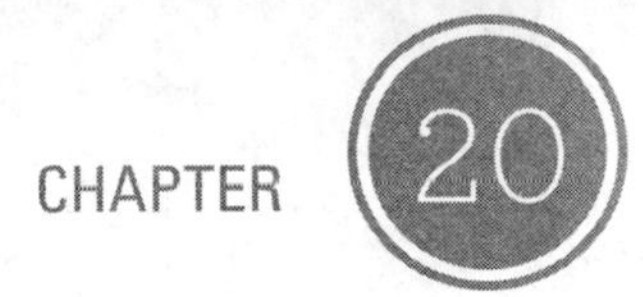


# Recipes for Stages Two and Three

All recipes in Stage One may also be used in Stages Two and Three of the Perfect 10 Diet. Some of the recipes in Stages Two and Three of the Perfect 10 Diet include whole grains or alcohol. If you have a history of alcohol abuse, please do not use recipes containing alcohol. Also, if you're having a hard time losing weight, cut down on grains, and limit or avoid recipes containing alcohol.

# Breakfast

## Mediterranean Avocado Boats

SERVINGS: 4
PREPARATION TIME: 30 min.

INGREDIENTS

1 tablespoon lime juice
2 ripe avocados, peeled and halved
½ teaspoon butter
5 medium eggs, beaten
2 green onions, minced
¼ cup chopped fresh cilantro
4 olives, chopped
Pinch salt and freshly ground black pepper

DIRECTIONS

1. Pour the lime juice on the avocado halves, and set aside.
2. Melt the butter in a large skillet over low heat.
3. Mix together the eggs, onions, cilantro, and olives, and place in a large skillet with the butter.
4. Cook for 5 minutes over medium heat, stirring often. Set aside.
5. Place the cooked egg mixture in the avocado halves. Add salt and pepper. Serve.

# Arugula Eggs with Salsa Verde

SERVINGS: 2 to 3
PREPARATION TIME: 20 min.

INGREDIENTS

2 cups chopped arugula
½ bunch chives, chopped
2 teaspoons extra-virgin olive oil
Pinch salt and freshly ground black pepper
4 medium eggs
1 teaspoon unsalted butter
1 cup mixed salad leaves
½ cup walnuts
¼ cup grated Parmesan cheese

DIRECTIONS

1. Place the arugula, chives, olive oil, and 2 tablespoons water in a blender. Blend until smooth. Add the salt and pepper.
2. Beat the eggs. Set aside.
3. Melt the butter in a skillet. Add the arugula mixture, and cook for 1 minute.
4. Add the beaten eggs, and cook until golden brown.
5. Divide up the mixed salad leaves among the serving plates. Sprinkle with walnuts, and place the cooked egg mixture on top.
6. Sprinkle with the Parmesan cheese. Serve.

## Scrambled Eggs with Goat Cheese

SERVINGS: 2 to 3
PREPARATION TIME: 15 min.

INGREDIENTS

6 medium eggs
4 ounces goat cheese
¼ cup cream
1 tablespoon fresh thyme or marjoram
Pinch salt and freshly ground black pepper
1 tablespoon unsalted butter

DIRECTIONS

1. Beat the eggs. Stir half the goat cheese into the beaten eggs, and add the cream, thyme or marjoram, salt, and pepper.
2. Melt the butter in a nonstick skillet, and add the egg mixture.
3. Continue to cook on low heat, stirring in the remaining goat cheese, until the mixture is firm. Serve warm.

## Zucchini Quiche

SERVINGS: 2 to 3
PREPARATION TIME: 1 hour

INGREDIENTS

2 tablespoons butter, divided
2 cups zucchini, cut into thin half-rounds
12 cherry tomatoes
2 tablespoons whole-wheat flour
2 large or 3 medium eggs
½ cup full-fat yogurt
1 teaspoon fresh oregano

8 ounces cream cheese
⅓ cup grated Parmesan cheese

DIRECTIONS

1. Preheat the oven to 375°F.
2. Coat a large ovenproof skillet with 1 tablespoon butter, and set aside.
3. In another skillet, sauté the zucchini in the remaining butter until soft. Add the tomatoes, and cook for 3 minutes. Remove from the heat, and let cool for 5 to 10 minutes.
4. Add the whole-wheat flour, and stir.
5. Spoon the zucchini mixture into the first skillet.
6. In a separate bowl, beat the eggs. Add the yogurt, oregano, and cream cheese.
7. Spoon the egg mixture on top of the zucchini mixture, and sprinkle with the Parmesan cheese.
8. Bake for 30 minutes at 375°F. Remove from the oven, and serve.

## Egg Wraps

SERVINGS: 1
PREPARATION TIME: 15 min.

INGREDIENTS

2 hard-boiled eggs
1 teaspoon extra-virgin olive oil
Pinch salt and freshly ground black pepper
1 whole-wheat wrap
1 slice pepper jack cheese

DIRECTIONS

1. Cut the boiled eggs into small pieces, and mix with the olive oil, salt, and pepper.
2. Place the mixture into the whole-wheat wrap. Add the cheese, and fold. Serve.

# Eggs Cocotte

SERVINGS: 4
PREPARATION TIME: 1 hour

INGREDIENTS

1 tablespoon unsalted butter
4 tablespoons grated Parmesan cheese, divided
1 teaspoon fresh thyme leaves, divided
Pinch salt and freshly ground black pepper
8 eggs
½ cup cream
4 fresh thyme sprigs
2 slices grilled whole-wheat or rye bread, for serving

DIRECTIONS

1. Preheat the oven to 325°F.
2. Brush a 4-compartment muffin pan with butter. Sprinkle the pan with half the cheese, and put ¼ teaspoon thyme leaves into each of the compartments. Season with salt and pepper.
3. Add 2 whole eggs and 2 tablespoons cream into each compartment of the pan. Sprinkle with the remaining cheese, and garnish each compartment with a thyme sprig.
4. Place the pan into a larger pan. Place the pans in the oven, and fill the larger pan with hot water reaching halfway up to the rim of the muffin pan.
5. Bake at 325°F for 8 to 10 minutes, until eggs are bubbly or lightly browned.
6. Serve on whole-wheat or rye bread.

## Strawberries with Cottage Cheese

SERVINGS: 1
PREPARATION TIME: 5 min.

INGREDIENTS

½ cup strawberries or any other berries of your choice
½ cup cottage cheese

DIRECTIONS

1. Cut the strawberries into small pieces, and mix with cottage cheese. Serve.

# Salads and Entrées

## Thai Salad

SERVINGS: 3 to 4
PREPARATION TIME: 1 hour

INGREDIENTS

12 ounces boneless skinless chicken breast
2 tablespoons reduced-salt teriyaki sauce
½ avocado
6 cups mixed greens (romaine, leaf lettuce, and iceberg)
½ cup chopped fresh cilantro
¼ cup chopped peanuts
4 scallions, chopped
½ teaspoon red pepper flakes
1 cup diced cucumber

DIRECTIONS

1. Place the chicken and teriyaki sauce in a glass container, and marinate for 30 minutes in the refrigerator.
2. Remove the chicken from the container, and pour the marinade into a small bowl.
3. Place the chicken on the grill, and cook each side for 5 minutes, brushing on the marinade as it cooks.
4. While the chicken cooks, slice the avocado.
5. Place the mixed greens over 2 to 3 serving plates. Add the cilantro, peanuts, scallions, red pepper flakes, cucumber, and avocado.
6. Place the chicken over the salads. Serve.

## Mexican Chicken Salad

SERVINGS: 2
PREPARATION TIME: 30 min.

INGREDIENTS

- 2 cups diced cooked chicken
- ¼ cup chopped red onion
- ½ green bell pepper, chopped
- 1 small tomato, chopped
- ½ avocado, sliced
- 2 tablespoons extra-virgin olive oil
- 2 tablespoons cider vinegar
- 2 packets of stevia or ½ teaspoon agave
- 2 tablespoons salsa
- ½ teaspoon cumin
- 1 clove garlic, chopped
- 1 head romaine lettuce
- 1 cup shredded Monterey Jack cheese

DIRECTIONS

1. Place the chicken, onion, pepper, tomato, and avocado in a large bowl.
2. Whisk together the olive oil, vinegar, stevia or agave, salsa, cumin, and garlic.
3. Place lettuce on the serving plates, and pour the olive oil mixture over it.
4. Place the chicken mixture on top.

## Mediterranean Lentil Salad

SERVINGS: 2 to 3
PREPARATION TIME: 1 hour

INGREDIENTS

10 cherry tomatoes
½ cup extra-virgin olive oil, divided
1½ cups brown lentils
1 lemon, juiced
1 fresh bay leaf
2 cloves garlic, crushed and chopped
2 medium red onions, chopped
Bunch parsley, chopped
½ cup olives, pitted
4 ounces grated Parmesan cheese

DIRECTIONS

1. Preheat oven to 250°F.
2. Place the cherry tomatoes in a baking tray with a touch of olive oil. Bake for 40 minutes at 250°F.
3. Place the lentils in a saucepan. Add the lemon juice, bay leaf, garlic, and water to cover. Cover, and cook for 40 minutes, or until the lentils are soft.

4. Drain the lentils, and transfer them to a large bowl. Add the cherry tomatoes, red onions, parsley, and olives.
5. Top with the Parmesan cheese. Serve.

## Shrimp in Coconut and Mango Sauce

SERVINGS: 1
PREPARATION TIME: 10 min.

INGREDIENTS

½ mango, peeled, stoned, and diced
¼ cup diced red pepper
1 teaspoon minced ginger
2 teaspoons minced red onion
2 teaspoons macadamia oil
Pinch salt and freshly ground black pepper
6 jumbo shrimp
3 ounces shredded unsweetened coconut

DIRECTIONS

1. Preheat the oven to 350°F.
2. Mix together the mango, red pepper, ginger, onion, and macadamia oil in a bowl. Add salt and pepper. Set aside.
3. Peel and devein the shrimp. Poach in hot water for 3 to 4 minutes. Remove from water, and chill.
4. Roll chilled shrimp in shredded coconut, and broil in the oven for 5 minutes at 350°F.
5. Serve hot with the mango sauce.

## Shrimp in Garlic Butter

SERVINGS: 1
PREPARATION TIME: 20 min.

INGREDIENTS

8 jumbo shrimp, in shells
2 tablespoons butter, divided
1½ cloves garlic, minced
1 tablespoon dry white wine
½ tablespoon snipped fresh chives or parsley, for garnish
Pinch salt

DIRECTIONS

1. If frozen, thaw shrimp. Peel and devein.
2. Rinse and dry shrimp.
3. Heat a large skillet over medium heat. Add 1 tablespoon butter and the garlic.
4. Cook, stirring, until butter is melted. Add the shrimp. Continue to cook, stirring frequently, for 1 to 3 minutes, or until the shrimp turns pink.
5. Loosen any browned bits, and stir.
6. Add the wine and remaining butter to the skillet. Pour over the shrimp.
7. Remove the shrimp from the skillet, and transfer to a platter.
8. Sprinkle with chives or parsley, add salt, and serve.

## Rabbit Stifado (Greek Village-Style)

SERVINGS: 4 to 5
PREPARATION TIME: 1 hour

INGREDIENTS

2 rabbits
½ ounces macadamia oil, divided

2 pearl onions
1 clove garlic, chopped
2 rosemary sprigs
2 thyme sprigs
1 bay leaf
2 black peppercorns
2 white peppercorns
2 Spanish onions, chopped
1 ounce red wine
1 whole tomato, chopped
1 (8-ounce) can tomato sauce
Dash sea salt

DIRECTIONS

1. Preheat the oven to 250°F.
2. In an ovenproof skillet, sauté the rabbits with half the macadamia oil over medium heat for 15 minutes. Add the pearl onions.
3. In a different skillet, add the remaining macadamia oil, garlic, rosemary, thyme, bay leaf, black and white peppercorns, and Spanish onions, and cook for 5 minutes. Add the red wine, and cook for an additional 5 minutes.
4. Add the tomato and tomato sauce. Cook for 15 minutes, and then add the sea salt, to taste.
5. Add the tomato mixture to the pan of sautéed rabbits, cover with aluminum foil, and bake for 1 hour at 250 °F. Serve hot.

## Sautéed Sole in Champagne

SERVINGS: 3
PREPARATION TIME: 15 min.

INGREDIENTS

3 large pieces sole fillets
Pinch salt and freshly ground black pepper

2 tablespoons butter
½ cup champagne
1 teaspoon dried oregano
2 tablespoons shredded Parmesan cheese
3 lemon wedges

DIRECTIONS

1. Season the sole fillets with salt and pepper.
2. Place in a skillet with the butter over medium heat, and sauté on each side for 7 to 10 minutes.
3. Pour the champagne in the skillet, but not over the fish.
4. Sprinkle the oregano over the fish, and cook for 5 minutes.
5. Sprinkle the fish with Parmesan cheese, and garnish with a lemon wedge. Serve.

## Grilled Tuna with Peanut Sauce

SERVINGS: 1
PREPARATION TIME: 20 min.

INGREDIENTS

6 ounces fresh or frozen tuna steaks or fillets
¼ cup unsalted peanuts, or all-natural ground peanut butter
½ scallion, cut into 1-inch pieces
1 teaspoon macadamia oil
1 teaspoon agave
½ teaspoon grated fresh ginger
½ clove garlic, quartered
½ teaspoon teriyaki sauce
1 sliced scallion, for garnish (optional)

DIRECTIONS

1. Preheat the grill.
2. Thaw fish if frozen. Rinse, dry, and set aside fish.

3. Combine peanuts, 4 tablespoons water, scallion, macadamia oil, agave, ginger, and garlic in a blender or food processor. Blend together thoroughly, and pour into a saucepan. Stir in 1 tablespoon water. Set aside.
4. Combine the teriyaki sauce and remaining water. Brush both sides of the tuna with the teriyaki mixture.
5. Place the tuna on a lightly greased, uncovered grill, and cook until the fish flakes easily with a fork (it can be light pink in the center). Turn once halfway through grilling.
6. Warm the peanut sauce over medium-low heat. Spoon the sauce over the tuna.
7. Garnish with the optional scallions. Serve.

## Coquille St. Jacques

SERVINGS: 6
PREPARATION TIME: 35 min.

INGREDIENTS

1 pounds scallops
1 bay leaf
Pinch of sea salt and freshly ground black pepper
Pinch of dried thyme
3 tablespoons butter
2 tablespoons minced onion
1 cup sliced mushrooms
3 tablespoons whole-wheat flour
¼ cup heavy cream
2 tablespoons dry sherry
⅓ cup buttered breadcrumbs
⅓ cup grated Parmesan cheese

DIRECTIONS

1. Preheat oven to 400°F.
2. In a saucepan, place 1 cup water, scallops, bay leaf, salt, pepper,

and thyme. Heat over medium heat and bring to a boil. Let boil 5 minutes.

3. Drain scallops, discarding the bay leaf and reserving the broth, and set aside.
4. In a separate saucepan, heat the butter, onions, and mushrooms; cook for 5 minutes. Add the whole wheat flour and 1 cup of the reserved broth to the mushroom mixture.
5. Add the heavy cream and cook, stirring until thick. Add the scallops and sherry, and mix together thoroughly. Transfer the scallops to a baking dish.
6. Mix the breadcrumbs and Parmesan cheese together, then sprinkle on top. Bake at 400°F for 15 minutes or until brown.

## Grilled Sea Bass in Tomato Fondue

SERVINGS: 2
PREPARATION TIME: 20 min.

INGREDIENTS

3 medium tomatoes, diced
12 ounces sea bass (or other similar fish)
Pinch salt and freshly ground black pepper
1 tablespoon butter
1 clove garlic, minced
1 large onion, chopped
2 teaspoons lime juice
1 tablespoon mix of fresh basil, sage, tarragon, and parsley
Lemon wedge (optional)

DIRECTIONS

1. Place the tomatoes in a bowl with hot water. Drain, and set aside.
2. Season the fish with salt and pepper.
3. Pan-fry the fish in the butter, 10 minutes on each side. Remove the fish to a plate, and cover with foil to keep warm.

4. Add the tomatoes, garlic, and onion to the skillet. Add the lime juice and herbs, and cook 4 minutes.
5. Spoon the tomato sauce over the fish; serve with a lemon wedge.

## Bouillabaisse

SERVINGS: 3 to 4
PREPARATION TIME: 25 to 35 min.

INGREDIENTS

3 pounds mixed fish, prawns, mussels, and squid rings
½ cup extra-virgin olive oil
1 clove garlic, chopped
1 leek, sliced
1 large onion, chopped
1 (14-ounce) can tomato paste, or 2 mashed tomatoes
1 tablespoon chopped fresh thyme
1 tablespoon orange zest
1 tablespoon chopped fresh basil
1 teaspoon fresh parsley
1 bay leaf
Pinch saffron
1 celery stalk, chopped
4 ounces dry white wine
4 ounces fish stock
Pinch salt and freshly ground black pepper

DIRECTIONS

1. Remove the bones and skin from the fish, and cut it into small cubes.
2. Peel and devein the prawns, but leave the tails intact. Set the fish and prawns aside.
3. Heat the olive oil in a large saucepan over medium heat; add the garlic, leek, and onions.

4. Cook until the onions are golden.
5. Add the tomato paste, thyme, orange zest, basil, parsley, bay leaf, saffron, celery, wine, and stock; bring to a boil.
6. Add the fish and prawns, and cook for 10 to 15 minutes, or until the mussels open and are thoroughly cooked.
7. Season with salt and pepper. Serve.

## Baked Fish with Mushrooms

SERVINGS: 2
PREPARATION TIME: 15 min.

INGREDIENTS

½ pound fresh or frozen fish fillets (½- to ¾-inch thick)
1 tablespoon butter
1 cup sliced mushrooms
2 tablespoons sliced green onion
½ teaspoon fresh, or ⅛ teaspoon dried, tarragon or thyme
Pinch salt

DIRECTIONS

1. Thaw fish if frozen. Rinse, dry, and set aside.
2. Preheat oven to 375°F. Arrange the fish in a baking dish. Sprinkle with salt.
3. Melt the butter in a small saucepan over medium heat. Add the mushrooms, onions, and half the herbs. Cook until the mushrooms and onions are tender. Spoon the mushroom mixture over the fish.
4. Sprinkle with additional herbs.
5. Bake, covered with aluminum foil, at 375°F for 12 to 15 minutes, or until the fish flakes. Remove from the oven, and serve.

## Grilled Salmon with Tomato–Pepper Relish

SERVINGS: 1
PREPARATION TIME: 15 min.

INGREDIENTS

½ medium red pepper, chopped
½ medium green pepper, chopped
½ medium red onion, chopped
1 tomato, peeled, seeded, and cut into strips
2 tablespoons extra-virgin olive oil, divided
1 teaspoon chopped fresh cilantro
1 (9-ounce) salmon fillet
Pinch salt and freshly ground black pepper

DIRECTIONS

1. Turn the oven to high broil.
2. Mix together the peppers, onion, tomato, 1 tablespoon olive oil, and cilantro in a large bowl.
3. Place the mixture in a skillet, and cook over medium heat for 30 minutes. Cool for 15 minutes, and set aside. Bring to room temperature before serving.
4. Season fish with salt and pepper, and cover with the remaining olive oil. Broil for 4 minutes on each side.
5. Transfer the fish to a plate, and top with the tomato–pepper relish. Serve.

## Grilled Halibut with Basil and Cherry Tomatoes

SERVINGS: 1
PREPARATION TIME: 10 min.

INGREDIENTS

½ bunch basil
½ cup plus 1 tablespoon extra-virgin olive oil, divided

5 yellow cherry tomatoes, halved
5 red cherry tomatoes, halved
1 (9-ounce) halibut fillet
Salt and freshly ground black pepper

DIRECTIONS

1. Preheat the grill.
2. Blanch the basil leaves by immersing them in hot water. Mix the basil with ¼ cup olive oil.
3. Add the halved red and yellow tomatoes to the basil mixture.
4. Season the fish fillet with salt and pepper, and rub it with ¼ cup olive oil.
5. Place the fillet on a grill for 8 minutes on each side. Transfer the fish to a plate, and spoon the tomatoes over the fish.
6. Drizzle with the remaining 1 tablespoon olive oil. Serve.

## Salmon Roll with Brown Rice

SERVINGS: 4
PREPARATION TIME: 45 min.

INGREDIENTS

1 cup uncooked short-grain brown rice
½ teaspoon sea salt
2 sheets nori (dried seaweed)
8 ounces goat cheese
6 (6-ounce) pieces salmon (thinly sliced)
½ cucumber, peeled, seeded and cut into matchsticks
½ medium-sized red onion, minced
2 hard-boiled eggs, whites and yolks shredded separately

DIRECTIONS

1. Rinse the rice well with water.
2. Bring the rice and 1 cup water to a boil and add the sea salt.
3. Reduce the heat to a very low simmer, and cover until the water is absorbed.

4. Remove the rice from the heat, and let it cool.
5. Lay a sushi mat on a flat surface, and place 1 sheet of nori on the mat.
6. Spread half the rice on to half the nori.
7. Flip the nori over, leaving the portion without rice facing you.
8. Spread the goat cheese on the portion of nori without rice, and place the salmon over the goat cheese.
9. Place the cucumber, onion, and hardboiled eggs on top of the salmon in any order.
10. Make a roll, and cut it into 6 small pieces with a sharp, wet knife.
11. Repeat the process to make a second roll. Serve.

## Creole Jambalaya

SERVINGS: 4 to 6
PREPARATION TIME: 4 to 6 hours

INGREDIENTS

20 minced clams with liquid
⅓ cup uncooked brown rice
¼ pound shrimp
¼ cup red or white wine
1 cup canned diced tomatoes
1 (8-ounce) can tomato sauce
1 onion, sliced
2 cloves garlic, minced
2 chicken base cubes
1 bay leaf
3 teaspoons Cajun seasoning
1 pound boneless, skinless chicken
½ pound fresh or frozen okra
¼ cup cream

DIRECTIONS

1. Place the liquid from the clams into a large slow cooker (do not add the clams).
2. Add the brown rice, shrimp, wine, tomatoes, tomato sauce, onion, garlic, chicken base cubes, bay leaf, and Cajun seasoning.
3. Place the chicken on top of the mixture.
4. Cook for 4 to 5 hours on low heat.
5. Add the okra in the last hour, if frozen.
6. Add the clams, cream, and okra (if fresh) in the last 30 minutes of cooking time. Remove the bay leaf, and serve.

## Cauliflower Wild Rice

SERVINGS: 2
PREPARATION TIME: 45 min.

INGREDIENTS

½ head cauliflower
1 teaspoon butter
¼ cup wild rice

DIRECTIONS

1. Place the cauliflower in a food processor or blender, and process until the cauliflower is well chopped.
2. Steam or stir-fry the cauliflower in the butter for several minutes. Avoid overcooking. Set aside.
3. Place the wild rice and 1 cup water in a covered pan, and cook on low heat for 30 minutes.
4. Toss the cauliflower over the wild rice, and season to taste. Serve.

## Shrimp and Wild Rice

SERVINGS: 2 to 3
PREPARATION TIME: 20 min.

INGREDIENTS

12 ounces wild rice
14 jumbo shrimp (peeled and deveined)
2 teaspoons paprika
Pinch salt and freshly ground black pepper
½ clove garlic, minced
1 tablespoon extra-virgin olive oil

DIRECTIONS

1. Cook the rice according to the package directions. Set aside.
2. Mix together the shrimp, paprika, salt, pepper, and garlic in a separate bowl.
3. Heat the olive oil in a skillet. Add the shrimp, and stir-fry for 2 to 3 minutes, until golden brown.
4. Serve over the wild rice.

## Whole Wheat Linguine with Seafood

SERVINGS: 3
PREPARATION TIME: 1 hour

INGREDIENTS

21 ounces whole wheat linguine
3 ounces extra-virgin olive oil
1 tablespoon garlic, sliced
2 tablespoons chopped parsley
5 ounces vegetable stock
8 ounces tomato sauce
1 tablespoon sea salt

½ teaspoon ground black pepper
6 ounces baby scallops
6 ounces calamari rings
6 ounces shrimp
18 mussels
18 Manila clams
8 ounces white wine
2 tablespoons basil, julienne

DIRECTIONS

1. Boil water and cook pasta for 12 to 15 minutes, stirring occasionally.
2. Drain the pasta in a colander and set aside.
3. Heat olive oil in a saucepan until hot. Add garlic, parsley, vegetable stock, tomato sauce, sea salt, and pepper. Mix well.
4. Add the scallops, calamari, shrimp, mussels, and clams, and cook for 5 minutes over medium heat.
5. Add the white wine and simmer for 5 minutes.
6. Add the pasta and mix well.
7. To serve, place the pasta mixture in a bowl and garnish with basil.

## Sautéed Vegetables

SERVINGS: 1 to 2
PREPARATION TIME: 40 min.

INGREDIENTS

6 ounces onion, diced
3 pieces green zucchinis, julienne
3 yellow squashes, julienne
4 ounces extra-virgin olive oil
2 cloves garlic, minced
1 teaspoon sea salt
½ teaspoon freshly ground black pepper

DIRECTIONS

1. Bring 1 cup water to a boil in a medium saucepan. Place the onion, zucchini, and squash in the pan and cook for 10 minutes.
2. Heat the olive oil in a medium pan. When hot, add the garlic and cook until brown.
3. Add the vegetables and cook until crunchy.
4. Add the salt and pepper, stirring to blend into vegetables.

## Duck Breasts in Grape Champagne

SERVINGS: 3
PREPARATION TIME: 45 min.

INGREDIENTS

1 teaspoon macadamia oil
3 (7-ounce) duck breasts, with skin
4 ounces unsalted butter
1½ shallots, minced
8 ounces seedless grapes, halved
12 ounces champagne
6 ounces vegetable stock
1 tablespoon agave
2 teaspoons sea salt
¼ teaspoon ground white pepper

DIRECTIONS

1. Preheat oven to 350°F.
2. Heat macadamia oil in a saucepan over medium heat.
3. In a saucepan, add 1 tablespoon of macadamia oil and heat until hot.
4. Add duck breast and cook until crispy and browned on both sides, 7 to 10 minutes.
5. Transfer the duck breasts to a baking dish, and bake at 350°F for 10 minutes.

6. Add the butter, shallots, and grapes to a pan. Cook 5 minutes or until tender. Add the champagne and raise the heat to cook off the alcohol.
7. Add the vegetable stock and simmer for 4 minutes, then add the agave, salt, and pepper. Mix thoroughly and remove from the heat.
8. To serve, slice the duck into ¼-inch slices and arrange on a plate. Drizzle the sauce over the duck. Spoon the grapes and shallots over the duck.

## Red Snapper in Cherry Tomato and Black Olive Sauce

SERVINGS: 3

PREPARATION TIME: 1 hour

INGREDIENTS

3 ounces macadamia oil, divided
3 (21-ounce) red snapper fillets
6 ounces cherry tomatoes
2 tablespoons basil, julienne
3 ounces black olives
2 tablespoons fresh lemon juice
½ teaspoon sea salt
¼ teaspoon ground black pepper

DIRECTIONS

1. Heat the oven to 350°F.
2. Heat 1½ ounces of macadamia oil in a saucepan over medium heat.
3. Add the red snapper fillets, skin side down, and cook until crispy. Flip and cook the other side for 2 minutes. Transfer to a baking dish.
4. Bake at 350°F for 5 minutes, or until the fish is white and flaky. Do not overbake.

5. In a separate bowl, rinse and dry the tomatoes. Add the basil, black olives, the remaining 1½ ounces macadamia oil, lemon juice, salt, and pepper.
6. To serve, place the fish on a plate and spoon the cold sauce over the fish.

## Chicken in Apple Cider

SERVINGS: 3 to 4
PREPARATION TIME: 45 min.

INGREDIENTS

1 tablespoon extra-virgin olive oil
1 onion, chopped
2 cloves garlic, crushed
10 shallots, chopped
4 boneless chicken breasts
1 tablespoon fresh tarragon leaves, chopped
1 cup apple cider
1 cup chicken broth
¼ cup dry white wine
1 cup full-fat yogurt (optional)
Salt and freshly ground black pepper, to taste

DIRECTIONS

1. Heat the olive oil in a large frying pan over medium heat. Add the onion, garlic, and shallots, and cook for 5 minutes, stirring occasionally.
2. Add the chicken, and cook for 10 to 12 minutes, or until golden on all sides.
3. Add the tarragon, cider, broth, and wine to the pan, and bring to a boil.
4. Reduce the heat. Cover and simmer for 30 minutes, or until the chicken is tender.
5. Remove the pan from the heat. Stir in the yogurt, and season to taste with salt and black pepper. Serve.

## Thai Duck Panang Curry

SERVINGS: 2 to 3
PREPARATION TIME: 45 min.

INGREDIENTS

½ roasted, boneless duck
1 cup coconut milk, divided
1 (8-ounce) can panang curry paste
1 tablespoon fish sauce
1 teaspoon agave
½ green or red pepper, chopped
3 to 5 fresh kaffir lime leaves

DIRECTIONS

1. Preheat the oven to 350°F
2. Roast the duck in the oven at 350°F for 45 minutes with 3 teaspoons coconut milk.
3. In a separate saucepan over medium heat, stir together the panang curry paste and remaining coconut milk until the mixture becomes smooth.
4. Add the fish sauce, agave, pepper, and lime leaves, and cook 15 minutes.
5. Place the sauce over the cooked duck. Serve.

## Stuffed Eggplant

SERVINGS: 3 to 4
PREPARATION TIME: 1 hour

INGREDIENTS

4 medium eggplants
4 tablespoons unsalted butter
1 small onion, chopped

2 tablespoons chopped shallots
1 pound shrimp, peeled, deveined, and cooked
½ pound white crab meat
2 tablespoons fresh parsley
1 egg, beaten
1 tablespoon lemon juice
1 tablespoon Worcestershire sauce
Pinch salt and freshly ground black pepper
½ cup grated Parmesan cheese

DIRECTIONS

1. Preheat the oven to 350°F
2. Cut each eggplant in half. Scoop out the pulp, and place in 1 cup boiling water.
3. Lower the heat, and cook for 5 minutes.
4. In a separate medium skillet, melt the butter and sauté the onion and shallots until soft.
5. Add the eggplant pulp, shrimp, crabmeat, parsley, egg, lemon juice, Worcestershire sauce, salt, and pepper to the skillet, and remove from heat.
6. Spoon the pulp mixture into the eggplant shells. Sprinkle the eggplant with the Parmesan cheese.
7. Place the dish containing the eggplant into a larger baking dish. Fill the larger dish with 1 inch of water, and bake at 350°F for 30 minutes. Serve.

## Shrimp Pizza

SERVINGS: 1
PREPARATION TIME: 30 min.

INGREDIENTS

1 (8-inch) whole-wheat pita bread shell
½ cup mozzarella cheese, divided
1 cup mixed salad greens
2 medium plum tomatoes, chopped
1 small red onion, chopped
10 chopped olives
6 cooked, peeled, and deveined shrimp
1 tablespoon feta cheese

DIRECTIONS

1. Preheat the oven to 450°F.
2. Top the pita with half the mozzarella cheese, and bake for 5 minutes at 450°F.
3. Combine the salad greens, tomatoes, onion, olives, and shrimp in a large bowl.
4. Top the bread shells with the shrimp mixture, and sprinkle with the feta cheese and the remaining mozzarella cheese. Cut into wedges, and serve.

## Lobster Fra Diavolo

SERVINGS: 4
PREPARATION TIME: 1 hour

INGREDIENTS

4 pounds ripe plum tomatoes, divided
¼ cup extra-virgin olive oil, divided
4 cloves garlic, peeled and minced

1 onion, minced
2 teaspoons red pepper flakes
Pinch salt and freshly ground black pepper
2 tablespoons tomato paste
1 teaspoon fresh basil
1 tablespoon chopped parsley
2 (2 pound) lobsters, split lengthwise
½ pound whole-wheat pasta

DIRECTIONS

1. Place the tomatoes in a large pot of boiling water. Cook for 1 minute. Transfer the tomatoes to a food processor or blender, and puree until soft.
2. Heat 1 tablespoon olive oil in a large saucepan over medium heat. Add the garlic and onion, and cook 3 minutes. Add the tomatoes, and bring to a simmer. Cover 30 minutes, stirring occasionally.
3. Add the pepper flakes, salt, pepper, tomato paste, basil, and parsley. Remove from the heat. Set aside.
4. Place the lobsters in a steamer for 5 minutes. When the lobsters are finished, remove the meat from the shells, and cut the meat into pieces.
5. Cover with the sauce, and cook for an additional 5 minutes. Add water if the sauce is too thick. Cook for another 5 minutes.
6. While the lobsters are cooking, cook the pasta until al dente, about 7 minutes, and then drain.
7. Serve the pasta with the lobster and sauce on top.

## Orange Duck

SERVINGS: 5 to 6
PREPARATION TIME: 1 hour 10 min.

INGREDIENTS

3 pounds duck
1 tablespoon extra-virgin olive oil

Pinch freshly ground black pepper
2 sprigs fresh rosemary
2 sprigs fresh thyme
1 clove garlic, chopped
1 tablespoon finely grated orange rind
1 tablespoon agave
2 tablespoons brandy
2 cucumbers, cut into small pieces, for garnish (optional)

DIRECTIONS

1. Preheat the oven to 350°F.
2. Pierce the duck skin, and brush the skin with the olive oil; season the meat with the black pepper, rosemary, thyme, and garlic.
3. Place the duck in a baking dish, and bake at 350°F for 1 hour, or until tender.
4. Remove from the pan. Cover, and set aside.
5. Skim the fat from the pan juices, and discard. In the same pan, add the orange rind, agave, and brandy. Cook for 10 minutes over low heat.
6. To serve, carve the duck, arrange it on a plate, and pour the sauce over it. Garnish the plate with the cucumber.

## Grilled Filet Mignon of Tuna

SERVINGS: 4
PREPARATION TIME: 4 hours

INGREDIENTS

2 cups reduced-salt teriyaki sauce
2 cloves garlic, minced
½ cup dry sherry
4 tablespoons freshly grated ginger
½ cup minced scallions
¼ teaspoon cayenne pepper

2 teaspoons freshly ground black pepper
¼ cup lemon juice or juice of 2 lemons
4 tuna steaks, sliced 2½ to 3 inches thick
2 tablespoons extra-virgin olive oil

DIRECTIONS

1. Combine the teriyaki sauce, garlic, sherry, ginger, scallions, cayenne pepper, black pepper, and lemon juice in a large bowl.
2. Place the tuna in the mixture, and marinate 3 hours, turning the steaks every 1 hour.
3. Drain the marinade 30 minutes before cooking.
4. Place the tuna on a stovetop grill, and brush on the olive oil. Grill for several minutes on each side.
5. Serve with a side salad.

## Snacks and Desserts

### Cauliflower au Gratin

SERVINGS: 2
PREPARATION TIME: 20 min.

INGREDIENTS

½ head cauliflower
1 tablespoon extra-virgin olive oil
2 tablespoons butter
1 cup sliced portobello mushrooms
1 clove garlic, crushed
3 tablespoons grated Parmesan cheese
1 tablespoon heavy cream

DIRECTIONS

1. Preheat the oven to 325°F.
2. Place the cauliflower in a food processor or blender, and chop.
3. Place the cauliflower in a covered dish with the 3 tablespoons water. Bake at 325°F for 5 to 6 minutes. Remove from the oven, and uncover.
4. Combine the olive oil with the butter in a large skillet over medium heat.
5. Add the mushrooms, and sauté 5 minutes or until cooked.
6. Add the garlic, cauliflower, and ½ cup water. If the sauce is too thick, gradually increase the amount of water used.
7. Add the Parmesan cheese and heavy cream.
8. Cook for an additional 10 minutes. Remove from the heat, and serve.

## Cauliflower Puree

SERVINGS: 2 to 3

PREPARATION TIME: 15 min.

INGREDIENTS

1 head cauliflower

3 tablespoons butter

1 teaspoon heavy cream

Pinch salt and freshly ground black pepper

DIRECTIONS

1. Preheat the oven to 325°F.
2. Bake the cauliflower at 325°F for 10 minutes, or until soft.
3. Place the cauliflower in a blender, and add the butter, cream, salt, and pepper. Puree until smooth.
4. Serve hot.

## Garlic-Cheese Stuffed Mushrooms

SERVINGS: 6
PREPARATION TIME: 40 min.

INGREDIENTS

6 small Portobello mushrooms
½ cup herbed cheese, such as Havarti with dill
2 cloves garlic

DIRECTIONS

1. Preheat the oven to 350°F.
2. Clean the mushrooms, and slice off the stems. Reserve the stems to be sautéed with olive oil as a side dish for a later lunch or dinner.
3. Divide the cheese among the mushroom caps.
4. Arrange the mushroom caps in a baking pan. Add the whole garlic cloves and ½ cup of water.
5. Bake at 350°F for 24 to 30 minutes. Remove from the oven, and serve hot.

## Pistachio Dark Chocolate

SERVINGS: 15
PREPARATION TIME: 75 min.

INGREDIENTS

15 (1-inch) pieces dark chocolate made with cocoa butter and reduced sugar
1 cup shelled pistachios

DIRECTIONS

1. Place the chocolate in a pan inside a larger pan filled with boiling water. Stir the chocolate until it melts.
2. Place the pistachios in the melted chocolate.
3. Refrigerate for 1 hour. Cut into small pieces, and serve.

## Strawberry Sorbet

SERVINGS: 5
PREPARATION TIME: 3 hours

INGREDIENTS

1 pound fresh strawberries, washed with the stems removed
1 small orange, peeled
1 teaspoon vanilla extract
¼ cup agave
2 teaspoons cinnamon

DIRECTIONS

1. Blend all the ingredients in a blender.
2. Strain the mixture through a mesh sieve to remove the strawberry seeds.
3. Place the strawberry mixture in a glass container in the freezer for 2 to 3 hours before serving.

## Brown Rice Pudding

SERVINGS: 6 to 8
PREPARATION TIME: 4 hours

INGREDIENTS

1½ cups cream or heavy cream
½ cup brown rice
¼ teaspoon salt
3 egg yolks
3 teaspoons agave
½ teaspoon ground cinnamon
1 tablespoon unsalted butter
2 teaspoons vanilla extract

DIRECTIONS

1. Combine the cream, rice, 1½ cups water, and salt in a saucepan. Bring the mixture to a boil over medium-low heat.
2. Reduce the heat. Cover and simmer 1½ hours until the rice is tender and the liquid is absorbed.
3. Mix the egg yolks, agave, and cinnamon in a bowl. Pour the egg mixture into the rice pan on the stove, stirring constantly for 6 minutes, or until the pudding is thickened.
4. Remove from the heat. Add the butter and vanilla, and stir. Leave in the pan, and let cool to room temperature. Refrigerate for at least 2 hours before serving. Serve cold.

## Orange Walnut Cake

SERVINGS: 16
PREPARATION TIME: 45 min.

INGREDIENTS

2 cups walnuts
1 cup whole-grain pastry flour
¾ cup whole-wheat flour
1 teaspoon baking powder
¼ teaspoon baking soda
8 medium eggs
1 cup unsalted butter
3 tablespoons agave, divided
½ cup buttermilk
3 tablespoons grated orange peel, divided

DIRECTIONS

1. Preheat the oven to 350°F.
2. Mix together the walnuts, flours, baking powder, and baking soda in a food processor or blender.

3. In a separate bowl, beat together the eggs, butter, 1½ tablespoons agave, buttermilk, and 2 tablespoons of the orange peel.
4. Combine the egg mixture with the flour mixture until it is completely blended into a smooth batter.
5. Pour the batter into a baking pan, and level the batter with a spatula. Bake for 25 minutes at 350°F.
6. As the cake bakes, add 1 cup water to the remaining agave and orange peel in a small pot.
7. Simmer on medium heat, 4 to 5 minutes.
8. Remove the cake from the oven, and let it cool completely. Drizzle with the orange syrup.

## Strawberry Flan

SERVINGS: 4
PREPARATION TIME: 1 to 2 hours

INGREDIENTS

3 eggs, beaten
1½ cups milk
½ cup agave, divided
1 teaspoon vanilla extract
¼ teaspoon ground cinnamon
2 strawberries cut into thin slices, for garnish

DIRECTIONS

1. Preheat the oven to 325°F.
2. Combine eggs, milk ¼ cup agave, and vanilla extract in a mixing bowl. Beat until well mixed but not foamy.
3. Mix remaining ¼ cup agave and cinnamon in small bowl.
4. Place 4 (6-ounce) custard cups in an 8-inch square baking dish.
5. Spoon 1 tablespoon of the agave-cinnamon mixture into each custard cup, then top with the egg mixture, dividing equally among the custard cups.

6. Place the baking dish on the middle rack of oven. Pour hot water into the baking dish around the custard cups to 1-inch depth.
7. Bake at 325°F for 40 minutes or until knife inserted near the center comes out clean.
8. Loosen the edges of the custard cups with a spatula or knife.
9. Invert the custard onto dessert plates, and serve cold. Garnish with cut strawberries.

## New York Style Cheesecake

SERVINGS: 4 to 6
PREPARATION TIME: 10 hours

INGREDIENTS

¼ cup unsalted butter, melted
1 cup whole wheat cracker crumbs
½ cup agave
40 ounces cream cheese, softened
½ cup heavy cream
3 large eggs
1 cup sour cream
1 teaspoon vanilla
¼ cup all-purpose whole wheat flour

DIRECTIONS

1. Preheat the oven to 350°F.
2. Grease the sides of a springform pan.
3. In a large bowl, combine the butter and cracker crumbs. Press into the bottom of the pan, and place the pan in the freezer for 1 hour.
4. In a large bowl, beat the agave and cream cheese for 4 minutes.
5. Blend in the heavy cream. Add the eggs, one at a time, mixing well after each egg is added.
6. Mix in the sour cream, vanilla, whole wheat flour until smooth. Pour the filling over the crust.

7. Bake at 350°F for 1 hour. Turn off the oven and let the cake cool in the oven for 5 hours.
8. Refrigerate for at least 4 hours before serving.

## Coconut Ice Cream

SERVINGS: 7 to 8
PREPARATION TIME: 4 hours

INGREDIENTS

6 egg yolks
3 tablespoons agave
2 cups heavy cream, divided
1 (13-ounce) can coconut milk
1 teaspoon vanilla extract
½ cup shredded, unsweetened coconut, lightly toasted

DIRECTIONS

1. Combine the egg yolks and agave in a medium bowl.
2. Bring the heavy cream to a simmer in a pot over medium-low heat.
3. Pour 1 cup of the cream into the egg yolk mixture, whisking constantly.
4. Pour the yolk mixture into the pot. Cook, stirring constantly, until the mixture is very thick.
5. Remove the pot from the heat; stir in the coconut milk, the remaining cream, and the vanilla extract.
6. Chill 4 hours.
7. Pour the mixture into an ice cream maker. Process according to the manufacturer's directions.
8. Scoop into bowls, and add shredded coconut on top. Serve.

## Kuai Buat Chi (Banana Cooked in Coconut, a Thai Dessert)

SERVINGS: 2 to 3
PREPARATION TIME: 5 min.

INGREDIENTS

2 to 3 small unripe bananas
4 cups coconut milk
1 to 2 teaspoons agave (optional)
Pinch salt (optional)

DIRECTIONS

1. Slice bananas lengthwise, and then halve the pieces.
2. Pour the coconut milk in a pan.
3. Add the agave and a pinch of salt, if desired.
4. Bring the mixture to a boil. Add the bananas.
5. Cook for 2 minutes, and remove from the heat.
6. Serve hot or cold, to taste.

## Strawberries Dipped in Chocolate

SERVINGS: 8 to 10
PREPARATION TIME: 15 min.

INGREDIENTS

12 ounces dark chocolate made with cocoa butter and reduced sugar
2 tablespoons heavy cream
1 pound strawberries

DIRECTIONS

1. Place the chocolate in a pan inside a larger pan filled with boiling water. Stir the chocolate until it melts.

2. Stir in the cream, and add 1 tablespoon water.
3. Keep the chocolate mixture hot, and dip the strawberries in the chocolate. Place the dipped strawberries on a sheet of parchment paper, and allow the chocolate to cool and harden. Serve.

## Stage Two on the Perfect 10 Diet Meal Plan

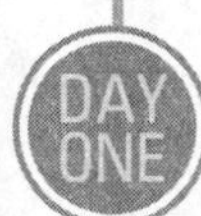


### A Typical Day on the Perfect 10 Diet, Stage Two

BREAKFAST: Mixed Fruit Salad and 1 Slice Rye Bread with Butter
OPTIONAL MIDMORNING SNACK: Vegetable Juice
LUNCH: Curried Cauliflower, Chick Peas, and Tomato Soup
OPTIONAL MIDAFTERNOON SNACK: Broccoli Florets with Cheddar Cheese
DINNER: Grilled Halibut with Cherry Tomatoes

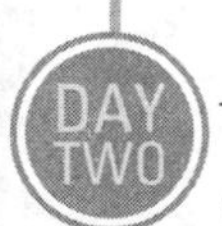


### A Typical Day on the Perfect 10 Diet, Stage Two

BREAKFAST: Yogurt with Sliced Kiwis
OPTIONAL MIDMORNING SNACK: Steamed Vegetables with Garlic
LUNCH: Bouillabaisse
OPTIONAL MIDAFTERNOON SNACK: Strawberries with a Wedge of French Camembert Cheese
DINNER: Barley Vegetable Soup

## A Typical Day on the Perfect 10 Diet, Stage Two

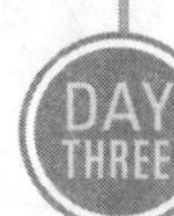


**BREAKFAST:** Eggs Cocotte

**OPTIONAL MIDMORNING SNACK:** Few Olives with Feta Cheese

**LUNCH:** Salmon with Stir-Fried Mushrooms, 1 Scoop Wild Rice

**OPTIONAL MIDAFTERNOON SNACK:** Lettuce with Full-Fat Almond Butter

**DINNER:** Grilled Sea Bass in Tomato Fondue

## A Typical Day on the Perfect 10 Diet, Stage Two

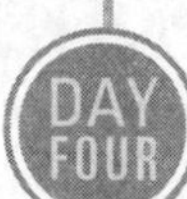


**BREAKFAST:** Natural Granola with ½ Cup Organic Milk

**OPTIONAL MIDMORNING SNACK:** 6 Ounces Tomato Juice

**LUNCH:** Turkey on Whole-Grain Wrap

**OPTIONAL MIDAFTERNOON SNACK:** Mixed Fruit Salad

**DINNER:** Fish in Champagne

## A Typical Day on the Perfect 10 Diet, Stage Two

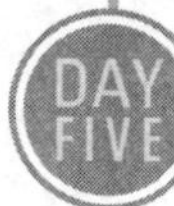


**BREAKFAST:** ½ Grapefruit and 1 Slice Rye Bread with Butter

**OPTIONAL MIDMORNING SNACK:** Vegetable Juice

**LUNCH:** Tomato Vegetable Soup

**OPTIONAL MIDAFTERNOON SNACK:** Three Steamed Asparagus Spears Dipped in Olive Oil

**DINNER:** Shrimp Jambalaya

### A Typical Day on the Perfect 10 Diet, Stage Two

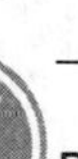


**BREAKFAST:** Eggs with Salmon
**OPTIONAL MIDMORNING SNACK:** Garlic-Cheese Stuffed Mushrooms
**LUNCH:** Thai Salad
**OPTIONAL MIDAFTERNOON SNACK:** Celery Dipped in Hummus
**DINNER:** Grilled Duck Breast with Cauliflower

### A Typical Day on the Perfect 10 Diet, Stage Two

DAY SEVEN

**BREAKFAST:** Turkey Slices on Pumpernickel or Whole-Grain Bread
**OPTIONAL MIDMORNING SNACK:** 1 Plum
**LUNCH:** Stir-Fried Chicken with 1 Scoop Brown Rice
**OPTIONAL MIDAFTERNOON SNACK:** 2 Pieces of Dark Chocolate with Reduced Sugar
**DINNER:** Squash Soup

## Stage Three on the Perfect 10 Diet Meal Plan

### A Typical Day on the Perfect 10 Diet, Stage Three

DAY ONE

**BREAKFAST:** Non-Instant Oatmeal with ½ Cup Organic Whole Milk
**OPTIONAL MIDMORNING SNACK:** Lettuce and Hummus Dip
**LUNCH:** Shrimp and Asparagus Bisque Soup
**OPTIONAL MIDAFTERNOON SNACK:** Banana and ½ Cup Coconut Milk
**DINNER:** Turkey Burger on Whole-Wheat Bread and a Side Salad with Pineapple

### A Typical Day on the Perfect 10 Diet, Stage Three

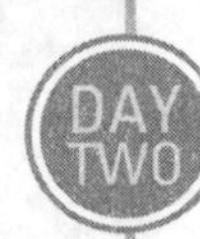


**BREAKFAST:** 1 Cup Barley with ½ Cup Unsweetened Almond Milk

**OPTIONAL MIDMORNING SNACK:** 2 Slices Salmon with Cream Cheese

**LUNCH:** Whole-Wheat Pasta with Shrimp and Marinara Sauce

**OPTIONAL MIDAFTERNOON SNACK:** Mixed Fruit Salad

**DINNER:** Mexican Salad

### A Typical Day on the Perfect 10 Diet, Stage Three

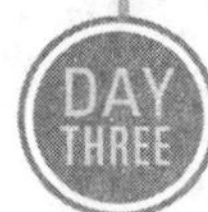


**BREAKFAST:** Vegetable Quiche and 1 Slice Rye Bread with Butter

**OPTIONAL MIDMORNING SNACK:** 1 Cup Cauliflower Puree

**LUNCH:** Grilled Chicken with Stuffed Eggplant

**OPTIONAL MIDAFTERNOON SNACK:** Berries in Full-Fat Yogurt

**DINNER:** Sautéed Salmon, Green Salad, and 1 Scoop Brown Rice

### A Typical Day on the Perfect 10 Diet, Stage Three

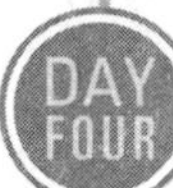


**BREAKFAST:** Rye Bread with Full-Fat Macadamia Butter

**OPTIONAL MIDMORNING SNACK:** Strawberries Dipped in Chocolate with Reduced Sugar

**LUNCH:** Tomato Eggplant Soup and 2 Whole-Wheat Crackers

**OPTIONAL MIDAFTERNOON SNACK:** Small Organic Decaffeinated Latte

**DINNER:** Lobster Fra Diavolo

### A Typical Day on the Perfect 10 Diet, Stage Three

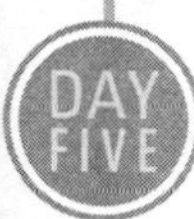


**BREAKFAST:** Mixed Fruit Salad with Natural Granola and Yogurt
**OPTIONAL MIDMORNING SNACK:** ½ Cup Nuts of Your Choice
**LUNCH:** Filet Mignon of Tuna with Mixed Greens
**OPTIONAL MIDAFTERNOON SNACK:** 1 Scoop Reduced-Sugar Coconut Ice Cream
**DINNER:** Stir-Fried Oysters, Side Salad, and 1 Scoop Brown Rice

### A Typical Day on the Perfect 10 Diet, Stage Three

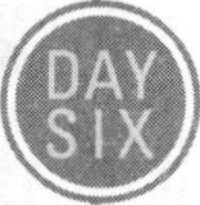


**BREAKFAST:** 2 Deviled Eggs with 1 Slice Rye Bread
**OPTIONAL MIDMORNING SNACK:** Broccoli Rabe
**LUNCH:** Grilled Fish with Caper Sauce, Brown Rice, and a Side Salad
**OPTIONAL MIDAFTERNOON SNACK:** Fruit Salad
**DINNER:** Stir-Fried Scallops and Asparagus

### A Typical Day on the Perfect 10 Diet, Stage Three

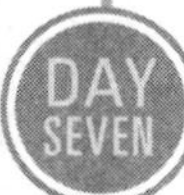


**BREAKFAST:** Zucchini Quiche
**OPTIONAL MIDMORNING SNACK:** 1 Apple
**LUNCH:** Liver Sautéed in Onions and 1 Scoop Wild Rice
**OPTIONAL MIDAFTERNOON SNACK:** Brown Rice Pudding
**DINNER:** Mixed Baked Seafood in Curry Sauce and Mixed Vegetables

# PART 5
## APPENDIXES

APPENDIX 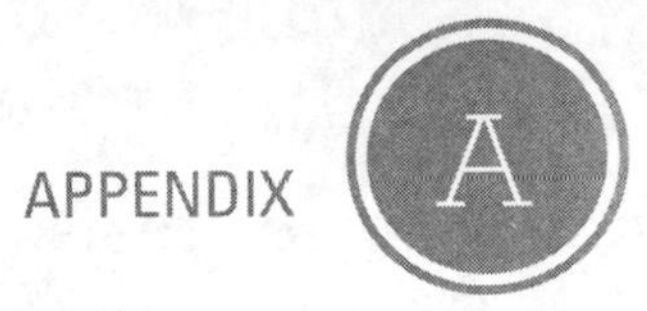


# Dietary Changes for Common Health Concerns

It's clear that everyone is different. Can the Perfect 10 Diet be adapted if you have a specific health issue? Absolutely. We can even break some rules for specific health concerns. These are the dietary changes I recommend to people who consult me for the following health conditions and illnesses.

## Allergy

- Eliminate milk products and gluten completely to see if you're allergic.
- Limit animal protein and replace with more plant protein sources, such as mushrooms, beans, and non–genetically modified soy.

## Anemia (Due to Iron Deficiency)

- Increase red meat to more than once every 3 weeks.
- Eat more beans and green leafy vegetables.

## Asthma

- Eliminate dairy products completely from your diet.
- Eat ginger and turmeric regularly for their anti-inflammatory effects.

## Atherosclerosis

- Drink pomegranate juice (it can really reverse atherosclerosis).
- Have melon extract regularly (in a pill form or as juice).
- Take fish oil regularly.

## Body Odor

- Eat more protein from plant sources and less from animal sources.
- Avoid caffeine.

## Bronchitis

- Eliminate dairy products completely from your diet.
- Eat more garlic regularly, for its natural antibiotic effects.
- Eat spicy foods, such as horseradish and wasabi (in Japanese food), to help liquefy bronchial secretions.

## Constipation

- Increase your consumption of fiber by eating more vegetables, fruits, and seeds.
- Drink much more water.
- Take extra fiber in a pill form.

## Diarrhea (Acute or Chronic)

- Avoid dairy products, raw vegetables, spices, caffeine, and alcohol.
- Eat more bland food and fewer spices.

## Eczema

- Increase your fish and other omega-3 fatty acids intake.
- Eat food rich in vitamin A, such as carrots.

## Eye Problems

- Eat plenty of fresh fruits and vegetables.
- Eat more pistachios, as they are rich in lutein.

## Fibrocystic Breasts

- Eliminate all sources of caffeine.
- Eat only hormone-free animal products.
- Eat organic, non–genetically modified soy.

## Fibroids

- Eat only hormone-free animal and dairy products.
- Eat plenty of iron-rich foods, such as green leafy vegetables and a little more red meat.

## Gout

- Avoid alcohol at all times.
- Reduce animal sources of protein, and eat more vegetable protein.

## Heartburn

- Eliminate all caffeine and alcohol.
- Avoid milk.
- Eat small, frequent meals (3 meals plus snacks).
- Avoid food high in carbohydrates, like rice and pasta, that can greatly distend the stomach and lead to reflux.
- Eat ginger regularly.

## Immune System Problems

- Eat more garlic and shiitake mushrooms.
- Eat more oranges, blueberries, and sweet potatoes.

## Kidney Problems

- Decrease protein intake.
- Replace animal protein sources with vegetable protein sources.

## Menstrual Pain

- Eat only hormone-free animal and dairy products.
- Eliminate caffeine.

## Migraine

- Avoid common dietary triggers, such as chocolate, red wine, cheese, sardines, fermented foods, cured meats, and pickled herring.
- Eliminate all sources of caffeine, including green tea.

## Mood Disorders

- Increase fish intake.
- Take in more omega-3 fatty acids in a pill form or from flaxseed oil.

## Osteoporosis

- Decrease dietary protein.
- Replace animal protein with vegetable protein as much as you can.
- Eat plenty of green leafy vegetables, as they are rich in vitamin K, which is good for the bones.

## Urinary Infections (Chronic)

- Avoid all caffeine.
- Avoid alcohol.
- Have cranberries every day.

## Varicose Veins

- Take horse chestnut extract.
- Eat lots of citrus fruits, which are rich in vitamin C.
- Eat blueberries and plums regularly.

APPENDIX 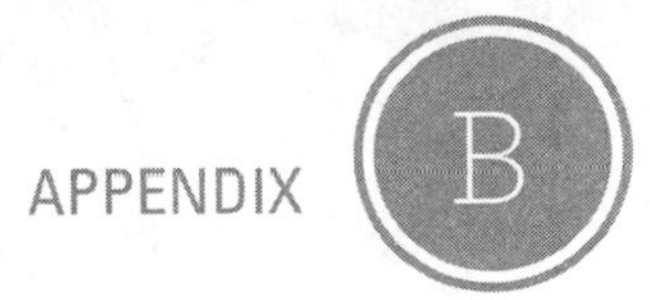


# Recommended Supplements

## Obesity

Obesity, America's most prevalent metabolic disturbance, is actually a manifestation of insulin excess and insulin resistance. To counteract this problem, I recommend supplements. Many nutrients can facilitate the weight-loss process. Researchers have found that chromium can help with stabilization of sugar levels and is optimal to reduce sugar cravings.

Conjugated linoleic acid (CLA) can help with weight loss. As I mentioned, CLA is found in butter and whole-fat dairy products. The supplementation of these two products enhances insulin sensitivity in muscle cells.

L-carnitine, which is manufactured naturally in the human body, can assist with the breakdown of fat; therefore, supplementation with L-carnitine may be beneficial. I also recommend vanadyl sulfate. Avoid many of the commercial fat-loss pills, as they usually contain caffeine and may cause palpitations.

### SUPPLEMENT WITH

- Chromium, 3,000 to 4,000 mcg/daily initially then reduce to 1,000 mcg/daily
- L-carnitine, 1,000 to 2,000 mg/daily

- Conjugated linoleic acid, 2 to 4 g/daily
- Vanadyl sulfate, 10 to 20 mg/daily
- Lipoic acid, 100 to 300 mg/daily

## Elevated Cholesterol

Cholesterol levels should improve on the Perfect 10 Diet through the elimination of refined carbohydrates and hydrogenated oils. If you still have a problem, some supplements can help improve cholesterol naturally.

### SUPPLEMENT WITH

- Omega-3 fatty acids, 2 to 3 g/daily
- Non-flush niacin, 1,500 mg/daily (in divided doses)
- Red yeast extract, 2,400 mg (in two divided doses)
- Pantothenic acid, 1,500 mg/daily
- Borage oil, 1,200 to 3,600 mg/daily

## Hypoglycemia

People with hypoglycemia are at risk of developing diabetes. Many will be advised to increase carbohydrate or sugar intake, due to a low blood sugar level. This will only worsen the condition; I definitely discourage increasing carbs. Hypoglycemia is a symptom of increased insulin secretion, which is related to high-carbohydrate diets. Decreasing sugar and increasing fat, or dividing protein throughout the day, is crucial to decreasing insulin secretion. The stabilization of sugar levels prevents hypoglycemic episodes and symptoms like dizziness, which occur as sugar levels fall. If you're hypoglycemic, have a small glass of whole milk when you feel dizzy rather than a glass of orange juice, which can lead to rapidly recurring symptoms.

### SUPPLEMENT WITH

- Chromium, 1000 to 3000 mcg/daily
- Zinc, 50 to 100 mg/daily
- Essential fatty acids, 4 g/daily
- Lipoic acid, 150 to 300 mg/daily

- L-carnitine, 500 to 1,500 mg/daily
- Coenzyme Q10, 100 mg/daily

## Candida and Yeast Infections

*Candida albicans* is a yeast that normally resides in our intestines. Low-fat diets, use of antibiotics, and immune suppression can all cause overgrowth of yeast, and that's bad for hormones. If you suffer from frequent yeast infections, avoid fermented products and limit fruit to 1 serving daily. If you suspect that you may be suffering from disseminated *Candida*, a test (D-arabinitol) can be performed to confirm the diagnosis.

### SUPPLEMENT WITH

- Beneficial bacteria, 1 to 3 teaspoons/daily
- Caprylic acid, 2 to 4 capsules/daily
- Oil of oregano, 2 to 4 drops/daily
- Olive leaf extract, 1 to 4 capsules/daily
- Panthothenic acid, 600 to 1,200 mg/daily

## Depression

Depression is related to a variety of factors: stress, disturbance in omega-3 to omega-6 ratio, deficiency in male or female sex hormones, and serotonin metabolism. You will need to seek professional help to determine the best course of treatment or therapy.

### SUPPLEMENT WITH

- St. John's wort (hypericum extract WS 5570), 300 mg 3 times/daily (the dose may increase to 1,800 mg/day for nonresponders)
- L-tryptophan, 50 mg, 2 to 3 times/daily

## Polycystic Ovary Syndrome

It's now believed that polycystic ovary disease is a disease of insulin resistance. The Perfect 10 Diet will help by decreasing insulin secretion. You can also use insulin-sensitizing drugs and fertility drugs if the condition isn't reversed by diet alone.

SUPPLEMENT WITH

- Chromium, 400 to 1,000 mcg/daily
- L-carnitine, 500 to 1,500 mg/daily
- Saw Palmetto, 160 mg, 2 tablets, 2 times daily

## Healthy Hair and Skin

When hair loss is accompanied by dandruff and itching, it's usually due to a fungus problem rather than a hormonal issue. Try avoiding milk products, bread, refined carbs, and sugar at all times. If your hair is losing its color, make sure you get enough nutrients that make melanin (the pigment hormone), such as cysteine, copper, thiamine, and vitamin $B_6$.

For healthy hair and skin, supplement the Perfect 10 Diet with a whole-food pill with the right supplements of vitamins, minerals, trace elements, and enzymes.

SUPPLEMENT WITH

- Vitamin A, 5,000 IU/daily
- Thiamine, 5 mg/daily
- Vitamin $B_6$, 25 mg/daily
- Riboflavin, 5 mg/daily
- Niacin, 10 mg/daily
- Pantothenic acid, 15 mg/daily
- Folic acid, 1 mg/daily
- Vitamin C, 500 mg/daily
- Vitamin E, 10 to 50 mg/daily
- Zinc, 100 mg/daily
- Copper, 0.8 mg/daily
- Iron, 25 mg/daily
- Manganese, 6 mg/daily
- Cysteine, 80 mg/daily
- Selenium, 25 mcg/daily
- Supeoxide dismutase, 25 mg/daily
- Catalase, 20 mg/daily

## HIV/AIDS

The HIV epidemic is not showing any signs of slowing. Many of the drugs developed have led to improved survival, but they also raise cardiovascular risk by increasing cholesterol levels. HIV lipodystrophy, or abnormal fat deposits in the neck and trunk and wasting of the face and extremities, is a condition of insulin resistance. Research suggests that the drugs that are used to treat the disease also play a role in such resistance.

Stavudine and most protease inhibitors have been implicated. The Perfect 10 Diet will help improve the cholesterol and sugar abnormalities associated with HIV lipodystrophy since it regulates insulin. If you're HIV positive, you should avoid hydrogenated fats or trans fats completely.

SUPPLEMENT WITH

- Coconut
- Mushrooms
- Selenium
- Green tea extract

## Osteoporosis

Osteoporosis is related to our modern diet, rather than to a lack of calcium. A diet high in refined carbs and deficient in fruit can lead to a deficiency in boron and magnesium, which are essential for normal bone health.

SUPPLEMENT WITH

- Calcium citrate, 1,200 mg/daily
- Vitamin D, 400 IU/daily
- Boron, 6 to 12 mg/daily

APPENDIX 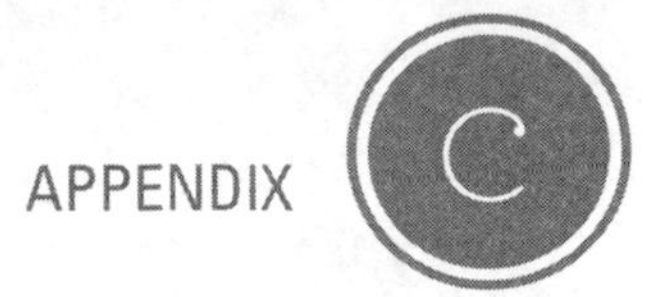

# Glycemic Index

The glycemic index is a tool that was designed by Dr. David Jenkins. It compares different carbohydrates to simple sugars with an ascending and descending scale. Most versions of the index give sugar a value of 100 and compare different blood groups to sugar.

## The Glycemic Index of Popular Foods

Low GI Foods . . . . . . . . . . Below 55
Intermediate GI foods . . . . . . . . . . Between 55 to 70
High GI Foods . . . . . . . . . . More than 70

## Breads, Muffins, and Cakes

Bagel . . . . . . . . . . 72
Croissant . . . . . . . . . . 80
Pita bread . . . . . . . . . . 57
Pumpernickel bread . . . . . . . . . . 51
Rye . . . . . . . . . . 55
Sponge cake . . . . . . . . . . 60
Waffles . . . . . . . . . . 76

## Breakfast Cereals

Kellogg's All-Bran . . . . . . . . . . 51
Kellogg's Corn Flakes . . . . . . . . . . 84
Kellogg's Rice Krispies . . . . . . . . . . 49
Special K . . . . . . . . . . 54
Oatmeal (old fashioned) . . . . . . . . . . 49

## Cookies

Chocolate chip . . . . . . . . . . 75

Oatmeal . . . . . . . . . . . . . . . . . 55
Shortbread . . . . . . . . . . . . . . . 64

## Grains

Bulgur . . . . . . . . . . . . . . . . . . 48
Rice
 Basmati . . . . . . . . . . . . . . 58
 Brown . . . . . . . . . . . . . . . 55
 White . . . . . . . . . . . . . . . . 72
Pasta
 Ravioli . . . . . . . . . . . . . . . 32
 Spaghetti . . . . . . . . . . . . . 43

## Vegetables

Beets . . . . . . . . . . . . . . . . . . 69
Carrots . . . . . . . . . . . . . . . . . 72
Peas . . . . . . . . . . . . . . . . . . . 48
Potatoes
 Baked . . . . . . . . . . . . . . . . 93
 Red-skinned . . . . . . . . . . . 88
 French fries . . . . . . . . . . . 75
Sweet potato . . . . . . . . . . . . 54

## Legumes

Chick peas . . . . . . . . . . . . . . 20
Lentils . . . . . . . . . . . . . . . . . 30
Navy beans . . . . . . . . . . . . . . 38
Soybeans . . . . . . . . . . . . . . . 18

## Fruits

Apple . . . . . . . . . . . . . . . . . . . 38
Banana . . . . . . . . . . . . . . . . . 55
Cantaloupe . . . . . . . . . . . . . . 65
Cherries . . . . . . . . . . . . . . . . . 22
Dates (dried) . . . . . . . . . . . 103
Grapefruit . . . . . . . . . . . . . . 25
Grapes . . . . . . . . . . . . . . . . . . 25
Kiwi . . . . . . . . . . . . . . . . . . . . 53
Mango . . . . . . . . . . . . . . . . . . 55
Orange . . . . . . . . . . . . . . . . . . 44
Papaya . . . . . . . . . . . . . . . . . . 58
Pear . . . . . . . . . . . . . . . . . . . . 38
Pineapple . . . . . . . . . . . . . . . 66
Plum . . . . . . . . . . . . . . . . . . . 38

## Snack Foods

Corn chips . . . . . . . . . . . . . . 72
Peanuts . . . . . . . . . . . . . . . . . 14
Nuts . . . . . . . . . . . . . . . . . . . . 30
Potato chips . . . . . . . . . . . . . 55
Pretzels . . . . . . . . . . . . . . . . . 83

APPENDIX 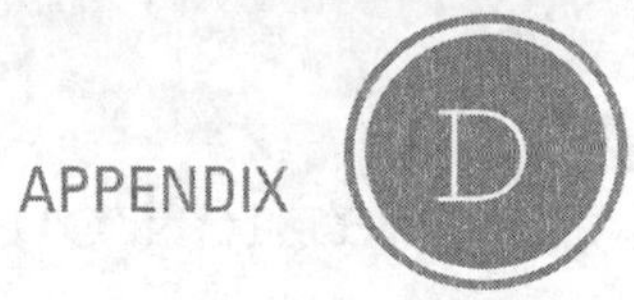

# Food Sources

Addresses, telephone numbers, fax numbers, and Web addresses are provided below for a small sampling of the many companies that offer healthy, organic foods. Many of the foods listed here are also available in whole-food and health-food stores, but some can be obtained only by mail order.

## Eggs

### Gold Circle Farms

INTERNET: www.goldcirclefarms.com

Gold Circle Farms provides organic eggs. Its eggs are available in many grocery and health-food stores.

## Organic Poultry and Red Meat

### White Egret Farm

15704 Webberville Rd., FM 969
Austin, TX 78724
Tel: 512/276-7408
Fax: 512/276-7489
INTERNET: www.whiteegretfarm.com

White Egret Farm offers natural beef and free-range turkey, as well as unprocessed goat and other dairy products. No hormones or antibiotics are used.

### Eat Wild

29428 129th Ave. SW
Vashon, WA 98070
Tel: 866/453-8489
Fax: 253/759-2318
INTERNET: www.eatwild.com

On the suppliers' page, you can find out how to purchase free-range poultry, beef, and lamb.

### Tropical Traditions

PO Box 333
Springville, CA 93265
INTERNET: www.tropicaltraditions.com

On the suppliers' page, you can find out how to purchase pasture-fed poultry, grass-fed beef, and whole-grain products.

### Oaklyn Plantation

1312 Oaklyn Rd.
Darlington, SC 29532
Tel: 843/395-0793
Fax: 843/395-0794
INTERNET: www.freerangechicken.com

Oaklyn Plantation offers free-range chicken and grass-fed beef from animals raised without antibiotics or growth hormones.

## Fish

### Barlean's Fishery

4936 Lake Terrell Rd.
Ferndale, WA 98248
Tel: 360/384-0485
Fax: 360/384-1746
INTERNET: www.barleansfishery.com

Barlean's Fishery offers ecologically friendly, wild-harvested salmon.

### Eco-Fish, Inc.

340 Central Ave.
Dover, NH 03820
Tel: 877/214-3474
INTERNET: www.ecofish.com

Eco-Fish offers ocean-caught salmon, halibut, tuna, and other seafood.

### Great Alaska Seafood

Tel: 866/262-8846
INTERNET: www.Great-Alaska-Seafood.com

Great Alaska Seafood offers ocean-caught fish and other seafood.

### Oregon Gourmet

201 SW Second St.
Corvallis, OR 97333
Tel: 541/752-7418
INTERNET: www.oregongourmet.com

Oregon Gourmet offers an assortment of wild northwest salmon.

## Whole Grains

### Diamond Organics

Tel: 888/ORGANIC
INTERNET: www.diamondorganics.com

Diamond Organics produces organic amaranth and whole-wheat flour.

### Homegrown Harvest

2260 Moonstation Ct., Suite 210
Kennesaw, GA 30144
Tel: 866/900-3321
INTERNET: www.homegrownharvest.com

Homegrown Harvest offers a wide variety of whole grains.

### The Baker

P.O. Box 528
60 Bridge Street
Milford, NJ 08848
Tel: 908/995-4040
Fax: 908/995-9669
INTERNET: www.the-baker.com

The Baker offers organic granola and whole grains.

## Oils

### Purity Farms

14635 Westcreek Rd.
Sedalia, CO 80135
Tel: 303/647-2368
Fax: 303/647-9875
INTERNET: www.purityfarms.com

Purity Farms offers organic ghee.

### Thai Kitchen

Tel: 800/967-8424 or 310/268-0209, ex. 103
INTERNET: www.thaikitchen.com

Thai Kitchen offers pure coconut milk, as well as other coconut products. You can find its products in many supermarket and health-food stores.

### Barlean's Organic Oils

4936 Lake Terrell Rd.
Ferndale, WA 98248
Tel: 360/384-0485
INTERNET: www.barleans.com

Barlean's Organic Oils offers organic, high-quality flaxseed, evening primrose, and fish oils.

### Omega Nutrition

6515 Aldrich Rd.
Bellingham, WA 98226
Tel: 360/384-1238
Fax: 360/384-0700
INTERNET: www.omeganutrition.com

Omega Nutrition offers organic flaxseed and olive oils.

### Spectrum

Spectrum Consumer Relations
The Hain Celestial Group, Inc.
4600 Sleepytime Dr.
Boulder, CO 80301
Tel: 800/434-4246
INTERNET: www.spectrumorganics.com

Offers a wide variety of cooking oils such as olive oil and flaxseed oil.

### Nutiva

P.O. Box 1716
Sebastopol, CA 95473
Tel: 800/993-4367
INTERNET: www.nutiva.com

Nutiva offers a wide variety of products, including coconut oil, hemp protein, and gluten-free products.

## Sweeteners

### Madhava Agave

Tel: 303/ 823-5166
INTERNET: www.madhavasagave.com

Offers agave sweetener.

### Volcanic Nectar

11382 North 5710 West
Highland, UT 84003
Tel: 801/492-6295
INTERNET: www.volcanicnectar.com

Offers agave sweetener.

## Water in Glass Bottles

Acqua Panna
777 West Putnam Ave.
P.O. Box 2313
Greenwich, CT 06830
Tel: 203/531-4100
INTERNET: www.nestle-watersna.com

### Mountain Valley Spring Company

150 Central Avenue
Hot Springs National Park, AR 71901
Tel: 501/624-1635
Fax: 501/623-5135
INTERNET: www.mountainvalleyspring.com

# Chocolate

## Dagoba Organic Chocolate

1105 Benson Way
Ashland, OR 97520
Tel: 541/482-2001
Fax: 800/482-5661
INTERNET: www.dagobachocolate.com

Dagoba offers dark organic chocolate with little sugar.

## Terra Nostre Chocolate

KFM Foods International, Inc.
P.O. Box 71054
Vancouver, BC V6N 4J9
Canada
Tel: 888/439-4443
Fax: 604/267-3582
INTERNET: www.terranostrachocolate.com

Terra Nostre offers organic dark chocolate with little sugar.

APPENDIX 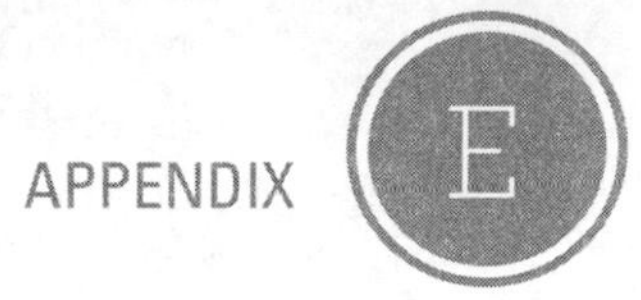


# Ingredients to Avoid

On the Perfect 10 Diet, it's crucial to stay away from processed foods at all times. However, if you do buy any products that are processed, you should avoid any products containing any of the following ingredients:

- artificial fats, such as Olestra
- artificial sweeteners
- artificial colorings
- brominated vegetable oil (BVO), a toxic additive found in some citrus sodas
- hydrogenated starch hydrolysate, a common sweetener
- hydrogenated or partially hydrogenated oils
- high-fructose corn syrup
- margarine
- monosodium glutamate (MSG)
- potassium bromate, a flavor enhancer in breads that is carcinogenic
- preservatives, such as BHA and BHT
- soy protein isolate
- sodium nitrite, found in processed meats
- sulfites, preservatives found in dried fruit, instant potatoes, and pizza
- vegetable shortening

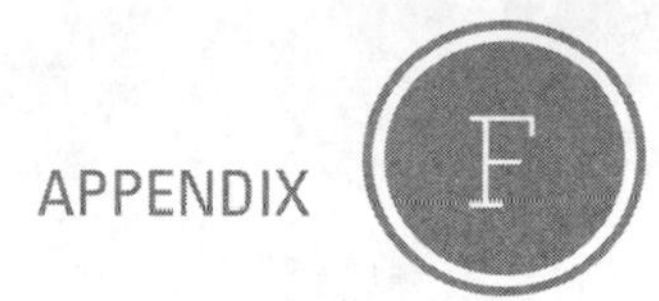

# Calorie-Burning Tips: Workouts and Housework

Weight loss means a healthier lifestyle. To lose weight, it helps to burn extra calories. Exercising more is one good strategy, and here's another: doing more chores around the house. You have to burn 3,500 calories to lose 1 pound. Aim to burn at least 1,400 calories a week on the Perfect 10 Diet.

To burn the amount of calories listed in the table, each activity should be performed for one hour at a moderate level of intensity.

| Exercise | Calories Burned |
|---|---|
| Bicycling | 290 |
| Dancing | 330 |
| Golfing | 330 |
| Hiking | 370 |
| Running | 560 |
| Stretching | 180 |
| Walking | 280 |

| Activity | Calories Burned |
|---|---|
| Gardening | 150 |
| Pushing a stroller | 300 |
| Raking leaves | 300 |
| Shoveling snow | 300 |
| Washing a car | 300 |

APPENDIX G

# Popular Diets

You either have perfection or you don't, and the Perfect 10 Diet has got it. However, the Perfect 10 Diet has plenty of competition. Many of these diet programs are well known and popular, but none of them will make you a perfect 10 in hormones or in health. In fact, these diets will disturb your hormones, and in turn, endanger your health. You see there is more than one way to go for weight loss, so don't be deceived. How do you know if you were previously on the right track or not? Read on. In this section, I review nine popular diets so you can understand their pros and cons as well as how greatly they differ from the Perfect 10 Diet, the only diet that balances all your hormones.

## 1. Jenny Craig

Technically, no food is forbidden because the Jenny Craig program relies on calorie counting. The program includes motivational and educational meetings with food counselors, and you can buy their packaged food.

THE ADVANTAGES: People lose weight when they reduce their calories and lower insulin demands.

THE DISADVANTAGES: Jenny Craig's food contains added chemicals and partially hydrogenated oils, which are bad for insulin, leptin, and sex hormones. Trans fats not only mess up hormones, but they can actually clog your arteries. There are long-term consequences when all food is valued only as calories.

## 2. NutriSystem

The NutriSystem program relies heavily on the glycemic index. You purchase processed food directly from the company by phone or online. The food is already prepared or requires little preparation.

THE ADVANTAGES: The glycemic index is a useful tool for losing weight, since it separates the good, slow-digesting carbs from the bad, rapidly metabolizing carbs. It's convenient for people with busy lifestyles who don't have time to spend in the kitchen.

THE DISADVANTAGES: You can't follow NutriSystem in the real world, since you can only eat the company's food. Their processed foods contain added chemicals, sugar, high-fructose corn syrup, and partially hydrogenated oils. All are toxic to the hormones and forbidden on the Perfect 10 Diet.

## 3. The American Heart Association Diet

The American Heart Association (AHA) recommends a low-fat diet, the same diet that is frequently recommended by physicians. The AHA condemns sugar and trans fats, but their numerous cookbooks include recipes made with refined white flour, sugar, and margarine. According to the AHA, the healthy fats are soybean and corn oils and tub margarine! Butter, coconut, and palm oils are condemned as atherogenic.

THE ADVANTAGES: The American Heart Association diet emphasizes fruits, vegetables, and whole grains as a part of a healthy diet.

THE DISADVANTAGES: The AHA has the wrong position on many fats. The recommended fats, such as soybean oil and tub margarine, have been linked to cancer. The low-fat recommendations overlook the effects of metabolized sugar on insulin and all other hormones discussed in the Perfect 10 Diet. Also, low-fat diets overlook the effects of excessive amounts of sugar on triglyceride levels, which are an independent risk factor for heart disease.

## 4. The Dean Ornish Diet

This is an extremely low-fat vegetarian diet designed by Dr. Dean Ornish. Roughly 70 percent of your calories will come from carbohydrates, 20 percent from protein, and 10 percent from fat. The Ornish diet encourages grains, legumes, vegetables, and fruits. Acceptable in moderation are fat-free dairy products and other fat-free products like crackers and salad dressings. Fats from nuts, seeds, olive oil, fish, and chicken are all to be avoided on this diet.

THE ADVANTAGES: A December 1998 short-term study on the Ornish diet, published in the *Journal of the American Medical Association* (*JAMA*) indicated that followers of the diet experienced a regression of arterial plaques. It's not known if the benefits seen were related to smoking cessation or the diet. The long-term effects of a very low-fat diet are unknown at this time.

THE DISADVANTAGES: This diet can dangerously raise your insulin levels, much more so than the average low-fat diets, and that spells more trouble for your other hormones. It's very low in fat, including essential fatty acids, which is dangerous to its followers and can lead to vitamin deficiencies, resulting in eczema and dandruff. The diet excludes many healthy fats with well-known benefits, such as olive oil and nuts. The diet is not suitable for diabetics or for the quarter of Americans who are on the verge of diabetes.

## 5. The Atkins Diet

This diet, designed by Dr. Robert Atkins, a cardiologist, is a high-fat/high-protein/very-low-carb diet. The Atkins Diet advises lots of protein—mostly in the form of meat, poultry, and processed meats—and restricts carbohydrates. Thirty percent of your calories will come from protein, 60 percent will come from fat, and the rest will come from carbs. You do not count calories; instead, you count net carbs, including those from vegetables, fruits, and whole grains. This forces the body to burn both fat and protein as a main source of fuel. You check your urine to make sure you remain in a state of ketosis (which means not utilizing any sugar), especially on the induction phase.

THE ADVANTAGES: The Atkins Diet correctly discourages refined carbs, sugar, and trans fats. It's very high in protein, which makes the diet optimal for people involved in heavy anaerobic activity, such as weight lifters. The Atkins Diet does appear to be beneficial for people with seizures.

THE DISADVANTAGES: This very high-fat diet can shut down HGH production. It's also very high in protein, which can lead to thyroid disease. The Atkins Diet also endorses products with soy protein isolate and Splenda. Both are forbidden on the Perfect 10 Diet. In addition, consumption of processed meats in any amount has been implicated in the development of many cancers.

## 6. The Flat Belly Diet

This is the latest diet to hit the market (in 2008). It was written by Liz Vaccariello, editor-in-chief of *Prevention* magazine. It is gaining ground rapidly since the diet targets belly fat. It advocates monounsaturated fats (such as those found in oils, olives, nuts and seeds, avocados, and dark chocolate) to lose weight. (Dark chocolate is included as a monounsaturated fat as part of the plan, but it is not a fat. It can contain cocoa butter, which is a saturated fat.) Acceptable food choices on the Flat Belly Diet include frozen meals, fat-free dairy, some fast food, replacement bars, Corn Flakes, Rice Krispies, pork, and ham.

THE ADVANTAGES: It is a diet that correctly tells readers to eat certain types of fats.

THE DISADVANTAGES: Processed food, ham, and frozen meals should never be part of your diet.

## 7. The Zone Diet

The Zone diet is a high-protein diet designed by Dr. Barry Sears, a biochemist. Acceptable protein choices on the Zone diet include veal, ham (deli style), Canadian bacon, egg whites, and eggs substitutes. The Zone diet advocates maintaining a strict ratio of calories: 30 percent from protein, 30 percent fat, and 40 percent carbohydrates at all meals in order to stabilize hormones like insulin, which triggers hunger. On the Zone diet, you divide your plate by 3 each and every time in order to get this exact ratio of carbs, fat, and protein. If you have trouble keeping this ratio straight at each and every single meal, you can just eat a processed Zone bar that contains soy protein isolate and some added sugar to reach this "favorable" hormonal zone. The Zone correctly discourages refined carbs.

THE ADVANTAGES: People lose weight on the Zone diet as they eliminate refined carbs from their diet.

THE DISADVANTAGES: The diet wrongly condemns saturated fats found in butter and egg yolks as dense and high in saturated fats. This dense, rich food is good for sex hormones. The Zone diet's protein choices are horrible for your health; for one thing, processed meats have been linked to cancer. The Zone diet is impractical to follow in the real world, with such a strict ratio for each and every meal. Worst of all, the Zone diet endorses processed products with added sugar, high-fructose corn syrup, and soy protein isolate. All are toxic to your body.

## 8. The South Beach Diet

The South Beach Diet was designed by a Miami cardiologist, Dr. Arthur Agatston. He initially developed this diet for his patients with heart disease; however, many patients showed another benefit: weight loss. The diet emphasizes the dangers of sugar and the low-fat diet dogma we've all bought into. It's moderate in fat and lower in carbohydrates. On the South Beach Diet, you avoid the saturated fats found in butter and animal products, such as bacon. You consume lean meats, such as veal and Canadian bacon, and low-fat dairy products. Vegetable oils and liquid margarine are acceptable fats.

THE ADVANTAGES: The diet emphasizes the dangers of refined carbs, which leads to weight loss.

THE DISADVANTAGES: Processed meats have been strongly linked to colon and prostate cancer. There is no difference between bacon and Canadian bacon. Both are processed, and both contain nitrites. The South Beach Diet has the wrong positions on many fats. The diet denounces saturated fats, such as butter, which are good for sex hormones, and advocates liquid margarine as a healthy substitute. The book denounces trans fats, yet includes recipes that use margarine and vegetable shortening. The diet endorses processed food and frozen entrées with added chemicals, soybean oil, nitrites, soy protein isolate, and partially hydrogenated fats. All damage your thyroid and leptin, and they can also clog your arteries and give you cancer.

## 9. Weight Watchers

This very popular program is a low-fat diet that relies on calorie restriction by counting points. About 50 percent of your calories will come from carbohydrates, 30 percent from protein, and 20 percent from fat. On Weight Watchers, you eat as you please: pizza, pasta, and even orange juice as long as it counts toward your total daily points. Technically, no food is forbidden. The program includes motivational and educational meetings in groups and online.

THE ADVANTAGES: Portion control is an essential component for the success of any diet.

THE DISADVANTAGES: There are long-term consequences when all food is viewed only as a source of calories. A low-fat diet is bad for all hormones discussed in the Perfect 10 Diet.

# Bibliography


Abbasi, F., T. McLaughlin, C. Lamendola, H. S. Kim, A. Tanaka, T. Wang, K. Nakajima, and G. M. Reaven. "High Carbohydrates Diets, Triglyceride Rich Lipoproteins and Coronary Heart Disease Risk." *Am J Cardiol* 1.85 (2000): 45–48.

Ajwani, Fatim, and Maria Ricupero. "What's the Skinny on Trans Fat?" *Geriatrics Aging* 9.5 (2006): 358–64.

Anderson, K. E., F. F. Kadlubar, M. Kulldorff, L. Harnack, M. Gross, et al. "Dietary Intake of Heterocyclic Amines and Benzo(a)pyrene: Associations with Pancreatic Cancer." *Cancer Epidemiol Biomarkers Prev* 14 (2005): 2261–65.

Appel, L. J., L. M. Bishop, B. A. Rosner, F. M. Sacks, J. F. Swain, V. J. Carey, J. Charleston, P. R. Conlin, T. P. Erlinger, N. M. Laranjo, P. McCarron, E. R. Miller, and E. Obarzanek. "Effects of Protein, Monounsaturated Fat, and Carbohydrate Intake on Blood Pressure and Serum Lipids: Results of the Omniheart Randomized Trial." *JAMA: The Journal of the American Medical Association* 294.19 (2005): 2455–64.

Bravata, Dena M., Lisa Sanders, Jane Huang, Harlan M. Krumholz, Ingram Olkin, and Christopher D. Gardner. "Efficacy and Safety of Low-Carbohydrate Diets: A Systematic Review." *JAMA: The Journal of the American Medical Association* 289 (2003): 1837–50.

Bray, G. A., S. J. Nielsen, and B. M. Popkin. "Consumption of High-Fructose Corn Syrup in Beverages May Play a Role in the Epidemic of Obesity." *Am J Clin Nutr* 79 (2004): 537–43.

Brehm, B. J., M. Briel, H. C. Bucher, U. Keller, A. Nordmann, A. J. Nordmann, and W. S. Yancy. "Effects of Low-Carbohydrate vs Low-Fat Diets on Weight Loss and Cardiovascular Risk Factors: A Meta-Analysis of Randomized Controlled Trials." *Arch Intern Med* 166.3 (2006): 285–93.

Burger, Albert G., John P. Monson, Anna M. Colao, and Anne Klibanski. "Cardiovascular Risk in Patients with Growth Hormone Deficiency: Effects of Growth Hormone Substitution." *Endocr Pract* 12.6 (2006): 682–89.

Calle, E. E., A. Chao, C J. Connell, W. D. Flanders, E. J. Jacobs, M. L. Mccullough, C. Rodriguez, R. Sinha, and M. J. Thun. "Meat Consumption and Risk of Colorectal Cancer." *JAMA: The Journal of the American Medical Association* 293.2 (2005): 172–82.

Cases, J. A., and N. Barzilai. "The Regulation of Body Fat Distribution and the Modulation of Insulin Action." *Int J Obes Relat Metab Disord* Suppl. 4 (2000): S63–66.

Cooper, D. S. "Clinical Practice. Subclinical Hypothyroidism." *N Engl J Med* 345 (2001): 260–65.

Cordain, L., and J. H. O'Keefe. "Cardiovascular Disease Resulting from a Diet and Lifestyle at Odds with Our Paleolithic Genome: How to Become a 21st-Century Hunter-Gatherer." *Mayo Clin Proc* 79.1 (2004): 101–8.

Cross, A. J., U. Peters, V. A. Kirsh, G. L. Andriole, D. Reding, et al. "A Prospective Study of Meat and Meat Mutagens and Prostate Cancer Risk." *Cancer Res* 65 (2005): 11779–784.

Dale, Krista M., Craig I. Coleman, Nickole N. Henyan, Jeffrey Kluger, and C. Michael White. "Statins and Cancer Risk: A Meta-Analysis." *JAMA: The Journal of the American Medical Association* 295 (2006): 74–80.

Dansinger, M. L., J. A. Gleason, J. L. Griffith, E. J. Schaefer, and H. P. Selker. "Comparison of the Atkins, Ornish, Weight Watchers, and Zone Diets for Weight Loss and Heart Disease Risk Reduction: A Randomized Trial." *JAMA: The Journal of the American Medical Association* 293.1 (2005): 43–53.

David, T., and N. T. Nash. "The Metabolic Syndrome, Early Clues, Effective Management." *Consultant* 99.6 (2004): 859–64.

Davidson, Michael, D. Hunninghake, K. Maki, P. Kwiterovich, and S. Kafonek. "Comparison of the Effects of Lean Red Meat vs. Lean White Meat on Serum Lipid Levels among Free-Living Persons with Hypercholesterolemia: A Long-Term, Randomized Clinical Trial." *Arch Intern Med* 159 (1999): 1331–38.

Ebbeling, Cara B., Michael M. Leidig, Henry A. Feldman, Margaret M. Lovesky, and David S. Ludwig. "Effects of a Low-Glycemic Load vs. Low-Fat Diet in Obese Young Adults: A Randomized Trial." *JAMA: The Journal of the American Medical Association* 297 (2007): 2092–2102.

Enig, Mary G. *Know Your Fats: The Complete Primer for Understanding the Nutrition of Fats, Oils, and Cholesterol*. Bethesda, MD: Bethesda Press, 2000.

Enig, Mary G., et al. "Dietary Fat and Cancer Trends—A Critique." *Fed Proc* 37.9 (1978): 2215–20.

Ford, E. S., and S. Liu. "Glycemic Index and Serum High-Density Lipoprotein Cholesterol Concentration among U.S. Adults." *Arch Intern Med* 161.4 (2001): 572–76.

Ford, E. S., and W. H. Giles. "Changes in Prevalence of Nonfatal Coronary Heart Disease in the United States from 1971–1994." *Ethn Dis* 13.1 (2003): 85–93.

Gapstur, Susan M., Peter H. Gann, William Lowe, Kiang Liu, Laura Colangelo, and Alan Dyer. "Abnormal Glucose Metabolism and Pancreatic Cancer Mortality." *JAMA: The Journal of the American Medical Association* 283 (2000): 2552–58.

Gardner, C. D., A. Kiazand, S. Alhassan, S. Kim, R. S. Stafford, R. R. Balise, H. C. Kraemer, and A. C. King. "Comparison of the Atkins, Zone, Ornish, and LEARN Diets for Change in Weight and Related Risk Factors among Overweight Premenopausal Women: The A to Z Weight Loss Study: A Randomized Trial." *JAMA: The Journal of the American Medical Association* 297.9 (2007): 969–977.

GISSI-HF Investigators. "Effect of N-3 Polyunsaturated Fatty Acids in Patients with Chronic Heart Failure (The GISSI-HF Trial): A Randomised, Double-Blind, Placebo-Controlled Trial." *The Lancet* 372.9645 (2008): 1223–30.

Grundy, S. M. "The Issue of Statin Safety: Where Do We Stand?" *Circulation* 111.23 (2005): 3016–19.

Harris, Ruth. "Leptin—Much More than a Satiety Signal." *Annu Rev Nutr* 20 (2000): 45–5.

Holmes, Michelle D., Donna Spiegelman, Walter C. Willett, JoAnn E. Manson, David J. Hunter, Robert L. Barbieri, Graham A. Colditz, and Susan E. Hankinson. "Dietary Fat Intake and Endogenous Sex Steroid Hormone Levels in Postmenopausal Women." *J Clin Oncol* 18.21 (2000): 3668–76.

Howard, B. V., L. Van Horn, C. E. Lewis, M. C. Limacher, K. L. Margolis, W. J. Mysiw, J. K. Ockene, L. M. Parker, M. G. Perri, L. Phillips, R. L. Prentice, J. Robbins, J. Hsia, J. E. Rossouw, G. E. Sarto, I. J. Schatz, L. G. Snetselaar, V. J. Stevens, L. F. Tinker, M. Trevisan, M. Z. Vitolins, G. L. Anderson, A. R. Assaf, J. E. Manson, T. Bassford, S. A. Beresford, H. R. Black, R. L. Brunner, R. G. Brzyski, B. Caan, R. T. Chlebowski, M. Gass, I. Granek, P. Greenland, M. L. Stefanick, J. Hays, D. Heber, G. Heiss, S. L. Hendrix, F. A. Hubbell, K. C. Johnson, J. M. Kotchen, S. Wassertheil-Smoller, L. H. Kuller, A. Z. LaCroix, R. D. Langer, and N. L. Lasser. "Low-Fat Dietary Pattern and Risk of Cardiovascular Disease: The Women's Health Initiative Randomized Controlled Dietary Modification Trial." *JAMA: The Journal of the American Medical Association* 295.6 (2006): 655–66.

Hu, F. B., Leslie Bronner, Walter C. Willett, Meir J. Stampfer, Kathryn M. Rexrode, Christine M. Albert, David Hunter, and JoAnn E. Manson. "Fish and Omega-3 Fatty Acid Intake and Risk of Coronary Heart Disease in Women." *JAMA: The Journal of the American Medical Association* 287 (2002): 1815–21.

Hu, F. B., M. J. Stampfer, C. H. Hennekens, W. C. Willett, E. B. Rimm, J. E. Manson, A. Ascherio, G. A. Colditz, B. A. Rosner, D. Spiegelman, F. E. Speizer, and F. M. Sacks. "A Prospective Study of Egg Consumption and Risk of Cardiovascular Disease in Men and Women." *JAMA: The Journal of the American Medical Association* 281.15 (1999): 1387–94.

Hu, F. B., and W. C. Willett. "Optimal Diets for Prevention of Coronary Heart Disease." *JAMA: The Journal of the American Medical Association* 288.20 (2002): 2569–78.

Hulley, S., C. Furberg, E. Barrett-Connor, et al. HERS Research Group. "Non-Cardiovascular Disease Outcomes During 6.8 Years of Hormone Therapy: Heart and Estrogen/Progestin Replacement Study Follow-Up (HERS II)." *JAMA: The Journal of the American Medical Association* 288 (2002): 58–66.

Kappagoda, C. Tissa, and Dianne A. Hyson. "Popular Diets and Coronary Artery Disease." *Geriatrics Aging* 8.10 (2005): 30–34.

Katan, M. B. "Effect of Low-Fat Diets on Plasma High-Density Lipoprotein Concentrations." *Am J Clin Nutr* 67.3 Suppl (1998): 573S–76S.

Kaushik, S., R. Wander, S. Leonard, B. German, and M. G. Traber. "Removal of Fat from Cow's Milk Decreases the Vitamin E Contents of the Resulting Dairy Products." *Lipids* 36.1 (2001): 73–78.

Kelleher, S., A. J. Conway, and D. J. Handelsman. "Blood Testosterone Threshold for Androgen Deficiency Symptoms." *J Clin Endocrinol Metab* 8 (2004): 3813–17.

Kelley, G. A., K. S. Kelley, and V. U. Tran. "Aerobic Exercise, Lipids and Lipoproteins in Overweight and Obese Adults: A Meta-Analysis of Randomized Controlled Trials." *International Journal of Obesity* 4.2 (Spring 2005): 73–80.

Keys, A., G. D. Foster, H. R. Wyatt, J. O. Hill, B. G. McGuckin, C. Brill, B. S. Mohammed, and B. Szapay. *Seven Countries: A Multivariate Analysis of Death and Coronary Heart Disease*. Cambridge, MA: Harvard University Press, 1980.

Larsson, S. C., and A. Wolk. "Meat Consumption and Risk of Colorectal Cancer: A Meta-Analysis of Prospective Studies." *Int J Cancer* 119 (2006): 2657–64.

Lopez-Garcia, E., M. B. Schulze, J. B. Meigs, et al. "Consumption of Trans Fatty Acids Is Related to Plasma Biomarkers of Inflammation and Endothelial Dysfunction" *J Nutr* 135 (2005): 562–66.

Mann, G. V., A. Spoerry, M. Gray, and D. Jarashow. "Atherosclerosis in the Masai." *Am J Epidemolo* 95.1 (1972): 26–37.

Miller, K. K., B. M. Biller, J. G. Lipman, G. Bradwin, N. Rifai, and A. Klibanski. "Truncal Adiposity, Relative Growth Hormone Deficiency, and Cardiovascular Risk." *J Clin Endocrinol Metab* 90 (2005): 768–74.

Mokad, A. H. et al. "The Spread of the Obesity Epidemic in the United States, 1991–1998." *JAMA: The Journal of the American Medical Association* 282.16 (1999): 1519–22.

Mozaffarian, D., and E. B. Rimm. "Fish Intake, Contaminants, and Human Health: Evaluating the Risks and the Benefits." *JAMA: The Journal of the American Medical Association* 296.15 (2006): 1885–99.

Mulligan, T., M. F. Frick, Q. C. Zuraw, A. Stemhagen, and C. McWhirter. "Prevalence of Hypogonadism in Males Aged at Least 45 Years: The HIM Study." *Int J Clin Pract* 60 (2006): 762–69.

Nielsen, S. J., and B. M. Popkin. "Changes in Beverage Intake between 1977 and 2001." *Am J Prev Med* 27 (2004): 205–10.

Parks, Elizabeth, and Marc Hellerstein. "Carbohydrate-Induced Hypertriacylglycerolemia: Historical Perspective and Review of Biological Mechanisms." *Am J Clin Nutr* 71.2 (2000): 412–33.

Pereira, M. A., D. R. Jacobs, J. J. Pins, S. K. Raatz, M. D. Gross, J. L. Slavin, and E. R. Seaquist. "Effect of Whole Grains on Insulin Sensitivity in Overweight Hyperinsulinemic Adults." *Am J Clin Nutr* 75 (2002): 848–55.

Platt, Michael E. *The Miracle of Bio-Identical Hormones: A Revolutionary Approach to Wellness for Men, Women and Children*. Palm Desert, CA: Clancy Lane Publishing, 2006.

Ridker, Paul M., Nader Rifai, Nancy R. Cook, Gary Bradwin, and Julie E. Buring. "Non-HDL Cholesterol, Apolipoproteins A-I and B100, Standard Lipid Measures, Lipid Ratios, and CRP as Risk Factors for Cardiovascular Disease in Women." *JAMA: The Journal of the American Medical Association* 294 (2005): 326–33.

Romero-Corral, Abel, et al. "Relationships Between Leptin and C-Reactive Protein with Cardiovascular Disease in the Adult General Population." *Nat Clin Pract Cardiovasc Med.* 5.7 (2008): 418–25.

Rossouw, J. E., G. L. Anderson, J. M. Kotchen, J. Ockene, R. L. Prentice, A. Z. Lacroix, C. Kooperberg, M. L. Stefanick, R. D. Jackson, S. A. Beresford, B. V. Howard, and K. C. Johnson. "Risks and Benefits of Estrogen Plus Progestin in Healthy Postmenopausal Women: Principal Results from the Women's Health Initiative Randomized Controlled Trial." *JAMA: The Journal of the American Medical Association* 288.3 (2002): 321–33.

Seftel, A. "Testosterone Replacement Therapy for Male Hypogonadism: Part III Pharmacologic and Clinical Profiles, Monitoring, Safety Issues, and Potential Future Agents." *Int J Impot Res* 19.1 (2007): 2–24.

Shai, Iris, Dan Schwarzfuchs, Osnat Tangi-Rozental, Rachel Zuk-Ramot, Benjamin Sarusi, Dov Brickner, Ziva Schwartz, Einat Sheiner, Rachel Marko, Esther Katorza, Joachim Thiery, Georg Fiedler, Yaakov Henkin, Matthias Bluher, Michael Stumvoll, Meir Stampfer, Danit Shahar, Shula Witkow, Ilana Greenberg, Rachel Golan, Drora Fraser, Arkady Bolotin, and Hilel Vardi. "Weight Loss with a Low-Carbohydrate, Mediterranean, or Low-Fat Diet." *N Engl J Med* 359.3 (2008): 229–41.

Shamsuzzaman, A. S., M. Winnicki, R. Wolk, A. Svatikova, B. G. Phillips, D. E. Davison, P. B. Berger, and V. K. Somers. "Independent Association between Plasma Leptin and C-Reactive Protein in Healthy Humans." *Circulation* 109.18 (2004): 2181–85.

Shulman, P., and D. Harari. "Low-Dose Transdermal Estradiol for Symptomatic Perimenopause." *Menopause* 11(1) (Jan-Feb 2004): 34–39.

Sierra-Johnson, J., et al. "Relation of Increased Leptin Concentrations to History of Myocardial Infarction and Stroke in the US Population." *Am J Cardiol* 100 (2007): 234–39.

Simopoulos, Artemis. "Essential Fatty Acids in Health and Chronic Disease." *Am J Clin Nutr* 70.3 (1999): 560S–69S.

Singh, I. M., M. H. Shishehbor, and B. J. Ansell. "High-Density Lipoprotein as a Therapeutic Target: A Systematic Review." *JAMA: The Journal of the American Medical Association* 298.7 (2007): 786–98.

Sinha, Rashmi, Amanda J. Cross, Barry I. Graubard, Michael F. Leitzmann, Arthur Schatzkin. "Meat Intake and Mortality: A Prospective Study of Over Half a Million People." *Arch Intern Med* 169(6) (2009): 562-71.

Smith, George, Yoav Ben-Shlomo, Andrew Beswick, John Yarnell, Stafford Lightman, and Peter Elwood. "Cortisol, Testosterone, and Coronary Heart Disease: Prospective Evidence from the Caerphilly Study." *Circulation* 112.3 (2005): 332–40.

Soderberg, S., et al. "Leptin, but Not Adiponectin, Predicts Stroke in Males." *J Intern Med* 256 (2004): 128–36.

Stephenson, Joan. "Low-Carb, Low-Fat Diet Gurus Face Off." *JAMA: The Journal of the American Medical Association* 289 (2003): 1767–73.

Stolzenberg-Solomon, Rachael Z., Barry I. Graubard, Suresh Chari, Paul Limburg, Philip R. Taylor, Jarmo Virtamo, and Demetrius Albanes. "Insulin, Glucose, Insulin Resistance, and Pancreatic Cancer in Male Smokers." *JAMA: The Journal of the American Medical Association* 294 (2005): 2872–78.

Surks, M. I., E. Ortiz, G. H. Daniels, C. T. Sawin, R. H. Cobin, J. A. Franklyn, J. M. Hershman, K. D. Burman, M. A. Denke, C. Gorman, R. S. Cooper, and N. J. Weissman. "Subclinical Thyroid Disease: Scientific Review and Guidelines for Diagnosis and Management." *JAMA: The Journal of the American Medical Association* 291 (2004): 228–38.

Taubes, Gary. "The Soft Science of Dietary Fat." *Science* 291.5513 (2001): 2536–45.

Whelton, S. P., J. He, P. K. Whelton, and P. Muntner. "Meta-Analysis of Observational Studies on Fish Intake and Coronary Heart Disease." *Am J Cardiol* 93 (9) (May 1, 2004): 1119–23.

Wolk, R., et al. "Plasma Leptin and Prognosis in Patients with Established Coronary Atherosclerosis." *J Am Coll Cardiol* 44 (2004): 1819–24.

Yancy, W. S., M. K. Olsen, J. R. Guyton, et al. "A Low-Carbohydrate, Ketogenic Diet vs. a Low-Fat Diet to Treat Obesity and Hyperlipidemia: a Randomized, Controlled Trial." *Ann Intern Med* 14 (2004): 769–77.

# Index

## R

## S

# About the Author

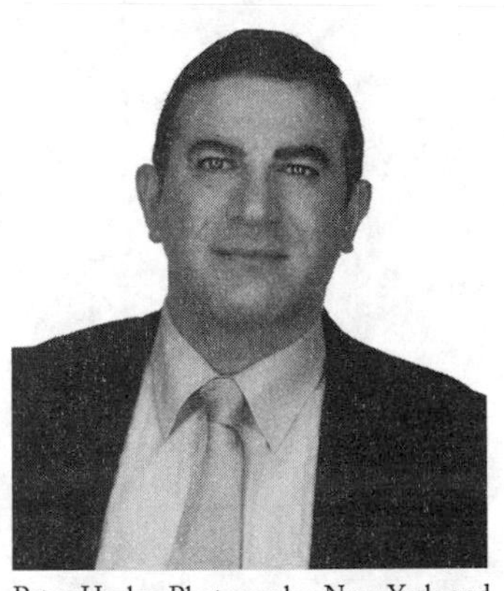

Peter Hurley Photography, New York and Los Angeles

Michael Aziz, MD, is board certified in internal medicine. He completed his training at Albert Einstein College of Medicine–Long Island Jewish Medical Center and Staten Island University Hospital in New York. He is a member of the American College of Physicians and the American Society of Internal Medicine, and he is also a fellow of the Royal Society of Medicine in the United Kingdom. He has appeared as a keynote speaker before prestigious groups nationally and internationally, including the American Academy of Anti-Aging Medicine. He is the founder and director of Midtown Integrative Medicine in New York City, a practice that focuses on traditional, complementary, and integrative medicine. Dr. Aziz lives in New York City.